7/2010

M000287816

Accessories to Modernity

Accessories to Modernity

FASHION AND THE FEMININE IN NINETEENTH-CENTURY FRANCE

Susan Hiner

UNIVERSITY OF PENNSYLVANIA PRESS *Philadelphia • Oxford*

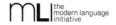

THIS BOOK IS MADE POSSIBLE BY A COLLABORATIVE GRANT FROM
THE ANDREW W. MELLON FOUNDATION.

Published by University of Pennsylvania Press
Philadelphia, Pennsylvania 19104–4112

Printed in the United States of America on acid-free paper

10 9 8 7 6 5 4 3 2 1

Library of Congress Cataloging-in-Publication Data

Hiner, Susan.
    Accessories to modernity : fashion and the feminine in
nineteenth-century France / Susan Hiner.
        p.   cm.
    Includes bibliographical references and index.
    ISBN 978-0-8122-4259-1 (hardcover : alk. paper)
    1. Fashion—France—History—19th century.
2. Clothing and dress—France—History—19th
century.   3. Women—France—History—19th
century.   4. France—Social life and customs—19th
century.   I. Title.
GT871.H56   2010
391.00944'09034—dc22
                                2010008119

CONTENTS

ILLUSTRATIONS

Accessories to Modernity

Prologue

In nineteenth-century France, modernity often operated precisely through what was most easily dismissed—the seemingly negligible fashion accessories of women. A cashmere shawl might obliquely refer to imperial conquest in Algeria but openly indicate married status in Parisian society. A silk parasol could whisper racial and cultural supremacy but loudly proclaim the delicacy of the fair sex. A painted fan might conceal aesthetic and social inauthenticity but also reveal the uncontested power of social status buttressed by wealth. Because of its trivialized status, the feminine fashion accessory could accomplish ideological work imperceptibly, both avowing and disavowing its connection to some of the most complex processes of modernity.

The hidden stories of fashion accessories come to light in the chapters that follow through an unearthing of their provenance, their histories, and their roles in both literary and extraliterary contexts.[1] Fashion accessories have been taken for granted, accepted as an inconsequential part of the décor of realist novels. Because they are taken to signify little beyond the discreet literary construction of reality, objects such as cashmere shawls, parasols, fans, and handbags have received little serious attention. Literary scholars have relegated the fashion accessory to the realm of the ornamental, the decorative, the feminine. Yet these accessories are far from secondary. They are the unmistakable armature of feminine seduction; more important still, as essential instruments in the production and presentation of respectability and virtue, they are crucial components of the bourgeois idealization of womanhood, which depended on women's objectifica-

1

tion—her becoming an aestheticized accessory in the social theater of male success and status.[2]

The accessory exemplifies one of the overarching paradoxes of the ideology of the feminine in nineteenth-century culture: the proper lady was required to carry on her person the social and moral hierarchies of a society in the process of reinvention while, at the same time, satisfying the imperatives of erotic seduction. As that *je ne sais quoi*, the subtle detail that pulls an outfit together and makes it all work in the fashion economy, the feminine accessory turns out to be a polyvalent cultural marker. The shawl, the parasol, the fan, and the handbag put on display in the pages of novels a wealth of social and historical meanings. By uncovering these links, *Accessories to Modernity* reveals the power of the seemingly frivolous fashion detail both to shape and reflect modern French culture.

Modernity in France refers to a confluence of phenomena occurring roughly from the period of the social and political upheavals unleashed by the Revolution of 1789 to the end of the Second Empire in 1870; it is marked in part by conflicts between and collusion among rapid social mobility and notions of legitimacy, colonialism and domestic retrenchment, and mass culture and elite aesthetics.[3] This book analyzes the complex ways in which women's fashion accessories became primary sites for the ideological work of modernity: the interplay of imperialist expansion and domestic rituals, the quest for authenticity in the face of increasing social mobility, gendering practices and their interrelation with social hierarchies, and the rise of commodity culture and woman's paradoxical, and fragile, status as both agent and object within it. The objects I analyze here "accessorize" these ideological impulses, naturalizing, domesticating, but sometimes also contesting them. These peripheral instruments of power moved into the indeterminate space created by postrevolutionary confusion when dress itself was an increasingly unreliable indicator of social position. Indeed, the accessory became improbably central to the project of social mobility.

While the term *accessory* may connote "marginal" or "peripheral," the fashion accessory is in fact laden with meanings pertinent to the cultural thinking of the time. I argue that by taking the novelistic items of women's fashion accessories literally and considering them in extraliterary contexts such as fashion journals, press illustrations, and sociohistorical documents (for example, court transcripts, *physiologies*, and manuals of *savoir-vivre*), we can discover the many cultural valences these objects possessed and cast fresh eyes onto some of the most widely read novels of Balzac, Flaubert, Zola, and Proust. For these objects contain histories not explicitly narrated in the plots of these novels, histories that may appear peripheral to the stories that contain them but that are fundamental to the larger cultural work in which these novels participate.

Yet *accessory* also bears another meaning often expressed in a legal context: the culpable support of or contribution to a crime. In this sense, both women and their fashion accessories aided and abetted what some might call the offenses of modernity. Whether through unthinking reliance on accessories to maintain their own social standing or through calculated wielding of them to manipulate social power, women were complicit, if unwittingly, in the very ideology that sought to suppress them—or at least those below them in social rank. The cultural pressure to possess certain accessories rendered these objects accomplices in an economy of subordination, and the close association between accessories and women caused an oscillating convergence and divergence of subject and object. However, as suggested above, precisely because these cultural artifacts played a crucial role in sustaining the dominant ideology, they could also be used to disrupt it; and this is exactly what some women did. The potential to dismantle the hierarchies of gender, class, and race always lay just below the surface, leading to an overinvestment in cultural symbols and a general malaise around their thinly veiled fragility.

By reading some of the central novels of nineteenth-century France in tandem with the cultural history of the objects they make such frequent use of, *Accessories to Modernity* aims to enrich our understanding of women's fashion accessories, demonstrating how literary, historical, and visual rhetorics inhere in them. Following an introductory first chapter that lays out the critical concepts and the cultural landscape to be explored, the book develops the rich metaphorical conceit of the *corbeille de mariage*, or wedding basket, both as object of analysis critical to understanding the cultural practices surrounding the feminine in nineteenth-century France and as structuring device—opening up, as it were, the treasure chest of luxury goods to be examined in the book. Each subsequent chapter considers a single accessory, the history of the object as well as its values in both literary and nonliterary contexts. These accessories relate simultaneously to key attributes in the conceptualization of idealized femininity in nineteenth-century France—virtue, delicacy, authenticity, and domesticity—and to the processes of modernity from which bourgeois and elite women were ostensibly excluded—colonialism, nationalism, industrialization, and commercialization. As my chapters show, the accessory negotiates a kind of commerce between these two fields, making both women and the objects that adorned them accessories to modernity.

Things, therefore, rather than texts structure this book, which aims to recover neglected objects and to present new insights into the texts and the culture that produced and exploited them. This organization offers a structural model of genealogy, proposing a project of recuperation of fashion accessories that have been constituted as marginal and placed outside of the power systems of modernity. Obviously, these objects existed and many were fashionable well before the nineteenth century; that history is all the more pertinent given their distinctive and distinctively modern function in nineteenth-century France, the supposed birthplace of fashion. As cultural signs of identity (class, race, gender), these accessories become vital documents in the construction of modernity itself. This book takes the accessory seriously and makes it central to an analysis of women as both subject and object—both producing and bearing the effects of the processes of modernity.

My first chapter, entitled "*La Femme comme il (en) faut* and the Pursuit of Distinction," theorizes the accessory as a principal marker of distinction for women in nineteenth-century France. I argue that the urge to classify and codify women through fashion was increasingly important just as class barriers became more fluid. Because of this fluidity, the pursuit of social distinction became ever more charged and nuanced, and the fashion accessory became an ever more crucial tool through which distinction could be produced and projected. This chapter offers an important overview of the complex cultural and social landscape of nineteenth-century France and an analysis of the feminine accessory as the key to distinction. To do this, I explore Balzac's 1840 essay "La Femme comme il faut" and Dumas's 1843 *Filles, lorettes et courtisanes*, along with several other protosociological texts, known as *physiologies*. Drawing also on an analysis of Balzac's short novel *Ferragus* from 1833, this chapter develops the complex category of the *femme comme il faut*, the proper lady, and the notions of respectability and distinction that both define her and that she redefines. I show that disciplining the female body through fashion reinstituted class distinctions that were becoming murky. My analysis also suggests, however, that mastery of the system—the proper deployment of fashion accessories—was the most nuanced and powerful path to individual distinction, and that by working the system, the fashion virtuoso could potentially disrupt the center from the margins.

In Chapter 2, entitled "Unpacking the *Corbeille de mariage*," I introduce and explore the *corbeille de mariage*, the gift basket filled with luxury accessories that the fiancé was required to offer his bride-to-be in exchange for the *dot* (dowry). The contents of the *corbeille* were most clearly luxury goods meant to seduce through their material opulence a marriageable *demoiselle*, thus reflecting and reinforcing her status of propriety and concluding the marriage contract. These seductive objects also contributed to the erotics of female fashion. The ritual of the *corbeille* thus institutionalized certain goods—silks, cashmere shawls, jewelry, lace, fans—as indices of respectability, their inclusion in the *corbeille* making them, theoretically, off limits to any but respectable women, while at the same time initiating the innocent into the erotic mysteries of marriage. This chapter explains how the *corbeille* came to be considered the criterion for distinction, the *über*-commodity of nineteenth-century French society. This encompassing symbol offers a contextualizing structure that justifies my choice of objects (all of which ended up in the *corbeille*) in the chapters that follow. I present the *corbeille de mariage* through the lens of Balzac's 1835 *Le Contrat de mariage*; Edmond Duranty's 1860 novel *Le Malheur d'Henriette Gérard*; Gyp's 1880 *Pauvres petites femmes*; and descriptions, illustrations, and advertisements in fashion journals, etiquette manuals, and popular plays. These many and varied documents nuance the category of respectability and its link to marriage that gripped nineteenth-century ideologies of upper-class and bourgeois women.

Chapter 3, "'Cashmere Fever': Virtue and the Domestication of the Exotic," discusses the rise of the cashmere shawl as a primary sign of both female virtue and social status in the first half of the century. This chapter charts the colonial context of the introduction of the *cachemire* into cultural practice and exposes the connections between imperial and domestic projects. With its reference to the double colonization of both exotic lands and women's bodies, the *cachemire* had real staying power. Originating in the exotic East and circulating to the West through trade routes opened by colonial exploits, this luxury textile became an ever more important conveyor of social value. It had to be included in every *corbeille de mariage*, even at the end of the nineteenth century when cashmere shawls were no longer considered particularly fashionable. A historical analysis of the *cachemire* in conjunction with readings of Balzac's *La Cousine Bette* (1846) and Flaubert's *L'Éducation sentimentale* (1869) shows the centrality of the circulating cashmere shawl to the production of both the plots of the novels and the conflicts over feminine virtue that govern those plots. Several popular texts and contemporaneous nonfictional documents make my case that "cashmere fever" was indeed endemic to the construction of nineteenth-century feminine respectability, even as the garment itself originated in the colonized lands of fantasized eroticism. By reevaluating the exploitation and economic value of cashmere and considering the ways in which certain exotic objects were assimilated in the service of sexual propriety, this chapter relocates the work of imperialism in the streets, drawing rooms, and boudoirs of Paris.

Chapter 4, entitled *"Mademoiselle Ombrelle*: Shielding the Fair Sex,"* focuses on the *ombrelle* (parasol) and takes up the question of idealized bourgeois femininity as constructed through whiteness, leisure, and social *savoir faire*. If virtue and propriety were signaled by the *cachemire*, protection of those components of feminine respectability was assured by the *ombrelle*. Used skillfully, the *ombrelle* produces an effect of light and shadow, a flattering frame and tool of idealization for its female subject that hinges on the contrast of transparency and opacity, visibility and invisibility, virtue and vice. The *ombrelle* had old associations with oriental royalty and by the nineteenth century was clearly linked to status and leisure. That the *ombrelle* also guaranteed whiteness further contributed to this accessory's participation in maintaining clearly demarcated social and cultural borders. I analyze this object in several literary texts, including Balzac's *Le Lys dans la vallée* (1836), Flaubert's *Madame Bovary* (1857), and Zola's *Nana* (1880). Parallel readings in vaudeville plays, children's literature, and etiquette manuals crystallize the *ombrelle*'s function in the ideology of the fair sex in nineteenth-century France.

Chapter 5, "Fan Fetish: Gender, Nostalgia, and Commodification," analyzes the *éventail* (fan) by a mapping of the fashion accessory that best represents Old Regime nostalgia onto social discourses. This chapter explores the gendering and fetishization of objects and their concomitant valorization as works of art or commodities. It thus bridges the concepts of virtue developed in earlier chapters and the move into the public sphere to be explored in the final chapter. More than any other women's fashion accessory, the fan works erotically and has a long history of association with female seduction; but this accessory also functions as hyperbolic art object, combining a variety of media and signifying the exotic. Just as the eighteenth-century fan brings the erotic into the social realm, it also marks the entry of the exotic art object into an economy, and by the nineteenth century, it began to signal a fetishizing nostalgia for the previous century. Flaubert's *Madame Bovary* and Balzac's *Le Cousin Pons* (1847) provide the primary vehicles for my literary analysis in the first part of this chapter, and I then turn briefly to Zola's *Au Bonheur des Dames* (1883) and Proust's *À la recherche du temps perdu* (1913-27) to demonstrate the later development of this commodity. Drawing also on popular literature and the fashion press, this chapter argues that this constantly resurfacing object, in the hands of the bourgeois subject, comes to mediate the developing tensions of modernity as both fans and women emerge as commodified objects of circulation.

In the final chapter, "Between Good Intentions and Ulterior Motives: The Culture of Handbags," I analyze the nineteenth-century explosion of female consumerism, perhaps the most striking transformation of modernity in terms of women's roles, by considering the object that best symbolizes woman's vexed relationship to money. The chapter outlines the rise of the handbag from its earliest incarnation in the First Empire as the *réticule*, a bag carried for the first time externally to the dress and necessitated by the sheer, clingy dresses of the Directory, to the handbag of the end of the century. From the *étuis*, or needlecases, to the embroidered *bourses* that ladies labored over and displayed to demonstrate their domestic prowess, the handbag evolved into a vehicle of consumption. As it came out from under the voluminous skirts formerly concealing the *poches* (pockets) of respectable ladies, so, too, did respectable ladies emerge in public as consumers with a newly visible relationship to money. Moving from an analysis of Balzac's 1832 novella *La Bourse* to a second reading of Zola's Second Empire novel *Au Bonheur des Dames*, alongside readings from the fashion press and fin-de-siècle women's magazines, this chapter addresses the emergence of the woman consumer and her entry into the marketplace in nineteenth-century France.

Accessories to Modernity analyzes the narrative and cultural functions of women's fashion accessories and argues that they served the ideological agendas of modernity in nineteenth-century France. While the problems of modernity treated here—imperialism, social mobility, authenticity, commodification—have been well documented in critical discourses, no study of these rich themes has been undertaken that analyzes them strictly through a focused attention on the crucial detail of the feminine fashion accessory. By examining these objects within a cultural context that includes both novels and fashion discourse of the period, my book reframes these accessories as key signifiers of modernity. And by viewing the themes of modernity, gender, and fashion through the particular lens of the feminine fashion accessory, *Accessories to Modernity* also makes a larger claim about the "accessory" status of nineteenth-century elite French women themselves, who both ornamented their husbands and signaled their wealth and standing and participated, however obliquely, in the ideological work of modernity. The feminine fashion accessory, as a bridge between erotic and exotic, domestic and other, mass production and work of art, uncovers the complicity of bourgeois and elite women in that ideological work. Through its linking of gender, social mobility, and imperial conquest, the fashion accessory actually proves to be central, and indeed an accessory, to modernity.

CHAPTER ONE

La Femme comme il (en) faut and the Pursuit of Distinction

Le glas de la haute société sonne, entendez-vous! Le premier
coup est ce mot moderne de femme comme il faut!

HONORÉ DE BALZAC

Alexandre Dumas *fils*'s 1848 novel *La Dame aux camélias* opens with the auction of the dead courtesan Marguerite Gautier's worldly goods. In her luxury apartment, prurient curiosity and rampant consumerism, combined with the practical reality of debt collection, produce the most jarring and scandalous of juxtapositions. The gasps are nearly audible as "Madame la duchesse de F . . . coudoyait Mlle A . . . , une des plus tristes de nos courtisanes modernes; Mme la marquise de T . . . hésitait pour acheter un meuble sur lequel enchérissait Mme D . . . , la femme adultère la plus élégante et la plus connue de notre époque. . . . Robes, cachemires, bijoux se vendaient avec une rapidité incroyable" (The Duchess of F. elbowed Mlle. A., one of the most melancholy examples of our modern courtesan; the Marquise de T. hesitated over a piece of furniture the price of which was being run high by Mme. D., the most elegant and famous adulteress of our time. . . . Dresses, cashmeres, jewels were sold with incredible rapidity).[1] Such commingling was scandalous indeed according to the prevailing ideology that kept respectable women and women of ill repute safely contained in their respective spheres. Respectable women belonged to and in *le monde*, while the fallen inhabited its shadowy opposite, *le demi-monde*.

Invented by Balzac and appearing in his *Autre étude de femme* in 1842, *la femme comme il en faut* is a pun on the common expression *la femme comme il faut*. With this pun, Balzac toys with the subtle yet crucial distinction between female types so important to the bourgeois ideology of female virtue. As his pun suggests, however, *femmes comme il faut* and *femmes comme il en faut* are perhaps less distinct than

9

that ideology would have it. In this context in French, the pronoun *en* serves to replace the partitive expression "d'elles" (of them) referring to an indefinite quantity: *femmes comme il faut en avoir*. Balzac puts this expression in the mouth of Blondet, who, anxious to instruct a Polish count among his interlocutors in the differences of Parisian women, is also keenly interested in impressing his initiated listeners with his wit: "Les femmes que vous verrez plus tard ayant un peu de leur air, essayant de les singer, sont des femmes *comme il en faut*; tandis que la belle inconnue, votre Béatrix de la journée, est la *femme comme il faut*" ("Later you will see women who look a bit like them, who try to imitate them. They are the 'femmes comme il en faut' [necessary women]. On the contrary, your beautiful stranger, your Beatrix by day, is the 'femme comme il faut' [proper woman]").[2] His differentiation turns on the mere absence or presence of a pronoun: *la femme comme il faut* is the proper lady, respectable and marriageable, while *la femme comme il en faut* is the kind of woman necessary to society, yet unmarriageable. The nearly invisible pronoun, the minuscule detail of grammar, like the fashion accessory in the grammar of clothing, makes all the difference, if one is capable of reading it.

In spite of the separation exacted by social arbiters of these worlds and the women who represent them, in many nineteenth-century literary texts as well as in nonfictional media, *monde* and *demi-monde*, *femmes comme il faut* and *comme il en faut* collide and combine, take stock of each other, and sometimes even shop together. Before the heyday of the department store in the latter half of the nineteenth century, during which the "democratization of fashion" triumphed, there were fashion spaces in which this commingling occurred on a regular basis, despite the anxiety this mixing produced. David Harvey, in his *Paris, Capital of Modernity*, links modernity with the opening of the first department store, the Bon Marché, in 1852; and it is not until the later years of the Second Empire (1830–70) that the department store begins to revolutionize consumer practices, as Rosalind Williams details in *Dream Worlds*. While Barbara Vinken places "the birthplace of fashion in modernity, in the Second Empire of Napoleon III," this book suggests that both fashion and modernity are already operative early in the century; and the paradoxical dilemmas Vinken associates with sociological fashion writers, such as Thorstein Veblen and Georg Simmel, were already being identified and analyzed by Balzac and Dumas in the first half of the nineteenth century, as we shall see (7). Some of these spaces of mixing were actual, such as the auction cited above[3] or the popular semipublic balls.[4] Others were discursive and visual, like the print pages and illustrated plates of fashion magazines, which had a broad readership, or the text and engravings of nonfictional, proto-sociological essays, such as the popular *physiologies* examined in this chapter. Others still were literary representations of a kind of circulation among women who were, in principle at least, meant to inhabit separate spheres.

In this chapter, I offer an overview of the urban feminine social landscape of nineteenth-century France and begin to point to the fashion accessory as a primary key to distinction. Distinction is that mechanism by which dominant class groups self-identify according to aesthetic value and behavior; fashion as taste became a key marker of distinction as the repeal of sumptuary laws legislating fashion clouded the visibility of social hierarchies.[5] The role of fashion as a circulating agent in the representation and interaction of the two apparently opposed social worlds of *monde* and *demi-monde* and of their respective female denizens became crucial as class barriers became more fluid.[6] It was through the fashion accessory in particular that distinction, so hotly pursued, would be forged, just as it was the accessory and its knockoffs that also disturbed the very boundaries that the concept of distinction sought to maintain.

The objects considered in this book were fashionable especially during the period from the July Monarchy through the Second Empire. This historical range is significant, for I am arguing that fashion, and specifically the pursuit of distinction through the accessory, takes on greater urgency in times of social instability. As anthropologist Aubrey Cannon has observed, "Change in the basis of prestige or status can undermine one's sense of position in relation to others, or create new means or new opportunities for achieving enhanced recognition. Either circumstance could lead individuals to seek new means of visible distinction."[7] From 1830 to 1871, France experienced two revolutions, a coup d'état, a foreign invasion, and a bloody internal uprising. Alongside this political volatility, and its concomitant social shifts, France also moved from a traditional economy to a modern, industrial one, a development that both reinforced the new hierarchies based on money and resulted in the explosion of the fashion industry onto the cultural scene. In the pages that follow, I read the woman's fashion accessory as cultural artifact and reposition it as central to critical discussions of cultural production in nineteenth-century France in order to clarify the role of bourgeois and elite women in French modernity.

MONDE AND *DEMI-MONDE*

The pursuit of distinction through the acquisition of fashionable accessories was both an endeavor by traditionalists to control and maintain
static social hierarchies and a pathway for the newly socially enfran-
chised. Consequently, neither "monde" nor "demi-monde" was easily
defined in mid-nineteenth-century Paris. According to historian Anne
Martin-Fugier, "le monde" of 1830 was "une nébuleuse de salons, so-
ciétés, coteries en expansion à partir de la cour" (a nebulous mass of
salons, societies, and groups expanding outward from the court). It had
its literal topography, familiar to readers of Balzac—"le monde parisien
se divise en quartiers" (Parisian society is divided by neighborhoods)—
the old aristocracy's faubourg Saint-Germain, the liberal aristocracy's
faubourg Saint Honoré, the banker and arriviste's Chaussée d'Antin,
and the musty, passé, commercial Marais ("La Vie élégante," 100–102).
The monolithic, court-centered "monde" of the Old Regime and the
Restoration was giving way to the kaleidoscopic, society-oriented model of the July Monarchy.[8] This produced a kind of social chaos deplored
by legitimists but welcomed by those who hoped to profit socially from
the new loopholes in the structure.[9]

"Le demi-monde," writes Dumas *fils* in the *Avant-Propos* to his 1855
play of that name, was a "terre nouvelle qui manquait à la topogra-
phie parisienne" (a new world that was missing from Parisian topography).[10] Dumas *fils* further insists that the "Demi-Monde ne représen-
te pas . . . la cohue des courtisanes, mais la classe des déclassées. Ce
monde se compose, en effet, de femmes, toutes de souche honorable,
qui, jeunes filles, épouses, mères, ont été de plein droit accueillies et
choyées dans les meilleures familles, et qui ont déserté" (11) (the *demi-monde* does not represent the crowd of courtesans, but the down-
graded class. Indeed, this world is composed of women, all from honorable backgrounds, who as young ladies, wives, mothers, had been by
all rights welcomed and pampered in the the best families, and who
deserted). The younger Dumas may have coined the provocative term,
but the notion of *demi-monde* obviously predated its naming and was
early on corrupted beyond his limited definition. It was and still is universally understood to contain precisely "la cohue des courtisanes."
In her social history of *le Tout-Paris* from 1815 to 1848, Martin-Fugier
connects the feminine underworlds described by Balzac and Nestor de
Roqueplan (famous for inventing the word *lorette*—a low-level courtesan) precisely through the term *demi-monde* and observes the absolute

exclusion of women of polite society from the gatherings of *demimon-daines*: "pas une dame de la bonne société, évidemment" (341) (not a single well-bred lady, obviously). In Second Empire France, as more attention was falling on public spaces with the explosion of boulevards, cafés, department stores, and public gardens, and as industry made the reproduction and acquisition of commodities less expensive, there was even greater potential for class mixing and thus a more acute urgency for displaying one's distinction.[11]

The opposing social categories embodied in the figures of the *femme comme il faut* and the *femme comme il en faut*, inhabitants respectively of *monde* and *demi-monde*, are the central focus of several protosociological *physiologies* and essays by authors such as Balzac, Dumas, Maurice Alhoy, and the Goncourt brothers, works included in the genre referred to as *la littérature panoramique*.[12] These *physiologies* contributed to the cultural construction of the socially indeterminate female figure and also registered the anxiety provoked by her indeterminacy. *Physiologies* were extremely popular, cheap little books, widely circulated from the 1820s through the 1850s, that occupied a discursive space somewhere between ethnography and literature, taking for subject social types and written with a dose of satire. They were often illustrated by famous lithographers (Gavarni and Daumier, for example) and frequently penned by the likes of Balzac in addition to less well-known journalists and *feuilletonnistes* (serial fiction writers). These short pieces offer piercing insights into the cultural phenomena they claim to represent but also often betray the cultural anxieties of their authors. Since they were so widely read, they exercised considerable influence in the very production of the "types" they supposedly represented.

From the *Physiologie du bas-bleu*, published in 1800, and the 1842 *Physiologie de la femme* to the 1868 *Physiologie de la femme la plus malheureuse du monde*, for example, texts in this genre were widespread and, if the majority of the titles are any indication, often centered on female types. The cultural work of reinventing a society in disarray seems to have been dealt with through various types of analyses of women. As Catherine Nesci points out in her study of women in Balzac, women shouldered the burden of "restoring" distinction to the new society: "C'est donc à l'être féminin que revient la lourde et double tâche de sauver la nouvelle société de la contingence de ses origines honteuses: il lui faut plaire pour enfanter et pour représenter. Comment peut-on à la fois se montrer et attiser le désir, et obéir aux convenances sociales qui imposent à la femme le silence et la pudeur?" (The burdensome double task of saving the new society from the contingency of its shameful origins thus falls to the female; she has to please in order both to give birth and to represent. How is it possible both to display oneself and stoke desire, and to obey the social rules that impose silence and prudishness on woman?).[13] The paradox expressed in Nesci's question underlies the bourgeois ideology of the feminine in nineteenth-century France. While men did the dirty work of capitalism, bourgeois women, protected from the brutal realities of an industrializing society, cultivated domestic ideals and clothed themselves in garments bespeaking demure innocence and leisure. Fashion accessories, as the luxurious trimmings of these costumes, signified wealth more pointedly than other articles of dress and so could indicate social status and thus refer, however obliquely, to the masculine world of capital. Yet, as feminine accoutrements, they also necessarily functioned in the feminine economy of respectability and virtue, values that came to signify taste.[14]

Controlling women's behavior and dress, dictating their social roles, and establishing related codes of morality were the unannounced aims of many of the physiological documents so popular at the time. Along with Balzac's essay on the *femme comme il faut*, the three *physiologies* dealing with the *lorette* that I will be drawing on here are Alexandre Dumas *père*'s 1843 *Filles, lorettes et courtisanes*, Maurice Alhoy's 1841 *Physiologie de la lorette*, and Edmond and Jules de Goncourt's 1852–53 *La Lorette*.[15] These two female types, the *femme comme il faut* and the *femme comme il en faut*, of which the *lorette* is one form, while presumably opposites, in fact exhibit many of the same qualities. Through detailed descriptions and explanations of the nineteenth-century French female social hierarchy as it is expressed primarily through dress, these texts illustrate both the blurring of feminine social hierarchies in nineteenth-century France and the desperate urge to reinscribe them. Fashion accessories, and in particular those luxury items associated with the interrelated concepts of respectability and social status, became the principal markers of distinction, as evidenced especially by their mandatory inclusion in the *corbeille de mariage*, the gift basket offered by the fiancé to his bride in order to cement the marriage contract.[16] At the same time, however, these items were erotically charged and increasingly accessible, making them extremely potent components of the fashion system, capable at once of marking off elites and allowing imposters to pass as elites themselves.

THAT *JE NE SAIS QUOI*

In the aftermath of the Revolution, writes Roland Barthes in a 1962 essay on dandyism, "la supériorité du statut, impossible désormais à afficher brutalement en raison de la règle démocratique, se masquait et se sublimait sous une nouvelle valeur: le *goût*, ou mieux encore, car le mot est justement ambigu: *la distinction*" ("the superiority of status, which because of the democratic imperative could no longer be advertised, was hidden and sublimated beneath a new value: *taste*, or better still, as the word is appropriately ambiguous, *distinction*").[17] Actually, as Barthes intimates, the idea was not in fact so new but had merely reached a specific articulation in nineteenth-century France. Distinction is, as Bourdieu has theorized, taste—a socially constructed tool of power. Summarizing Bourdieu's social theory of distinction in his *Sociology of Taste*, Jukka Grownow explains Bourdieu's configuring of the relationship between taste and social dominance: "the taste of the ruling class is always the legitimate taste of a society. But in his [Bourdieu's] opinion this legitimate taste is not genuine good taste: in fact, there could not possibly be any genuine good taste. Legitimate taste pretends to be the universally valid and disinterested good taste, whereas in reality it is nothing more than the taste of one particular class, the ruling class."[18] Distinction, then, according to Bourdieu, was and is socially constructed but passed off as natural, or innate, as it were, to use the idiom of nineteenth-century notions of aristocracy, and it functioned to maintain class distinction by producing and maintaining an aesthetic elitism that would mirror social elitism. This mechanism of power was in full force in the era of Balzac but was theorized by later sociologists. Both Simmel and Veblen, social theorists of the late nineteenth and early twentieth centuries and the first sociologists to articulate fashion's social function, argue that pressure from inferior classes in the form of imitation is what drives fashion to reinvent itself.[19] The sartorial signs of distinction were ever changing because they could be co-opted and manipulated by social inferiors. Fashion's transformative properties thus reinforced the democratizing impulses of the revolutionary period, which subverted the notion of an essential identity, whether noble or otherwise. Correlatively, its very mutability imposed a new need for subtlety and finesse on elite efforts to maintain social superiority.

The paradoxical function of fashion, expressing both social rigidity and social mobility, harks back to Walter Benjamin and Baudelaire, who both wrote extensively about nineteenth-century fashion and recognized it as emblematic at once of change and fixity.[20] Separated by nearly a century, both authors, captivated by the modern transformations of nineteenth-century Paris, seized upon the notion of fashion as a modern phenomenon. As Peter Wollen reminds us, reading through Benjamin, "Baudelaire . . . developed his 'taste for modernity' in an obsessive concern for the details of dress" (139). Baudelaire's anonymous *passante*, one of his most iconic images, figuring modernity's transience, for example, is characterized by the minute details of her garments: "Une femme passa, d'une main fastueuse / Soulevant, balançant le feston et l'ourlet" (a woman passed, and with a jeweled hand / gathered up her black embroidered hem).[21] Benjamin, too, in his vast promenade through the nineteenth-century cultural arcade, cites fashion ninety-one times, interweaving these discussions with historical, political, and social observations (131). Baudelaire and Benjamin insist upon the dialectical nature of fashion both to convey a fixed social meaning and to change and reinvent itself to survive; it is the agent of both hierarchy and its subversion. Simmel, too, develops his influential theory of fashion according to a similar dialectical model:

> The vital conditions of fashion as a universal phenomenon in the history of our race are circumscribed by these conceptions. Fashion is the imitation of a given example and satisfies the demand for social adaptation; it leads the individual upon the road which all travel, it furnishes a general condition, which resolves the conduct of every individual into a mere example. At the same time it satisfies in no less degree the need of differentiation, the tendency towards dissimilarity, the desire for change and contrast. (296)

The nineteenth century, on which all of these theorists of modernity and fashion draw, was the laboratory for this dialectical vision of the operations of fashion, since it was during this period that rigid historical links between social class and clothing, reinforcing status and fashion as a form of belonging, were questioned and undermined both legally and in social practice even as dress continued to be used to signal status and hierarchy.

Already by the mid-eighteenth century, traditional sumptuary laws, based originally on medieval morality codes that explained social status by divine ordinance, had been challenged by wealthy bourgeois who imitated their social superiors in dress; but the Revolution would "radically and legally overturn clothing's hierarchical and statutory signs."[22]

In his classic study of the rise of bourgeois fashion, Philippe Perrot traces the history of the dissolution of the sumptuary laws and the rise of new vestimentary codes implemented primarily by the rising bourgeois class. He argues that a "moral ideology of good taste" emerged alongside the refinement of consumption as "purchasing know-how," thus producing the collusion between fashion and distinction that would become vital to nineteenth-century self-representation (20). While modernity is a fluid concept whose origins and reach are subject to debate, its impact in the nineteenth century comes into view precisely though this intersection of fashion and distinction that occurred in the years following the French Revolution, when fashion achieved greater and more flexible signifying power.

With the "freedom of dress" decree of 1793, which states that "[e]veryone is free to wear whatever clothing and accessories of his sex that he finds pleasing," the Revolution successfully legitimized a consumer economy that had been emerging throughout the eighteenth century.[23] Note, however, the gendered prescription of this decree of freedom in dress: while the decree seems to initiate a release from the restrictions dictated by social class on luxury consumption and display, it very clearly qualifies clothing and accessories according to gender. Even if class could be shown to be mutable and delinked from the concept of essential identity, gender, however, remained fixed. According to Vinken, the most radical shift to emerge was what she calls a "new post-revolutionary (1792) sexual politics" in which clothing worked to gender people, and fashion became "a synonym for femininity" (7, 11). The frequently noted status of the bourgeois woman as the adornment of her husband and the reference to his wealth bears out Vinken's observation. Furthermore, fashion became a double repository: both for a misogynistic discourse about the frivolity and decadence of women and for an idealizing discourse linking women's dress to virtue and respectability.

"By 1797," Cissie Fairchilds writes, after a hiatus in the period of the Terror, the "dressmakers had reopened their shops, the fashion press was back in business and the fashion industry in its modern form had been born. Clothes no longer were thought to make the man and citizen; instead, they had become, by default, what they are today, an expression of an individual's personality and a way he differentiates himself from others" (429).[24] However significant the cultural shift regarding fashion was in the last days of the eighteenth century, with the disruption of traditional social hierarchies and the consumer boom, fashion as readable text became ever more subtle, more diffused, and more laden with meaning in the nineteenth century.[25] Fairchilds concludes her essay with the claim that "after 1794 clothes would symbolize what someone was or aspired to be, but they would not make him so" (430). While it is true that the repeal of the sumptuary laws disrupted the essentializing impulse of the *Ancien Régime*, the belief in or yearning for this kind of "essence," the notion of innate "taste" linked to aristocratic heritage, persisted, sometimes in the form of nostalgia and sometimes in the urge to pass from one class to another.

Already in early to mid-nineteenth-century France, Balzac and others recognized that "good taste" could be acquired and was not an essential quality of elites. It thus facilitated social climbing, circulation, even imposture; and yet details of dress remained signals of distinction and were used as key markers of exclusivity, thus reproducing elite structures. Once simply a reflection of one's status, fashion and *élégance*, as prerequisites for admission to *le monde*, were now becoming important elements in the production of status.[26] According to Balzac, fashion's threat, especially as it pertained to women, was that it did indeed have performative power, and increasingly so over the course of the century, thus potentially presenting a challenge to fixed notions of identity, like gender or class.[27] It is precisely fashion's capacity to "make [one] so" that the *physiologies* point to and attempt to expose. They reveal fashion as such not to celebrate it in a Butlerian way, however, but rather to demonstrate the perils and/or ridiculousness of modern society; the discourses subtending these texts are not willing to abandon the idea of fixed, stable identity, and yet they signal the performativity of identities in crucial ways.

Vinken has taken issue with what she considers to be a one-sided sociological approach to fashion inaugurated by Simmel and developed by Bourdieu, which she claims does not fully account for the performative power of fashion, because their theories overemphasize the claim that fashion "*represents* class and gender" (my emphasis), falling back, as she suggests, into a reinforcement rather than subversion of the social order. For Vinken, however, "Fashion not only confirms and economically functionalizes the division of gender and class; it constructs and subverts them by stripping them bare . . . and reveals them as an effect of construction" (4). By privileging this paradoxical nature of fashion as an expression of both conformity and individualism, a paradox originating with Simmel in the early twentieth century, Vinken takes the dialectical nature of fashion to a further degree, stressing its subversive and performative capacities. It is the performative, as well as the representational, power of fashion that Vinken wishes to emphasize. While not contesting the legitimacy of the representative power of fashion in nineteenth-century France, my argument also builds and elaborates on Vinken's by illustrating this fashion dialectic in the socially charismatic but troubling figure of the *femme comme il faut*. The physiologies reveal the deep grasp of as well as the fear inspired by the laying bare of social categories—whether classed or gendered—that fashion can accomplish.

This two-sidedness of fashion, on the one hand its capacity to erect and maintain systematic hierarchies and on the other its vulnerability to co-optation and subversion of the hierarchy by "social inferiors," is a key to understanding the increased value of distinction in nineteenth-century France. These dueling capacities are of a piece, however: in the hands of aristocratic consumers, fashion must self-subvert to continually reinforce hierarchy. As a product in a modern economy, fashion must also self-subvert to maintain a market, among both aristocrats and rising imposters. Thus, fashion's capacity for self-subversion can be exploited for both hierarchy and profit, which will sometimes work together but sometimes be at odds.

Distinction had become a complex and shifting code, legible only to those who possessed the skills to decipher it. As Barthes maintains, "La *distinction* engage en effet la signalétique du vêtement dans une voie semi-clandestine: car d'une part le groupe auquel elle s'offre en lecture est réduit, et d'autre part les signes nécessaires à cette lecture sont rares et malaisément perceptibles sans une certaine connaissance de la nouvelle langue vestimentaire" ("Dandysme," 99) (*"Distinction* takes the signaling aspect of clothes down a semi-clandestine path: for, on the one hand, the group that reads its signs is a limited one, on the other the signs necessary for this reading are rare, and without a particular knowledge of the new vestimentary language, perceptible only with difficulty") ("Dandyism," 66). The signs that become most pertinent in the nineteenth-century vestimentary code are the details of dress that can more pointedly signal luxury—"superfluous" fashion accessories. The fashion accessory—linked to the tradition of the *marchande des modes* and the *magasin de nouveautés*—becomes the fetishistic and nuancing detail that most effectively constitutes and marks distinction in nineteenth-century France.[28]

Balzac's notion of distinction, echoed in Dumas *père* and in many other contemporary observers, and which in many ways anticipates

Bourdieu's, provides a useful framework for the analyses of the objects and novels addressed in this book and will help piece together the links between fashion accessories and the social commentary that their stories illustrate in later chapters. The texts I analyze in the pages that follow are deeply conservative in their approach to fashion, women, and society and decry fashion's performative power by attempting to expose the fashionably disguised as opposed to the authentically elegant.[29] The humor in these texts notwithstanding, implicit in their project is a nostalgia for the strict hierarchies of the *Ancien Régime* and for the transparency of meaning and identity that fashion had conveyed, as well as a troubled recognition of and a grudging admiration for the new, modern, potentially subversive function of fashion.

VIRTUE AND VIRTUOSITY

Two representative nonfictional texts loosely modeled on the popular genre of the *physiologie* illustrate the social poles of *monde* and *demi-monde* discussed above and express the nuanced value of fashion accessories in the production of distinction. Balzac's 1840 essay "La Femme comme il faut" reveals the highly structured feminine social world of mid-nineteenth-century Paris and focuses on the staging of social position through dress and manners. Dumas *père* undertook a similar enterprise in his short study of 1843, *Filles, lorettes et courtisanes*. In these exemplary texts, both Dumas and Balzac set forth rigid feminine social hierarchies that paradoxically also point to the growing fluidity of the social structure and reveal the alarm produced by such mobility. These texts demonstrate that fashion served social mobility and social exclusion at once. In both "La Femme comme il faut" and *Filles, lorettes et courtisanes*, continuous references to elements of fashion, their circulation, and potential imitation of them are more than mere descriptive details. The discourse on fashion is in fact a cover for the social anxieties underlying both texts: anxieties that distinctions are dissolving and with them the entire social order.

Both texts indicate a distinct separation between *monde* and *demi-monde* and propose rigid hierarchies within those opposite realms. Both texts also allude to the erosion of social hierarchy and express anxiety over the increased social mobility of post-Restoration society. In these two sociological texts, the impulse to recreate hierarchy is set in motion by the effacement of hierarchy, lamented by both works. Balzac's hierarchy is somewhat fluid, as he focuses on one central social figure and relates other types only to her. Dumas's is more rigidly drawn, and within his tripartite structure corresponding to the established social order, we find further subcategories, suggesting a zeal for classification that borders on obsession. While presumably depicting two mutually exclusive social realms, dominated by women of opposite social standing, both texts claim to perform a comparable function: to instruct male readers in the nuances that might help to reinforce the fragile, if not crumbling, hierarchy by offering them a key to deciphering the mysteries of fashion. Both texts explicitly state that, if armed with enough information, the newcomer to Paris will be able to distinguish proper ladies from their inferiors and will thus be safe from the clutches of the grasping *lorette*, the *femme comme il en faut*, and her kin. The newcomer is, of course, a cover for those insiders who ought already to be in the know, since taste is presumed to be innate, but who nonetheless need some help navigating the complexities of Parisian society. This vital information is oriented almost exclusively to fashion, and the accessory assumes a crucial role in the legibility of the new society.

"La Femme comme il faut" is a short piece first written in 1840 as part of *Les Français peints par eux-mêmes* and appearing again in 1842 as part of the short fictional piece entitled *Autre étude de femme*. It appears thus first as a physiological essay and then as a fragment of the larger work in the form of a portrait by the dandy Blondet of the "fille posthume de la législation napoléonienne" (the posthumous daughter of Napoleonic law).[30] The context is significant, as Blondet's audience includes an outsider, a Polish émigré, who needs some instruction in the social labyrinth of Paris. As signaled above, the "outsider" doubles and covers for those Parisian insiders who need instruction on negotiating the new society. In this sense, the outsider or newcomer is a ruse. References to Napoléon's *Code Civil* locate the social "problem" alluded to by the text as emanating from the repeal of the law of primogeniture and thus announce the fragmentation of the monolithic fortunes of the *Ancien Régime* as the origin of contemporary social chaos.[31] Dumas's *Filles, lorettes et courtisanes* also appears to have a didactic and scientific purpose. In his acknowledgments, the author refers directly to the work of Alexandre Parent-Duchâtelet, who famously classified prostitutes for the Parisian government, alongside "quelques-uns de [s] es amis, forts savants sur la matière" (several of his friends, particularly well versed in the matter).[32]

In Balzac's and Dumas's *physiologies*, fashion serves the paradoxical function observed by Baudelaire and Benjamin and described above by

Simmel, Vinken, and Perrot: it both reinforces and threatens social hierarchies. There are remarkable similarities between these two texts, the one squarely situated in the *monde* and the other portraying the *demimonde*, "un coin du grand panorama parisien que personne n'a osé peindre" (11) (a corner of the large Parisian panorama that no one has dared paint).[33] Both texts embed their discussions of the presumably frivolous and feminine topic of fashion within a sociopolitical context, thus begging a deeper, indeed a political, reading of fashion. In spite of their apparently divergent subject matter, both texts express the urge to erect a hierarchy and depict the fashion virtuoso as a "modern" and troubling heroine. Balzac's *femme comme il faut*, always striving for distinction, and her *demi-mondaine* double, Dumas's *lorette*,[34] the consummate imitator and would-be courtesan, are both modern creatures springing from uncertain origins and are defined primarily through their relationship to dress. They represent a sociopolitical threat precisely because of their lack of claims to authenticity and their clever pursuit of its signs.

LA FEMME COMME IL FAUT

In post-Revolutionary France, which saw the effacement of the official language of dress, the pursuit of distinction was paramount to maintaining social hierarchy. Women were the blank page on which this hierarchy was to be reinscribed, and the language to be used was fashion. How could a woman satisfy the representational goals of an ideology that demanded that she be both sexually virtuous and erotically appealing? One response to this paradox of the idealized feminine is the modern figure of the *femme comme il faut*, who through her virtuosity manages to be both respectable and fashionably sexy. By the time Balzac is writing, the expression "comme il faut" was already a cliché linked to social discourse. In his recently published doctoral dissertation, written in 1948, *La Mode en 1830*, Algirdas Greimas describes the linguistic connection between fashion and the social:

> Les expressions déjà anciennes "il est de bonne compagnie," "il est de bon genre," "il est de bon ton" font directement allusion au caractère social de la mode. Il en est de même de la qualification de *comme il faut*, qui, partie d'un jugement à caractère moral et surtout social, devient une expression à la mode et qui, après une période d'usure, tendra à désigner communément un certain type d'élégance et d'appartenance sociale assez mal déterminé qui dominera plus tard la société de la monarchie de Juillet. (11–12)

[The already old expressions "he is well-mannered," "he is proper," "he is suitable" allude directly to the social character of fashion. It is the same for the qualification "comme il faut," which, emerging from a moral and especially social type of judgment, becomes a fashionable expression and which, after a period of overuse, would lean toward commonly designating a certain type of elegance and vague social belonging that would later dominate July Monarchy society.]

Greimas's explanation of the idiom illuminates the links between the fashionable and the moral, and Balzac capitalized on this social and moral convergence in the expression. Famous for his proto-Darwinian classification of social species, Balzac lays out a crucial distinction between two types of Parisiennes that wittily turns on the absence or presence of a pronoun and that hinges on the social currency of "comme il faut." *La femme comme il faut*, the proper lady, is distinguished from *la femme comme il en faut* by her style:

La distinction particulière aux femmes bien élevées se trahit surtout par la manière dont elle tient le châle ou la mante croisés sur sa poitrine. Elle vous a, tout en marchant, un petit air digne et serein, comme les madones de Raphaël dans leurs cadres. . . . Le chapeau, d'une simplicité remarquable, a des rubans frais. Peut-être y aura-t-il des fleurs, mais les plus habiles de ces femmes n'ont que de nœuds. La plume veut la voiture, les fleurs attirent trop le regard. Là-dessous vous voyez la figure fraîche et reposée d'une femme sûre d'elle-même sans fatuité, qui ne regarde rien et voit tout, dont la vanité, blasée par une continuelle satisfaction, répand sur sa physionomie une indifférence qui pique la curiosité. Elle sait qu'on l'étudie, elle sait que presque tous, même les femmes, se retournent pour la revoir. Aussi traverse-t-elle Paris comme un fil de la Vierge, blanche et pure. (*Autre étude de femme*, 68)

[The distinction peculiar to a well-bred woman betrays itself, especially in the way she holds her shawl or cloak crossed over her bosom. Even as she walks she has a little air of serene dignity, like Raphael's Madonnas in their frames. . . . Her bonnet, remarkable for its simplicity, is trimmed with crisp ribbons; there may be flowers in it, but the cleverest of such women wear only bows. Feathers demand a carriage; flowers are too showy. Beneath it you see the fresh unworn face of a woman who, without conceit, is sure of herself; who looks at nothing, and sees everything; whose vanity, satiated by being constantly gratified, stamps her face with an indifference which piques your curiosity. She knows that she is looked at, she knows that everybody, even women, turn around to see her again. And she threads her way through Paris like a gossamer, spotless and pure. (*Balzac's Works*, 36–37)]

Balzac's *femme comme il faut* is twice sacralized in the narrator's discourse: first, she is likened to Raphael's Madonnas; and second, her promenade through Paris is as delicate and fragile as the "fil de la Vierge," a gossamer thread so perfect it must have been spun by the Virgin Mary herself. The *femme comme il faut* thus leaves a trail of saintliness in her wake even as she turns every head. For Balzac, "good" taste is apparently a moral characteristic.

This sacralization is not without irony, however, for Balzac's narrator has also asserted that the *femme comme il faut* is a modern invention, a pale imitation itself of the *grande dame* who has disappeared from French society. Michel Butor explains:

> On assiste, à travers une immense série de personnages, à la dégradation de la "grande dame" en "femme comme il faut," ce qui va d'ailleurs produire une fermentation féminine extraordinaire. La femme comme il faut est encore plus mystérieuse que la grande dame. Cette expression "comme il faut" implique toute une façade à préserver. Comme elle n'a plus le même pouvoir que la grande dame, cette préservation devient à la fois plus nécessaire et plus difficile.
>
> [Through a vast series of characters, we witness the degradation of the "great lady" into "femme comme il faut," which will produce an extraordinary fermentation of the feminine. The "femme comme il faut" is even more mysterious than the "grande dame." This expression "comme il faut" implies a whole façade to maintain. Since she no longer has the same power as the "grande dame," this preservation becomes at once more necessary and more difficult.] [35]

The *femme comme il faut* must try to recreate the cachet of the *grande dame* in a social climate that is beginning to admit wealthy inferiors to the tribe, thereby undermining forever the divine right to status previously reserved for the aristocracy. A paradoxical figure, descended from the aristocratic *grande dame*, she is also quintessentially modern, as Balzac makes clear from the first of his many descriptions of this "fleur rare." The *femme comme il faut* evokes for the narrator the image of "un monde de choses élégantes" (66) (a world of elegance and refinement [35]). The key terms are all here: *monde, choses, élégantes*: she is the incarnation of chic. Balzac then announces the other key feature of the *femme comme il faut* with an oxymoron: her "exquise simplicité" (67). From here he elaborates, detailing each accoutrement and accessory of the *femme comme il faut*, who, because she possesses "beaucoup de goût" (71), knows just how to drape her shawl, just how to walk so that her lace will flutter, just how to contrive a studied naturalness.

Her ease of dress translates into sociopolitical terms. Of uncertain provenance, the *femme comme il faut*, "sortie des rangs de la noblesse ou poussée de la bourgeoisie, venue de tout terrain, même de la province, est l'expression du temps actuel, une dernière image du bon goût, de l'esprit, de la grâce, de la distinction réunis, mais amoindris" (65) (issuing from the ranks of nobility or sprouting from the citizen class, and the product of every soil, even the provinces, is the expression of these times, a last remaining embodiment of good taste, wit, grace, and distinction, all combined, but dwarfed [34]). In spite of Balzac's enumeration of her many noble qualities, however, the adjective "amoindris" (dwarfed) stands out and dilutes her aristocratic pretentions. The *femme comme il faut* is poised to usurp the position of the *grande dame*, thus replacing name and lineage with brand and look, coats of arms with coats of cashmere; in short, she represents tradition supplanted by the modern.

Her rivals and social inferiors, the *bourgeoise* and the *femme comme il en faut*, are defined solely in relation to her and through their own appropriation of the fashion language she masters. The *bourgeoise*, for whom Balzac reserves most of his satire, may be summed up by her overdressing in every sense: "en hiver, [elle a] un boa par-dessus une pèlerine en fourrure, un châle et une écharpe en été" (70) (in winter, she wears a boa over her fur cloak; in summer, a shawl and a scarf [38]). The sartorial excess of the *bourgeoise* betrays ostentation and social climbing, a "trying too hard" that is the strict antithesis of the *femme comme il faut*, who is always "à l'aise dans sa toilette" (71) (at ease in full dress [39]) and who, it follows, would never overtly display her social aspirations. Like the *bourgeoise*, the *femme comme il en faut*, the nocturnal and *demi-mondaine* opposite of the *femme comme il faut*, also borrows elements of her respectable model's style; but whether intentionally or not, she never achieves the "natural" air of the *femme comme il faut*. The "*femme comme il en faut*" can only *imitate* the proper lady, and she most certainly cannot deceive the true Parisian, whose discerning eye will immediately spot the "agrafes mal cachées, des cordons qui montrent leur lacis d'un blanc roux au dos de la robe par une fente entrebâillée, des souliers éraillés, des rubans de chapeau repassés, une robe trop bouffante, une tournure trop gommée" (69) (hooks ill fastened, strings showing loops of rusty-white tape through a gaping slit in the back, rubbed shoe-leather, ironed bonnet-strings, an over-full skirt, an over-tight waist [37–38]). The *femme comme il en faut* draws attention to her seams, her buttons, her laces—in short, the very elements that suggest her *un*dress, rather than her dress. Balzac's detailed enumeration of the discreet elements of female dress here not only points to the lapses in decorum and faking of identity of the *femme comme il en faut*, however, but also, by dint of her close resemblance to her more refined double, this language suggests the inauthenticity of the *femme comme il faut* as well. The metaphor of clothing, and in particular the problematic visibility of the seams, indicating artifice, helps to articulate the anxieties surrounding crumbling notions of identities and hierarchies.[36]

Parisians are presumably well equipped to spot these lapses, but not so the uninitiated traveler (covering for the ignorant Parisian), who may well mistake them for the proper women they are aping. Balzac thus uses the discourse of fashion to categorize and stratify his society, and he also stresses the new value of appearance and costume in the production of status: "Autrefois une femme pouvait avoir une voix de harengère, une démarche de grenadier, un front de courtisane audacieuse, les cheveux plantés en arrière, le pied gros, la main épaisse, elle était néanmoins une grande dame; mais aujourd'hui, fût-elle une Montmorency, si les demoiselles de Montmorency pouvaient jamais être ainsi, elle ne serait pas femme comme il faut" (66) (Formerly, a woman might have the voice of a fish-seller, the walk of a grenadier, the face of an impudent courtesan, her hair too high on her forehead, a large foot, a thick hand—she was a great lady in spite of it all; but in these days, even if she were a Montmorency, if the Montmorency would ever be such a creature—she would not be a lady" [34]). This is perhaps as close as Balzac comes to both expressing and contesting the complex powers of essentialized identity so precious to aristocratic values. While Balzac's narrator expresses admiration for the virtuosity of this new woman, she also clearly represents the disturbing ascendency of a new society. With his emphasis on her social performativity, her subtle iterations of aristocratic identity reveal this figure to be both the flashpoint of a nostalgic conformity, through a reinscription of distinction, and an exposure of the mechanisms of that presumed innate, but culturally constructed, identity. While set up as strictly antithetical figures, the *femme comme il faut* and the *femme comme il en faut* both participate in this class performance; and as we shall see, they are in large measure rather more like sisters than opposites.

A fictional illustration of the antithesis between the *femme comme il faut* and the *femme comme il en faut* occurs in Balzac's early short novel

Ferragus, written in 1833. We first observe the heroine Madame Jules (the name given to Clémence Desmarets, wife of Jules Desmarets) through the eyes of her jealous admirer Auguste de Maulincourt as she alights from a carriage in a seamy street and enters into an unseemly apartment house. "A huit heures et demie du soir . . . dans la direction de la rue Soly, la plus étroite et la moins praticable de toutes les rues de Paris. . . . Elle dans cette crotte, à cette heure!" (At half past eight one evening . . . [toward] the rue Soly . . . one of the narrowest and least practicable thoroughfares in Paris. . . . She in that filthy neighborhood, at that hour of the night! [12–13]).[37] The incongruity of the situation is heightened as we are treated to a description of this woman: "A son bas de soie gris, pas une mouche, à son soulier, pas une éclaboussure. Le châle était bien collé sur le buste, il en dessinait vaguement les délicieux contours, et le jeune homme en avait vu les blanches épaules au bal; il savait tout ce que le châle couvrait de trésors" (39) (Not a speck on her grey stockings, not a trace of mud on her shoes. The shawl clung tightly around the outlines of her bust, vaguely moulding its exquisite contours; but the young man had seen those white shoulders in the ballroom, and he knew what a wealth of beauty was hidden beneath the shawl [14]). After her mysterious detour, Madame Jules returns to the right side of the tracks, still trailed by Auguste, who observes as she enters a flower shop in the rue Richelieu and purchases an eminently appropriate hair ornament for that evening's soirée—des marabouts. Nothing could be more proper, the text tells us, than the white plumage of the exotic marabout: "—Madame, rien ne va mieux aux brunes . . . les marabouts prêtent à leur toilette un flou qui leur manque. Madame la duchesse de Langeais dit que cela donne à une femme quelque chose de vague, d'ossianique, et de très comme il faut" (41) (Nothing could be more becoming, madam, to a brunette; . . . the marabouts impart just the mysterious touch they lack. Her Grace, the Duchess of Langeais says that the feathers lend something vague and Ossianic, and a certain distinction to a woman [16]).[38] Later, when Madame Jules arrives at the ball where Auguste will begin his investigation into his idol's secret life, we discover the effect of her toilette: "vêtue de blanc, simple et noble, coiffée précisément avec ces marabouts que le jeune baron lui avait vu choisir dans le magasin de fleurs" (47) (dressed in white, simple and noble, wearing those very feathers which the Baron had watched her choose in the shop [22]). The simplicity of her dress is equated with nobility, and the emphasis on simplicity is further developed by the uniformity of color—white—symbolically reinforcing her virtue. Finally, this simplicity is mirrored in the text by the brevity of the description itself:

the value of *comme il faut* seems to be organized around the principle of "less is more."

Juxtapose this brief but meaningful description with the lengthy introduction to Madame Jules's apparent foil, Ida Gruget, who arrives shortly after the evening of the ball at the Desmarets' residence and accuses Clémence in the presence of her husband of having unseemly *rapports* with a certain Ferragus. Just as it was incongruous, indeed scandalous, to find Clémence in the rue Soly, so it is inconsonant to find Ida in the Desmarets' drawing room. But in contrast to the single sentence he allots to the physical description of Madame Jules, Balzac devotes a full two and a half pages to the description of Ida, even before she opens her mouth to repeat verbally what we have already deduced visually about her style. Ida is the exemplary Parisian *grisette*.[39] Lovable though she may be, Ida is the picture of impropriety—because of her sudden intrusion into Madame Jules's drawing room, because of her inappropriate attire, which indicates her low social status, and because of what she has come to say:

> La jeune femme qui se trouvait en présence de monsieur et madame Jules avait le pied si découvert dans sa chaussure qu'à peine voyait-on une légère ligne noire entre le tapis et son bas blanc. Cette chaussure, dont la caricature parisienne rend si bien le trait, est une grâce particulière à la grisette parisienne; mais elle se trahit encore mieux aux yeux de l'observateur par le soin avec lequel ses vêtements adhèrent à ses formes, qu'ils dessinent nettement. Aussi l'inconnue était-elle, pour ne pas perdre l'expression pittoresque créée par le soldat français, ficelée dans une robe verte, à guimpe, qui laissait deviner la beauté de son corsage, alors parfaitement visible; car son châle de cachemire Ternaux, tombant à terre, n'était plus retenu que par les deux bouts qu'elle gardait entortillés à demi dans ses poignets. (104–5)

> [The young woman now meeting M. and Mme. Jules wore shoes that displayed so much white stocking that they looked almost like an invisible black boundary against the carpet. That kind of footwear, so neatly rendered by French comic drawings, is one of the Parisian grisette's peculiar charms of dress. But she betrays herself even more blatantly to observant eyes by how tightly she wears her clothes, which show clearly her curves. Thus the visitor was "tightly wrapped" in a green dress, to use the picturesque expression coined by a French soldier, a dress with a chemisette, which revealed a fine bosom, then fully displayed, for her Ternaux shawl had all but slipped down to the floor. She had only kept its ends loosely wrapped around her wrists. (71–72)][40]

What distinguishes Ida from Madame Jules is her excess, in contrast to the noble simplicity of Madame Jules, an abundance of garish detail, which in turn signals a lack of decorum. Ida's lack of propriety is marked by the indecorous manner in which she wears her many adornments, in contrast to the uniform respectability of Madame Jules's attire, organized and crowned by the white marabouts. These marabouts, the genuine article, we are led to assume from the chic address of the florist, are vestimentary signs of *comme il faut* and luxury all at once. And naturally, they have their counterpart in the costume of the *grisette*—the "châle de cachemire Ternaux" (a "Ternaux" shawl).

Recall Balzac's method of determining a woman's social standing: the *femme comme il faut* is superior to the *femme comme il en faut* by simple virtue of "la manière dont elle tient le châle ou la mante croisés sur sa poitrine" (*Autre étude*, 68) (the way she holds her shawl or cloak crossed over her bosom [37]). Ida's shawl is doubly inappropriate. First, she wears it like an open curtain at a bedroom window, repeating the metaphorical offenses in costume of the *femme comme il en faut* of the *Autre étude*. Gaping and trailing on the floor, the shawl leaves little to the imagination. Ida's manner of wearing her shawl directly contrasts with Balzac's decorously draped proper lady, *la femme comme il faut*, to whom shawl draping comes "naturally." But second, Ida's shawl also reveals a more subtle indication of her inferior social status. Hers is a shawl of "cachemire Ternaux," inauthentic, a French copy of the genuine article, mass produced and of lesser quality than the original, the *cachemire de l'Inde*, and therefore significantly less expensive.

When we compare their ornaments, the opposition of Madame Jules and Ida Gruget seems to emerge as a contrast of authenticity (unique) and imitation (mass produced). In *Ferragus*, this opposition becomes clouded as the text's and characters' secrets are revealed (Ferragus proves to be Mme Jules's father, a relationship that tarnishes her respectability and brings her much closer socially to Ida), thus raising an essential question that haunts nineteenth-century novels of society: what happens when the *femme comme il en faut* begins to have access to the fashion signs of the *femme comme il faut*? One result is that social and their associated moral hierarchies are obscured. The codes of distinction begin to falter, and with them social lines begin to blur. The hierarchy produced and maintained by distinction is undone by the impulse toward imitation. This phenomenon also opens up onto a crucial ideological obsession of the nineteenth century illustrated by the cashmere plots in the novels analyzed in detail in Chapter 3: the anxiety over authenticity and its link to increasing social mobility. Again, Walter Benjamin is helpful, this time for his discussion of "aura" and its loss in the age of "mechanical reproduction." While Benjamin's context was different (he was writing about photography), his theory may be applied to the drama of cashmere:

> The situations into which the product of mechanical reproduction can be brought may not touch the actual work of art, yet the quality of its presence is always depreciated. . . . In the case of the art object, a most sensitive nucleus—namely, its authenticity—is interfered with. . . . The authenticity of a thing is the essence of all that is transmissible from its beginning, ranging from its substantive duration to its testimony to the history which it has experienced. Since the historical testimony rests on the authenticity, the former, too, is jeopardized by reproduction when substantive duration ceases to matter. And what is really jeopardized when the historical testimony is affected is the authority of the object.[41]

The fashionable accessories, in this example, hair ornaments and cashmere shawl, clearly carry moral value. But as both of Balzac's texts demonstrate, in spite of her proper status, the *femme comme il faut* was already compromised, for her authenticity was only performed, staged, and not innate.

LA LORETTE

Just as the "grande dame d'autrefois" is marked for extinction in Balzac's essay, so the courtesan is excised from Dumas's. But while Balzac writes from the top down, first identifying the *femme comme il faut* as the nearest modern equivalent of the *grande dame* and then descending the social ladder as he considers her various imitators, Dumas writes from the bottom up. *Filles, lorettes et courtisanes* is a faithful title, reflecting the three-tiered hierarchy Dumas observes in the *demi-monde* that corresponds more or less to the familiar broad social categories of working class, bourgeois, and aristocratic. The preface promises a treatment "en trois classes distinctes, en trois catégories progressives, en trois échelons ascendants, qui conduiront successivement le lecteur du coin de la borne où la prostituée des rues guette le nocturne passant, jusqu'au boudoir princier où l'élégante courtisane, qu'on a envoyé chercher dans une voiture sans armoirie, est introduite par un valet sans livrée" (11–12) (in three distinct classes, three progressive categories, three ascending echelons, which will lead the reader successively from the corner of the boundary stone where the streetwalker waits for the nocturnal passerby, all the way to the princely boudoir into which the elegant courtesan, who has been sent for in an unmarked carriage, is introduced by an ununiformed valet). Dumas does not, however, represent these categories equally. His first chapter on "filles" (prostitutes) borrows extensively from the contemporary work of medical bureaucrat Parent-Duchâtelet, famous for instituting the regulation of prostitution in nineteenth-century Paris and for writing the monumental *De la prostitution dans la ville de Paris* in 1836.[42] Strangely, Dumas's final chapter on "courtisanes," so tantalizingly advertised in the preface, offers instead only a displacement of the discourse on the contemporary courtesan. For here, Dumas refers almost exclusively to courtesans of antiquity[43] and of eighteenth-century France, thus suggesting that like Balzac's *grande dame*, the idealized courtesan survives in the modern age only in a degraded form, characterized almost exclusively by her prodigality: "à qui deux millions de rentes ne suffisaient pas pour ses capricieuses fantaisies et qui trouvait encore moyen, avec ce revenu royal, de faire 500,000 fr. de dettes" (127) (for whom two million in income wasn't enough for her capricious fantasies and who always found a way, with this royal revenue, to be 500,000 francs in debt). The effacement of the courtesan in this text is in itself an expression of the anxiety over social mobility referred to in such lighthearted terms, but so frequently, throughout. In fact, as Jann Matlock has documented, "the courtesan was the most dangerous of all prostitutes because one could not tell her apart from women of polite society."[44] An *insoumise*, that is, not listed on the police rolls, the courtesan was not regulated by the police as were her socially inferior sisters, and because of her access to wealth, she also had easy access to the worldly accoutrements of her respectable foils. Perhaps the courtesan was beyond the reach of Dumas's project, just as she was outside of the law. The *lorette*, however, a dangerously new phenomenon, could still be exposed and demystified.

In mid-nineteenth-century Paris (1841), journalist and fashionable man-about-town Nestor Roqueplan first identified and named this new species of woman the *lorette*. A *lorette* was an aspiring courtesan, a kind of female equivalent of a Balzacian rags-to-riches hero, a working-class girl who refused traditional work and who chose instead to lead a life of luxury borrowed on credit and paid for by a number of "Arthurs"—the nickname given to her lovers and benefactors. The *lorette*, then, was also the incarnation of bourgeois culture's worst fears over the corruption of female virtue, the breakdown of social distinctions, and the resulting dissolution of male fortune. It is no surprise perhaps that she was a wildly popular figure in contemporary literature and imagery.[45] And given the primacy of fashion in the construction and restriction of female identity in the nineteenth century, it is even less surprising that she should be represented most consistently in her relationship to fashion.

The period in which the *lorette* texts appear spans the second half of the July Monarchy and the first part of the Second Empire. This is an important context to recognize as it was during this period (originating well before Haussmann) that the urban geography of Paris was being transformed to encompass heretofore uninhabited areas, thus provoking new constructions, property speculation, and modernization (boulevards, circulation of both goods and people, shopping, etc.). The *lorette* was linked to the rising industrial society, embodying capitalism at the expense of the earlier, premodern society, incarnated by the *grisette*.[46] The *lorette* would eventually evolve into the Second Empire *cocotte* and *cocodette*, who openly advertised their sexual availability and their kept condition through their luxury garments in the public spaces of high society such as Longchamp and the Bois de Boulogne.[47]

The link between the *lorette* and modernization is visible in the changing Parisian geography she inhabited. Her milieu was the recently socialized quartier situated in northwestern Paris in the area around the newly built church Notre-Dame de Lorette in what is now the ninth arrondissement. Martin-Fugier explains the significance of this neighborhood especially in relation to the faubourg Saint Germain, the quartier of the old aristocracy, in the emerging society of the July Monarchy: "La Chaussée d'Antin possède l'argent et la puissance mais le 'noble faubourg' détient le prestige qui légitime. Dans cette configuration, la Chaussée d'Antin fait figure de parvenue . . . symbole de dynamisme et de modernité, par sa proximité avec le Boulevard, [elle] avait aussi une image tapageuse de quartier où s'exhibent la richesse et la mode" (103– 6). (The Chaussée d'Antin has money and power, but the "noble" Saint Germain neighborhood retains the prestige that legitimates it. In this configuration, the Chaussée d'Antin represents the upstart . . . symbolic of dynamism and modernity, by its proximity to the Boulevard, it also had the flashy image of an area where wealth and fashion were displayed). When in 1841 Roqueplan named "the more or less young women who devote themselves to ruining sons of [good] families" *lorettes*, he was associating this figure with the particular space and circumstances of Parisian modernity.[48] Fashionable young kept women inhabited this area rent free presumably because they were the mistresses of wealthy landlords who had yet to find tenants for their newly constructed apartments. But its proximity to the new financial center (the Bourse) and to the new center of fashionable social activity (the Opéra) as well as to the modern commercial spaces of the grands boulevards would eventually make this most profitable of Parisian situations the place where the *lorette* could best locate and secure her "investors."[49]

Novelist Henry Murger, in his *Scènes de la vie de bohème*, also contributes to the growing mythology surrounding this new Parisian figure, defining the type of the *lorette* as a "race hybride, créatures impertinentes, beautés médiocres, demi-chair, demi-onguents, dont le boudoir est un comptoir où elles débitent des morceaux de leur cœur, comme on ferait des tranches de rosbif. La plupart de ces filles, qui déshonorent le plaisir et sont la honte de la galanterie moderne, n'ont point toujours l'intelligence des bêtes dont elles portent les plumes sur leurs chapeaux" (a hybrid race [of] impertinent creatures, mediocre beauties, half-flesh, half-perfume, whose boudoir is a deli counter where they sell pieces of their hearts as if they were slices of roast beef. Most of these women, who bring dishonor to pleasure and modern gallantry, don't even always have the intelligence of the animals that provide the feathers for their hats).[50] Murger scorns the *lorette* for her embodiment of hybridity, implicitly critiquing her for applying masculine codes of commerce to the feminine realm of the sentimental. If she were to acknowledge herself as a prostitute, perhaps this would not be so troubling; but she gets herself up as a proper lady and demands all the accoutrements of bourgeois luxury, and here is where the trouble lies. While there is much to say about the explicit misogyny of Murger's text, the most telling detail is his damning reference to hat feathers. Balzac, too, had condemned the use of feathers in "La Femme comme il faut" as being too flashy. Only a Madame Jules, with her perfectly simple and monochromatic marabouts, could wear feathers with elegance. Murger's use of a fashion detail, an accessory, to illuminate the woman's character is consistent with both the physiologists' portrayal of the *lorette* as fashion crazed (and thus dim) and their use of the theme and discourse of fashion to express the *lorette*'s disconcertingly flexible position in society.

Dumas *père* devotes his attention throughout his text to the category Balzac had defined as the *femme comme il en faut*, the opposite of the proper lady, and, as in Balzac, his text raises the specter of social instability through an anecdotal discourse on fashion. When the prostitute was expelled from her covered haunts of the Palais Royal and into the muddy streets of Paris, Dumas recounts, she had to don new dress, more suitable to the streets than her usual brightly colored, lightweight "indoor" wear. As a result of her relocation, she began to resemble the "femme honnête," as she was now forced to use both of her hands to "relever sa robe" (lift her skirt) and "retenir son châle" (hold her shawl), thus miming decorum and presumably distracting her from other, more inviting gestures. "La prostituée, grâce à son nouveau costume, pourrait encore tromper quelque provincial nouvellement arrivé, qui la prendrait pour une comtesse égarée, ou quelque bourgeoise" (21) (The prostitute, thanks to her new costume, could deceive some bumpkin newly arrived from the provinces, who would take her for a lost countess or a bourgeoise). This potential confusion was a source of great consternation and required an immediate remedy, which, according to Dumas's chronology, was where Parent-Duchâtelet and the work of regulation came in. Likewise, the "filles à numéros" (the so-called aristocracy within the "filles" category), who were generally "assez élégamment mises" (fairly well dressed), could deceive hapless tourists and students into the fiction that they were "baronnes,... comtesses... et marquises" (48).[51] Dumas's anecdotes repeatedly declare the theme of social imposture through sartorial skill.

Bracketing the courtesan, the *lorette*, designated by Dumas as the "bourgeoise" of the *demi-mondaine* hierarchy, represents the greatest potential threat to social stability. She is Dumas's emblem for the modern—fashionable and fleeting—and thus embodies the structural counterpart of Balzac's *femme comme il faut*: she is her *demi-mondaine* double. Like her more respectable cousin, the *lorette* is hard to classify, having only recently appeared on the social stage.[52] Whether the offspring of a colonel of the empire or a porter's daughter, like Balzac's *femme comme il faut*, the *lorette*'s origins are murky: "Ne cherchons pas ses origines," Dumas warns, "si son origine est destinée à rester plongée dans les ténèbres du doute ou dans les mystères de l'inconnu" (63) (let's not look for her origins... if her origin is destined to remain plunged in the darkness of doubt or the mystery of the unknown). As with Roqueplan and Murger, for Dumas *père*, the problem of the *lorette*'s indeterminacy is central. *Lorettes* are "de charmants petits êtres propres, élégants, coquets, qu'on ne pouvait classer dans aucun des genres connus: ce n'était ni le genre fille, ni le genre grisette, ni le genre courtisane. Ce n'était non plus le genre bourgeois. C'était encore moins le genre femme honnête" (58) (charming little beings, clean, elegant and coquettish, which we cannot classify in any of the known types: she is neither a "fille," a "grisette," nor a courtesan. She is not a bourgeoise either, and is even less a respectable lady). In spite of these caveats to classification and his claimed disavowal of interest in origins, Dumas makes every effort here to pin down the new species through the containing and classifying project of his essay.

Dumas's chapter on the *lorette* recounts shopping and fashion anecdotes to elucidate her "rapports sociaux, politiques et intellectuels" (social, political, and intellectual relations), which the author describes with the express aim of arming his readers better to "combat" her. Her lovers are numerous, at least as numerous as her fashion needs: "l'un fournit les gants, l'autre les chapeaux, celui-ci les étoffes, celui-là les façons" (65) (one furnishes gloves, the other hats, this one cloth, the other sewn pieces). Taking a stylistic cue here from the fashion journal, Dumas refers to the breadth of the fashion industry and suggests also the masquerade of honesty in which the *lorette* engages through her dress. Gloves and hats are the accessories of outer extremities without which proper ladies could not be seen publicly.[53] Fabrics (*étoffes*) and cuts (*façons*) are the raw materials of garment creation, but these too carry moral weight, as both terms may also refer to ethical properties— substance and manners. The *lorette*'s most important relationships are apparently with her *fournisseurs*, or merchants, for they are both her creditors and the suppliers of the tools of her trade.[54] Dumas's enumeration of the *lorette*'s many *fournisseurs* and their goods mimics the list of her lovers, making explicit the parallel between material and sexual consumption:

> Ce sont eux qui lui confectionnent ses chapeaux à la lionne, si relevés par derrière, si inclinés par devant, qui laissent voir le chignon, et desquels s'échappe ce joli nœud de rubans qui flotte coquettement jusqu'au bas de son dos. Ce sont eux qui lui fournissent ses crispins de velours ou de satin, qui tombent si carrément jusqu'aux genoux, et qui sont si coquettement garnis de franges. Enfin ce sont eux qui lui livrent les manchons qui imitent si admirablement l'hermine, la martre et le renard bleu, qu'il faut l'œil d'une femme jalouse pour reconnaître la contrefaçon. (67)

> [The merchants are the ones who create her rakish hats, so high in the back, so low in the front, which reveal the chignon and from which trails the pretty knot of ribbons that float flirtatiously down her back. They are the ones who provide her velvet and satin coats, which fall just to her knees and are so coquettishly fringed. Finally, they are the ones who deliver the muffs that so cleverly imitate ermine, mink and

blue fox that it would take the eye of a jealous woman to perceive the counterfeit.]

The merchant is the *lorette*'s partner in sartorial seduction and social masquerade, and it thus stands to reason that he should expect to profit from her social and sexual conquests. Dumas's litany reads like a fashion reporter's description of the latest trends and could be quite convincingly compared to a passage from a *journal de mode*, as he clearly borrows the tropes of fashion reporting. His text is rich in detail and visually suggestive, both characteristics imperative for print descriptions of fashions. Dumas ends, however, on the theme of imitation or forgery ("la contrefaçon"), which is, of course, the crux of the matter.

The *lorette*'s relative elegance reveals her shifting financial status, and the *fournisseur* is quick to recognize the signs of a new love and to capitalize on it:

> A peine voit-il poindre à l'horizon de la rue Lafitte les crispins de velours, la pèlerine d'hermine, et le Bibi excentrique, dans leur fraîcheur primitive, qu'il devine qu'il s'est fait un changement dans la position de sa cliente. Aussitôt il reparaît sur le carré, la figure souriante, sonne aussi modestement qu'il sonnait fort, et en échange du châle de mérinos, qu'il a souvent insolemment arraché de dessus ses épaules, il vient humblement lui offrir le cachemire de l'Inde. (84)

> [As soon as he spots the velvet gloves, the ermine cape, and the eccentric Bibi [a hat], all in their primal freshness, appearing on the horizon of the rue Lafitte, he instantly guesses the change in his client's position. Just as quickly, he reappears smiling at her doorstep and rings as modestly now as he rang loudly before, and in exchange for the merino wool shawl that he had so often insolently wrenched off her shoulders, he now humbly offers her an Indian cashmere].[55]

The text presents a metonymy: the clothes make the woman. Gloves, cape, and stylish hat—all three accessories and protective coverings for the elegant lady—indicate the *lorette*'s social and financial ascendancy. Not only does the merchant now treat the newly gentrified *lorette* with the respect due a proper lady, he also treats her to the single garment that most clearly denotes respectability.

The *cachemire de l'Inde*, as we learned in Balzac's *Ferragus*, is the authentic cashmere worn by the *femme comme il faut*, a sign not only of wealth but of standing, even virtue, representing economic, cultural, and moral capital at once. In the Frédéric Bouchot engraving pictured in Figure 1, the caricaturist seizes upon the value of this prized acces-

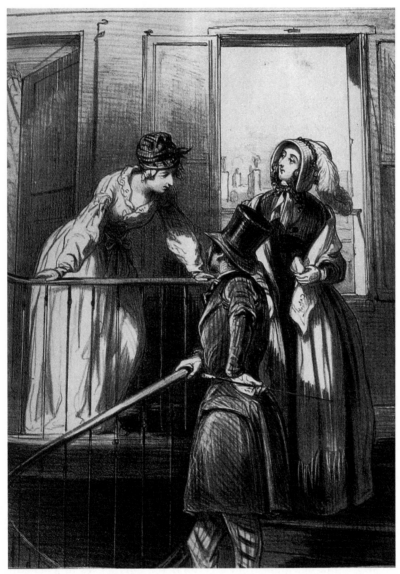

Figure 1. "La rue Notre Dame de Lorette," Frédéric Bouchot, Maciet Collection, Bibliothèque des Arts décoratifs.

sory to illustrate the venality of the *lorette*. Situated in an apartment stairwell in the rue Notre Dame de Lorette, with a view of the cityscape visible through the open window, one *lorette* declines the invitation of another, who is on her way with a fashionable male companion to the Bois de Boulogne. The speaker, clad in a housedress and kerchief, instead of the shawl and feathered hat of her friend, will stay home for her English lesson, which, she informs us, will be brief as she only needs to learn how to ask for a *cachemire*. The reduction of the *lorette*'s raison d'être to the acquisition of a cashmere shawl reinforces the cultural perception of these women's venality: the well-dressed *lorette*, wrapped in her shawl, has arrived and can now be presented on the public stage of the Bois, which played host to aristocrats and courtesans alike, on the arm of her companion. Her less fortunate friend will have to hone her skills before she can achieve the coveted goal of the cashmere—which, as we shall see in a later chapter, accorded respectability for its association with marriage as much as for its association with luxury.

The *lorette* thus insinuates her way up the social ladder through a careful appropriation of sartorial signals—her masterful imitation may eventually pay off with the passage to authenticity, as the shawl exchange and illustration both suggest. Dumas appropriates the discourse of the fashion journal to designate the fluid position of the dangerous *lorette*. By observing the minutest shift in sartorial detail, the *fournisseur*, who has perhaps the most to gain from a mobile social hierarchy, reads social change and responds in turn with new clothes. The real "man-eater" is, of course, the *fournisseur*, for it is the merchant who profits from the *lorette*'s association with wealth and her endless need to appear fashionable in order to pass as a lady of leisure. The very imperative of fashion, conceived and maintained by the merchant, traps the *lorette* in her cycle of spending and speculation.

The *lorette* produces and performs a self-perpetuating fiction of luxury, and her most valued props are, naturally, her garments. Alhoy's *Physiologie de la lorette* deconstructs the *lorette*'s "luxury effect" in an illustration of her flight from creditors. The *lorette* lives in a state of perpetual deferral that mimics modern credit practices. As long as she can maintain the luxury effect, she avoids paying her bills. Along with her toothbrush and her iron, when a *lorette* decamps clandestinely the moment the bill comes due, she layers her dresses on her body, like so many possible disguises. "Elle revêt d'abord trois jupons de toutes nuances qu'elle recouvre d'une robe de chali indigo; la robe de chali reçoit en surcharge une robe de crêpe Rachel orange; le crêpe Rachel est surfoulé par une robe Kabaïle tricolore; la robe Kabaïle s'étreint sous un cachemire agonisant et un tartan dans la force de l'âge: un manteau couvre le tout. La Lorette dit au portier qu'elle va au bain, et l'oiseau s'envole" (36) (First she puts on three underskirts of different colors which she covers with an indigo chali dress; the chali dress gets an overload of an orange "Rachel" crepe dress; the Rachel crepe is then trampled by a tricolored Kabaïle dress, which is then squeezed under a cashmere on its last legs and a robust tartan: a coat conceals everything. The *lorette* tells the doorman that she's off to the baths, and the bird flies the coop!). She escapes her exasperated landlord and other creditors by foregoing a valise and arrives in her new digs in an apparently unfortunate state, which she quickly reverses by undressing—not to display her body, but rather her capital, signaled by her wardrobe. Her striptease ends at the first and most fashionable layer of clothing. Her new landlord, once he sees her "richesses vestimentaires" (vestimentary riches) is reassured: "Tiens! cette dame a beaucoup d'effets" (37) ("this lady has got lots of stuff"). The *lorette*'s manipulation of the material of luxury points to a cultural shift in value lamented by many of the physiologists and novelists of the period: her identity resides in her display of luxury and not in the cult of origins to which luxury used to refer; her capital is her costume—the fragile and fleeting ephemera of fashion—and lacks the stable value of the traditional standards of gold and land.

Alhoy's *physiologie* describes the *lorette* attempting to pass not only as a respectable woman, thus transgressing social boundaries, but also, more disturbingly, we learn, as a man, moving into the public sphere of capital. Alhoy's text makes an important digression into what he calls the "excentricités" of the *lorette*, in which he outlines her curious penchant for transvestism. She likes to smoke cigars, but that is not all: "La Lorette éprouve très-souvent l'envie de changer sa couturière contre un tailleur" (86) (very often she likes to exchange her seamstress for a tailor), that is, she likes to dress in men's clothing, claiming, according to Alhoy, that "dans la loi naturelle, tel ou tel vêtement n'appartient pas plus à un sexe que tel ou tel autre" (86) (in nature, no article of clothing belongs more to one sex than to the other). Cross-dressing outside of carnival was prohibited without written permission from the authorities. What follows in Alhoy's description is a hilarious series of petitions from *lorettes*, demanding permission to dress as men for various reasons. One wishes to use a cane to beat someone who has insulted her, another wants to drink her coffee at the bar, and a third still, unable to successfully pluck her moustache, would rather grow a beard "comme vous, monsieur le préfet" (88) ("like you, monsieur le préfet"). While the entire episode is farcical, each request nonetheless expressly states an interest in occupying spaces or exerting agency reserved for men, and each request is, of course, summarily denied.

That *lorettes* dressed up as men has been documented and explained in part by their proximity to and association with the theater but also by their desire to enter restricted spaces such as gambling halls and the Bourse itself.[56] Alhoy describes one legally cross-dressed *lorette* who seems to have "porté chapeau toute sa vie et qu'elle est née avec des bottes" (90) (worn a hat all her life and been born wearing boots). She knows how to twirl a cane and make off with the best cigar. Further, at the theater, she steals the seat reserved by a yellow glove by pocketing the very glove. If the glove is the metonymy of the fashionable man, she has now absorbed him. On the one hand, her donning of male garb facilitates her passage into male space and her approximation of male behavior, which here can only be seen as far from honest.[57] But on the other hand, her cross-dressing seems only to have served to further exaggerate her femininity and was thus put in the service of her primary occupation. We are reminded of Flaubert's Rosanette disguised as a soldier at the masked ball, whose tight pants reveal better than her voluminous skirts her feminine contours, or of Emma Bovary in the frenzy of her adulterous affair with Léon, whose cross-dressing emblematizes her struggle against patriarchal social structures (Czyba 115, V. Thompson 135). Once unmasked, Alhoy's *lorette* exclaims indignantly to the arresting officer, "Je ne suis pas une femme!" (90) ("I am not a woman!"). And this is in fact precisely the problem—that is, by her very performativity, she undermines the notion of a stable feminine ideal. By masquerading as masculine just as elsewhere she performs respectability, she disrupts ideological structures working to shape society. The *physiologie*'s comic representation of this "eccentricity" of the *lorette* betrays the serious anxiety surrounding this female type, who not only usurps the appearance of feminine respectability in her assumption of the accessories of bourgeois luxury but also literally dresses as a man, thus presenting an affront to the gender hierarchy that makes the notion of female respectability pertinent in the first place. This literal gender imposture, shocking though it may have been, suggests a more subtle subversion: the *lorette* brazenly functions commercially as a woman, effecting a scandalous blending of private and public spheres, the feminine ideal corrupted by capital.

The *lorette* is fully reduced to her pure commercial essence in the

Goncourt brothers' *La Lorette*. Gone are the endearing and entertaining anecdotes of the earlier *physiologies*, and the *lorette* as social type, produced by this very discourse that claims merely to represent her (the Goncourts dedicate their work to Gavarni), is strangely void of both body and soul. "Toutes n'ont n'y [*sic*] esprit, ni gorge, ni cœur, ni tempérament. Toutes ont le même dieu: le dieu Cent-Sous" (42) (All of them have neither spirit, cleavage, heart, nor personality. They all have the same god: the god of Money). The style of this text, with its repetitive enumerations of possessions and payments, introduced always either by the anonymous singular pronoun "elle" or the plural "toutes," strips the *lorette* of any existence outside of the commercially signifying. "Elle ne paye pas son propriétaire; elle ne paye pas sa couturière; elle ne paye pas sa crémière; elle ne paye pas son porteur d'eau. Elle paye sa lingère. Son coiffeur se paye" (40) (She doesn't pay her landlord, she doesn't pay her dressmaker, she doesn't pay the dairyman, she doesn't pay her water carrier. She pays her laundress. Her coiffeur "gets paid."). Disembodied and soulless, what she does still have is a corset. And her corset "à la paresseuse," which doesn't require lacing by a husband or a maid from behind, speaks volumes.[58] Her autonomy and her venality are matched in her transgressive adaptation of the undergarment designed precisely to contain, restrict, and shape the feminine silhouette and indeed the ideology of the feminine in the nineteenth century.[59] Her favorite lover is known by the title "Monsieur de l'Ambassade des Cachemires," for he alone procures for her the indispensable accessory:

> Une chose est pour la Lorette ce qu'est une montre pour un enfant de treize ans, la possession d'une actrice pour l'enfant de dix-sept, l'Académie pour le jeune homme de soixante; une chose à fond rouge, ou noir, ou vert, chargée de différentes couleurs: une chose faite avec la laine des chèvres de l'Ourna-Dessa;—cette chose est un cachemire de l'Inde. (55)

> [One thing is for the Lorette what a watch is for a thirteen-year-old, possession of an actress for a seventeen-year-old, the Académie for the young man of sixty; a thing with a red, black, or green background, filled with different colors; a thing made with the wool of goats from Ourna-Dessa;—this thing is an Indian cashmere shawl.]

The accessory that most frequently defined female respectability—the cashmere shawl—was the most coveted "capital" the *lorette* could acquire, for it facilitated her slippage into polite society.

The *lorette* is a type associated with a specific time and place who serves to crystallize anxieties surrounding political and social upheavals in mid-nineteenth-century France. The *physiologies* and illustrative series that purport to represent her functioned to identify, classify, decipher, and, indeed, contain her within their pages. This discursive gesture that claims to describe, however, is actually itself constitutive of the figure and thus helps to manage the anxieties circulating about the upheavals of modernization as they emerge in mid-nineteenth-century Paris. The *physiologies* work hard to define and classify this type, especially with respect to her potential social subversion. Her most readable form of transgression is expressed in her relation to fashion, and so these texts focus on fashion anecdotes to suggest both her contamination of the feminine ideal and her intrusion into the masculine domain of the market. These texts inscribe her subversion through their focus on fashion, but they also suggest the limits of her subversion, as evidenced in her containment and reproduction in discourse and illustrations.

As Victoria Thompson points out, the *physiologies* propose that the *lorette* uses fashion subversively to pass both as a respectable woman and as a man (metaphorically and literally) in order to practice a form of speculation (in lovers) and thus to secure power (access to money). Her very real cross-dressing, however, serves essentially to reinscribe her femininity; and as these texts also detail, her commerce in fashion ultimately expresses the impossibility of her consolidation of wealth. It is this metaphorical passing as masculine that earns her the disrepute represented by her illustrators and physiologists. The story of the *lorette* is, then, the story of women's oblique participation in and visible exclusion from modern capital and bourgeois enrichment.[60] Related to this is the sense in which she embodies an essential paradox of fashion—which is at once a tool of female subjugation and conformity and an expression of difference, agency, and creativity. As Balzac suggested of the *femme comme il faut*, the *lorette* appears in these texts as pure signifier, pure performativity, and is ultimately dissociated from any authentic account of identity: this is why she so potently subverts the contemporary social order.

CONCLUSION

As the protosociological texts examined here make clear, fashion was both a mirror of and a two-way street between *monde* and *demi-monde*. The fashion accessory was the key component in the construction and performance of social status. These texts also express the growing anxiety over the potential reversibility of proper and venal through the vehicle of fashion. Readings of fiction contemporary to the *physiologies* further deepen the theme of the erasure of distinction between *monde* and *demi-monde* so feared by the authors of the sociological texts. Balzac's proper lady, the *femme comme il faut*, emblematizes the correct use of fashion details in the service of distinction. However proper she may be, she nonetheless resembles her *demi-mondaine* doubles in her careful manipulation of fashion signs toward the production of status. Balzac's characters suspect the imminent passing of an era: "Le glas de la haute société sonne . . . le premier coup est ce mot moderne de *femme comme il faut!*" (*Autre étude*, 65) (The knell of the highest society is tolling . . . the first stroke is your modern word *lady!* [34]); and by 1867, in the *A propos de La Dame aux camélias* (the play), Dumas *fils* tells of its death by indistinction, first signaled by a loss of differentiation in fashion and then spreading to other domains: "[on] se prêta des patrons de robe entre courtisanes et femmes du monde, . . . [n]on seulement on eut les mêmes toilettes, mais on eut le même langage, les mêmes danses, les mêmes aventures, les mêmes amours, disons tout, les mêmes spécialités. . . . Nous allons à la prostitution universelle" (372) (courtesans and society women would lend each other dress patterns, . . . not only did they wear the same clothes, but had the same language, the same dances, the same adventures, the same affairs, let's say it, the same "specialities". . . . We are headed for universal prostitution). The anxiety expressed in these works is one of social indeterminacy, but it is characterized by a preoccupation with a loss of moral distinction among women. The fashion accessory, the fetishistic detail of fashion, was promoted in these texts as the principal marker of distinction. As Vinken has provocatively asserted, "the modern depends upon the fetish . . . because in fashion the fetish arrives at its ancestral realm: the stuff of which dreams are made, the realm of the accessory. . . . Already in its etymological sense of 'making, producing, manufacturing,' the fetish is a product of art, associated with artificiality. The female body must then also count as such a product of art" (27).[61] The accessory as exemplary fetish object negotiated the material and the fantasized, the woman as object and subject of modernity. From the cashmere shawl to the *Bibi excentrique*, it was the fashion accessory that most clearly delineated the nuanced modes of distinction that were becoming increasingly necessary as more and more women had access to fashion. By focusing on the ornamentation of women, who in turn were the ornaments of men, these texts deflect onto a seemingly frivolous topic serious anxieties underpinning nineteenth-century social and sexual politics.[62] The fetishized accessory served to complicate the codes of respectability and status that modernity was threatening to efface.

In nineteenth-century France, *monde* and *demi-monde* appeared to be worlds apart. Yet, as I have demonstrated in the works analyzed in this chapter, as in the nineteenth-century France they describe, the virtual space of fashion is a busy crossroads of *monde* and *demi-monde*. For there was indeed imitation on both sides of the social border: women of Balzac's *demi-monde* strove to pass for proper ladies, clothing themselves in the wardrobe of respectability, while by the Second Empire, respectable women were taking their fashion cues from courtesans, the logical heiresses of the *lorettes*.[63] Not only was the courtesan versed in nineteenth-century theories of *élégance*, but she had also mastered what the aristocrats of earlier days had always understood: the sartorial *je ne sais quoi* that bestows the first prize of French society, distinction. The nineteenth-century courtesan's emergence as fashion plate is thus emblematic of a society's reinvention just as surely as it exemplifies the transgressive blurring of *demi-monde* and *monde*, of *immonde* and *mondaine*.

The back stories of the fashion accessory, present in so many nineteenth-century texts, however, and the struggles of modernity they reveal point to gender hierarchy and to the deeper threat posed by women, the nineteenth-century male's accessory par excellence. This book focuses in large part on the complex figure of the paradoxical *femme comme il faut*—who was at once the souvenir of *Ancien Régime* elite values and herald of modern social flux—and the set of fashion accessories that helped her perform her *comme il faut* role. Those accessories, so crucial to the performance of respectability and the social production of female propriety, were also essential elements in the passage from girlhood to marriage in nineteenth-century France. In the next chapter, I will examine in detail the marriage gift basket, offered by the fiancé to his bride—the *corbeille de mariage*. Through its association with marriage, the *corbeille* institutionalized the links between respectability and luxury, between virtue and erotics, that the objects it contained, the accessories to modernity, incarnated. Like the *physiologies* examined in this chapter, the *corbeille de mariage* was an order-making enterprise, distilling and ritualizing into a single auspicious moment in the life of a *jeune fille*, the moment of the marriage contract, the notion of feminine respectability.

CHAPTER TWO

Unpacking the *Corbeille de mariage*

*On avait eu l'idée de remplacer la corbeille par quelque mil-
liers de francs, insérés dans une enveloppe, mais cette innovation a
froissé la délicatesse de sentiment du plus grand nombre des fian-
cés, et la vieille mode a prévalu, nous en sommes bien aise.*

LA BARONNE STAFFE

In September 1874, in the first issue of the fashion magazine *La Dernière
Mode*, Marguerite de Ponty wrote ecstatically and meticulously about
the ideal *corbeille de mariage*. Her fantasy *corbeille* would contain a
wide assortment of diamonds and other jewels to befit every social occasion; fine laces, sprung "des mains des fées elles-mêmes" (from the
hands of the fairies themselves) and of every variety, to provide trim
for gowns, handkerchiefs, parasols, and other accessories; exquisitely
painted fans, all crafted with superlative skill and from the most opulent of materials. This vision of splendor is enveloped in one final, but
indispensable, luxury garment, the staple of every *corbeille*:

> Une corbeille de mariage!. . . . Tout cela étalé un instant sous votre
> regard, mesdames, entre, à divers titres, dans la corbeille: et un
> cachemire des Indes d'un prix quelconque, ce vêtement nécessaire ne
> se portant que très rarement (car la mode ne l'admet plus comme ha-
> billé). Qu'il glisse, ce châle, des épaules avec ses plis orientaux et envel-
> oppe d'autres merveilles: tout le délicieux écrin que nous avons, pierre
> à pierre ou perle à perle, raconté.[1]

> [A *corbeille de mariage*!. . . . All this that we have been glimpsing must
> for various reasons have its place in the *corbeille* and an Indian cash-
> mere shawl, of a certain price—indispensable, even if only very rarely
> worn. (Fashion having declared it not to be formal dress.) Let it (this
> shawl) slip from the shoulders, with its oriental folds, and envelop oth-
> er marvels—all that jewel box which, stone by stone or pearl by pearl,
> we have been recounting.][2]

Marguerite de Ponty was the pseudonym of poet Stéphane Mallarmé, who for four months in 1874 was also "the editor, the designer and the author" of *La Dernière Mode*, a women's fashion magazine that ran until 1875 (4). That the notably abstruse poet could have expressed such a devotion to and flair for writing about the subject of fashion is curious and compelling in itself.[3] But more compelling still are those undeclared "various reasons" for the inclusion of these particular objects in the *corbeille*. The poet–fashion writer expresses in this text, intended for an upper-class female audience, the conflation of woman and luxury object. Using the shawl as metaphor, he manages to poeticize fashion and to link the *corbeille*, repository of *merveilles*, to the well-bred young lady, virtuous and respectable, the *trésor* of her father's house. For here, *corbeille* and woman are expertly enmeshed through the fashion writer's clever and exotic draping of the imaginary shawl over both eroticized feminine flesh and the jewel box of treasures that the bride-to-be receives from her fiancé on the day her marriage contract is signed. The text makes clear, albeit subtly, the connection between the enumerated gems and pearls of the *corbeille* and the discreet "jewels," those "autres merveilles," of the female body.[4]

The contents of the *corbeille* were at once luxurious goods meant to seduce through their material opulence a marriageable *demoiselle*, reflecting and reinforcing her status of propriety and concluding the marriage contract, and also seductive objects in their contribution to the erotics of female fashion. The *corbeille* thus signifies both literally and symbolically the notion of *trésor*, so frequently used to describe both the *corbeille* contents and the young lady for whom they are destined. The cultural significance of the *corbeille* comes into focus by studying not only the object itself and its contents but also its representation in literary and nonliterary documents of the nineteenth century. *La Corbeille, journal des modes*, founded in 1836 and running through the 1870s, was a popular women's fashion journal of the nineteenth century covering, like much of the feminine fashion press, social events, the latest fashions, serialized fiction, and advice for women. Its frontispice image pictures the object spilling over with tantalizing accessories and at the same time conflates a material embodiment of luxury fashion with the discursive engine through which this object would gain importance (Figure 2). The *corbeille* would graft directives of female behaviors and ideologies of female value onto the literal object and its discursive doubles. The literal treasure contained in the chest, with its heirloom quality and oriental provenance, is equivalent to the *trésor* of the young lady

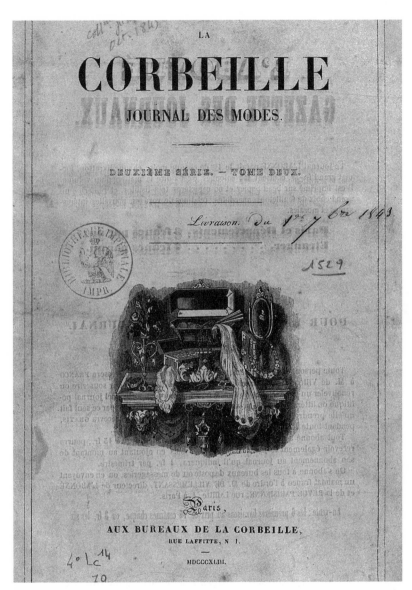

Figure 2. "Page de titre avec corbeille," *La Corbeille, journal des modes*, 1843, Bibliothèque nationale de France.

herself, the virtuous and sheltered minor of her father's house and symbolic capital of bourgeois respectability. The *corbeille* classified certain objects as markers of respectability: because they were included in the *corbeille*, an object deeply tied to marriage and its rituals, these luxury goods were, in principle at least, not permitted to women of ill repute.

How the contents of the *corbeille* came to be considered the criteria for distinction, the *über*-commodity of nineteenth-century French society, is the subject of this chapter, which contextualizes my choice of objects in the chapters that follow. The fashionable luxury goods required to fill a *corbeille* were essential to the production of respectability in part because they were designed and marketed to seduce women into marriage, but they also had to be deployed with restraint—that is, female desire for fashion had to be kept in check and satisfied only as a compensation for filling the respectable role of wife. The gendering of luxury fashions was embodied in the custom of the *corbeille*, offered by the groom, who in a sense endowed the bride with her new status by endowing her with the raiments of that role. By taking up the *corbeille*, this chapter explores the fraught relations around women as guarantors of respectability, as desired objects doubling the accessories that adorn them, and as agents whose own desire is mediated and infiltrated by fashion.

In this chapter I present the *corbeille de mariage* and its gendered negotiation of symbolic and literal capital through a detailed analysis of Balzac's 1835 novella *Le Contrat de mariage*, along with references to other literary texts, including Edmond Duranty's 1860 novel *Le Malheur d'Henriette Gérard* and Gyp's dialogue entitled "La Corbeille de mariage" from her 1888 collection entitled *Pauvres petites femmes*. These literary readings are interwoven with an exploration of descriptions and advertisements in fashion journals, etiquette manuals, and popular plays, as well as several illustrations from contemporaneous publications, all of which nuance the category of respectability that gripped nineteenth-century ideologies of women in France. Before I pass to the figurative unpacking of the *corbeille*, I consider the object itself and some of its contents, in order to restore this now largely forgotten object to its position of vital importance in the marriage transaction of nineteenth-century France, heeding victorianist Elaine Freedgood's call that we must "literalize [objects] in order to re-figure them, that is, we need to re-materialize them in order to understand their value differently" (28). Understanding why these objects were associated with feminine propriety and indeed how they contributed to its very fabrication is the overarching aim of this book, and in this chapter I will make some preliminary claims on which subsequent chapters will build. The *corbeille de mariage* was the object that contained all the others, so it is logical to begin here.

LA CORBEILLE

The *corbeille de mariage*, or *corbeille de noces*, was a gift basket filled with luxury accessories that the intended was required to offer his bride in exchange for the *dot* (dowry).[5] Its monetary value was generally equivalent to between 5 and 10 percent of the value of the dowry and grew ever greater during the nineteenth century, but its sociocultural value was incalculable.[6] The *corbeille* itself during the nineteenth century was practically a piece of furniture, "un secrétaire, un bonheur-du-jour, ou un coffre susceptible de contenir beaucoup plus de gâteries que par le passé" (Bricard 310) (a secretary, a little desk, or a trunk able to contain many more treats than in the past), and is illustrated in the advertisement from an 1860 number of the fashion journal *Psyché* for Lavigne's "Corbeille parisienne" pictured in Figure 3. The *corbeille* as functional furniture transformed the promise of luxurious bliss offered by the previously held notion of *corbeille* as treasure chest into an emblem of bourgeois domesticity. With the *corbeille* came marriage and a young lady's entry into the role of mistress of the *foyer*. Likewise, the following excerpt from *La Mode illustrée* of 1880 confirms the combined ornamental value and functionality of the nineteenth-century *corbeille*: "La classique et traditionnelle *corbeille de mariage* est actuellement remplacée par un joli meuble, destiné à orner le salon, le parloir ou la chambre de la jeune femme qui la reçoit. On place sur les tablettes les tissus, les dentelles, les fourrures, dans les petits tiroirs on dispose les écrins" (150) (The classic and traditional marriage box is now replaced by a pretty piece of furniture, destined to dress up the drawing room, the parlor or the bedroom of the young woman who receives it. On its shelves, you place fabrics, laces, furs, and in the little drawers, you put jewelry cases).

But even early in the century, it could be quite extravagant and was intended for display to friends and family, marking the young lady's entry into *le monde*. In the 1815 edition of the collection of "observations sur les mœurs et les usages parisiens au commencement du XIXe siècle" known as *l'Hermite de la Chaussée d'Antin*, Étienne de Jouy describes the adventure of a young man accompanied by an older friend, the nar-

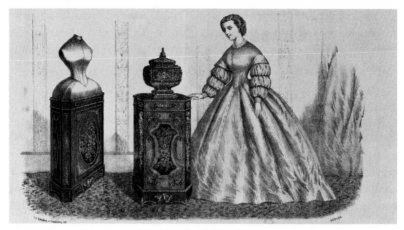

Figure 3. *Psyché: journal de modes*, 1860, Bibliothèque nationale de France.

rator, as they shop for the *corbeille* and its contents for the young man's impending marriage:

> La corbeille, en forme d'autel antique, n'était pas moins remarquable par l'élégance que par le fini du travail: des miniatures allégoriques d'un goût exquis, peintes sur velours par les artistes les plus distingués, et encadrées dans des bordures de perles, ornaient les parois extérieures; le dedans, tapissé d'aromates précieux, exhalait à-la-fois tous les parfums de l'Arabie. Robes, diamans [*sic*], schalls, dentelles, tout fut enfermé dans cette brillante enveloppe. (117)

> [The *corbeille*, shaped like an ancient altar, was no less remarkable for its elegance than for its workmanship: allegorical figures of exquisite taste, painted on velvet by the most distinguished artists and framed in borders of pearls, decorated the exterior edges; from inside, embroidered with precious spices, wafted all the perfumes of Arabia at once. Dresses, diamonds, shawls, laces. Everything was held in this brilliant envelope.][7]

Whether reconfigured as furniture for the bourgeois household or replicating an ancient altar, the *corbeille* was the literal and figurative treasure chest containing the props and costumes of the married lady and rewarding her with its riches as well as its respectability.

Typically offered on the day the marriage contract was signed and carefully scrutinized before any signatures were made, the *corbeille* embodied the rite of passage to female adulthood. Significantly, it was the groom who offered the *corbeille*, thus enabling the *jeune fille* to make

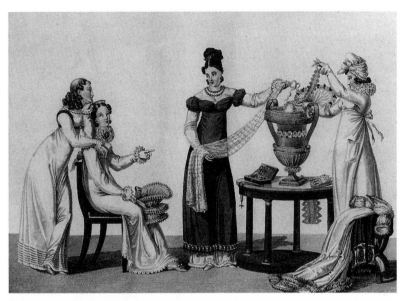

Figure 4.   *Le Bon Genre*, 1820, Bibliothèque nationale de France.

this transition, all the while remaining legally a minor under the *Code Civil*.[8] It was, essentially, a hierarchizing as well as a containing object, for in it lay all the accoutrements of respectable womanhood. *Corbeilles* were universal among members of the bourgeois and upper classes in nineteenth-century France and were available for a range of budgets. They were widely advertised and illustrated in the fashion press throughout the century, as the plates pictured in Figures 4–5 from early to late century attest.

Many images such as these stage the moment of unpacking the *corbeille* and examining its contents. The bride is attended by other women who assist her with this inspection and who seem at times to share in the sensual pleasure of viewing and touching the treasured material accoutrements of married femininity. Some standard items are visible in several of the images—laces, jewelry, colored fabrics suggestive of shawls. In the "Bulletin des Modes" column from March 1847 in the fashion journal *La Mode*, an anonymous fashion correspondent confirms, however, that *corbeilles* were available for a range of budgets and that, in spite of a wide variation in cost, certain key elements were always de rigueur:

Nous avons vu cette semaine, dans les salons de la Maison de commis-

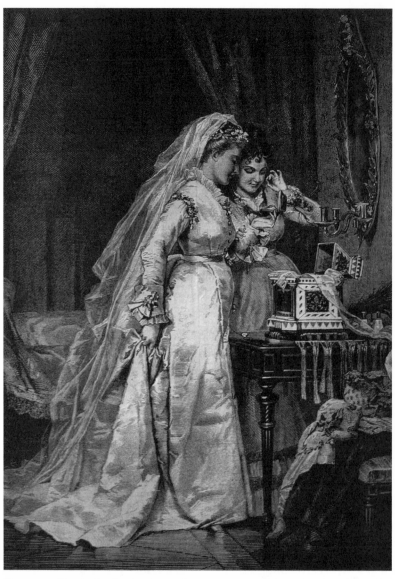

Figure 5. "La Corbeille de mariage," 1880, Maciet Collection, Bibliothèque des arts décoratifs.

sion Lassalle et Compagnie, deux corbeilles de mariage, dont l'une lui avait été fixée à 12.000 fr., et l'autre à 3.000 fr.

La première ... était composée d'un superbe cachemire des Indes long, fond noir, d'un second cachemire des Indes carré multicolore ... d'un admirable mouchoir brodé avec les armes, d'un paroissien en velours cramoisi avec ornemens en or découpés ..., d'un nécessaire de travail avec pièces ciselées, d'un éventail ancien, d'une boîte à gants, d'une boîte à mouchoirs en bois de rose....

La corbeille de 3.000 fr. était composée d'un cachemire des Indes carré gros vert, d'un châle français à quatre faces ..., d'un paroissien en velours gros bleu avec fermoir et chiffres en argent, d'un mouchoir brodé garni de valenciennes, d'un carnet de visites, d'un éventail, d'un flacon, d'une bourse, d'une boîte à gants avec une douzaine de paires de gants. (385)

[This week, in the salons of the Maison de commission Lasalle et Compagnie, we have seen two *corbeilles de mariage*, one of which priced at 12,000 francs and the other at 3,000 francs.

The first one ... contained a superb long Indian cashmere shawl, black background, a second Indian cashmere shawl, square and multicolored ... an admirable handkerchief embroidered with the arms, a prayer book in crimson velvet with ornaments in cut gold ..., a sewing bag with sculpted pieces, an antique fan, a glove box, a rosewood handkerchief box....

The 3,000 franc *corbeille* contained a square Indian shawl in dark green, a French shawl with four sides ..., a prayer book in dark blue velvet with clasp and monogram in silver, an embroidered handkerchief decorated with *valenciennes* [a type of lace], a card holder, a fan, a bottle, a purse, a glove box with a dozen pairs of gloves.]

Regardless of budget, present in both *corbeilles* are the essential ingredients of propriety, albeit fabricated from materials of varying quality: cashmere shawls, laces, handkerchiefs, fans, gloves, and purses. The inclusion of the prayer book in both *corbeilles* testifies to the valuation of the other objects and legitimizes certain fashions as belonging—alongside the object connoting feminine domesticity, the sewing bag—to respectability. In the social theater of nineteenth-century France, the *corbeille* contained the costumes of the married lady and, hence, of propriety.

Although the Revolution had officially dispensed with sumptuary laws, it is quite clear from the importance and ubiquity of the *corbeille* and its contents that sumptuary customs associated with moral hierarchies remained intact and constant throughout the nineteenth century.

The *corbeille* signified precisely the prohibiting impulse surrounding improper premarital conduct and could thus logically serve as a reward, in effect, for good behavior. But it could equally be manipulated as a bribe, a payoff as it were, for a dutiful daughter's agreeing to a less than pleasing match. As Bricard explains: "Jouant de l'attrait irrésistible de ces présents, des mères peu scrupuleuses ont quelquefois obtenu le consentement de leur fille en leur faisant miroiter les splendeurs de la corbeille qu'on leur destinait" (310) (Playing on the irresistible charm of these gifts, unscrupulous mothers sometimes got their daughters' consent by flashing before them the splendors of the *corbeille* they would receive). The *corbeille* thus functioned as both literal capital—luxurious fashion items connoting pleasure that could, if necessary, be pawned or sold in the used-clothing market—and symbolic capital, as the goods it contained figured the treasured daughter who would receive them and referred, through a set of complex sartorial conventions, to the respectability of marriage.

DANGERS OF THE *CORBEILLE*

Reaching excessive proportions in nineteenth-century France, the *corbeille de mariage* also suggested the conflicts inherent in nineteenth-century concepts of marriage—which ranged from pure financial transaction to idealized social institution.[9] It could appease women through fashionable luxury items permitted to them only as married ladies, securing both their status of respectability and their access to pleasure. But it could also prove insufficient, either literally unequal to the female prize (and her dowry) it was purchasing, a scenario to be discussed shortly, or symbolically deficient, for instance, to a girl who was unable to blind herself to the financial and sexual transaction concealed by the beautiful envelope of the *corbeille*'s treasures.

Indeed, a glittering *corbeille* was not bribe enough for the fictional Henriette Gérard to consent without struggle to marrying an elderly tycoon, for in Edmond Duranty's 1860 novel, Henriette uses the *corbeille* and what it signifies to exact vengeance on her greedy, heartless family as well as her lustful, elderly spouse. Forced to renounce her true love and to marry the rich old Mathéus so that her parents can profit from his wealth and properties, Henriette schemes until the very last minute to find a way to escape her horrific fate. But when the *corbeille* arrives and her mother puts it on display for all to see, Henriette understands the inexorable nature of her position:

Madame Gérard disposait de son côté les magnificences de la corbeille, riche en bijoux, en fourrures et en autres dentelles, ainsi qu'en
châles de l'Inde et de la Chine. Le blanc de la soie, le blanc du linge, le
blanc des dentelles, s'étalait en grands plis et en grandes masses, dra-
pés avec une sorte de négligence qu'on aurait pu dire inspirée par la
quantité; le rouge, le bleu, le noir, le lilas, le vert, des châles et des robes,
les chamarrages fous des Chinois, ressortaient luisants, vigoureux, et
égratignaient l'œil. Le fauve sombre ou clair des fourrures ressemblait à
des bordures de cadre en bois doré ou en bois noir auprès des peintures
chaudes simulées par les étoffes. Du milieu de ces draperies jaillissaient
comme des fusées les colliers, les bracelets, les boucles d'oreilles, les
flacons.

Les paysannes considéraient cet étalage avec le respect consacré aux
objets religieux. (346)[10]

[Mme Gérard arranged at her side the wonders of the *corbeille*, rich in
jewels, furs and other laces, as well as Indian and Chinese shawls. The
white of the silk, the white of the linens, the white of the laces, spread
out in big folds and great masses, draped with a kind of negligence that
might have been said to have been inspired by quantity; the red, blue,
black, lilac of the shawls and dresses, the wild patterns of the Chinese
shawls, stood out gleaming and robust and scratched the eye. The fe-
line orange of the furs, dark and light, looked like the edges of golden
or black wood frames around the ardent paintings simulated by the
cloths. From the midst of these draperies the necklaces, bracelets, earrings, and bottles shot out like rockets.

The peasants considered this display with the respect due to reli-
gious objects.]

Unlike the peasants, steeped in the conventions of bourgeois marriage as idealized institution, Henriette, who has been privy to the financial realities of her family's negotiations, views this *corbeille* with
dread. Representative of her entry into female adulthood, its description is characterized by violence. On the level of color, in particular, the
movement of the description of Henriette's *corbeille* imitates the transformation of the innocent girl into the sexually experienced woman.
From the excess of whites in the display of luxurious undergarments,
the text passes to an explosion of strong colors, red first and foremost,
that strike the eye and jewels that are phallically determined. Through
her equivalence with the treasured *corbeille*, the treasured daughter is
displayed in all of her erotic potential just as the garments that will envelop her are spread out for public viewing. Capable of discerning the
crude truth behind the idealizing conventions surrounding marriage,

Henriette understands that her virginity is the price of the luxuries of the *corbeille*.

Duranty's peasants' reverence for the *corbeille* and its contents is tied to their understanding of its traditional meaning. The *corbeille* signifies the groom's valuing of his bride, and the rare and treasured qualities of its contents refer symbolically to the *trésor* of the bride's purity, which ostensibly only the *mari* will enjoy. Henriette's *corbeille* overflows with the white laces, contrasted with the rich tones of the shawls, the jewels, and the dress materials befitting a married lady. But the text itself suggests a more complex understanding of the *corbeille*, one that Henriette comes to grasp only too well. For this *corbeille* tells us that she is to become the sexual prey of an old man she does not love. The descriptive display of the bride's intimate apparel, as well as the text's passage from these to the vigorous and dark colors of marriage shot through with an unmistakable vocabulary of violence (*égratignaient, jaillissaient, fusées*), points to the erotic subtext of the *corbeille*'s ostensible meaning. The reds, blues, and blacks may even suggest bruising, further implying the potential violence associated with marriage.[11] Duranty's novel in fact probes the *malheur* of marriage for young girls and goes so far in this passage as to suggest that Henriette's wedding night will prove just short of rape. By deemphasizing the *corbeille*'s association with respectability, the text exposes, rather, the violent reality of a marriage against one's will.

Realizing there is no escape from the financial and sexual transaction that her parents have orchestrated, legally arranged so that they and Henriette's brother, and not their daughter herself, will receive most of Mathéus's wealth, Henriette finally accepts her plight and marries the old man, thinking that, once married, she might at least be able to offer financial help to her impecunious former lover. The gift of the *corbeille* and its ostentatious display force Henriette to realize her powerlessness in the face of the marriage plot—the *corbeille* is tantamount to the marriage contract. And yet, the day after her marriage, when Henriette learns that her true love has committed suicide, in a fit of violent rage she attacks her husband, threatening him with a *corbeille* "en porcelaine . . . suspendue au-dessus de la tête de Mathéus" (380) (made of porcelain . . . dangling over Mathéus's head). Symbolically seizing control of the *corbeille de mariage* and the wealth it represents, wielding it as a weapon to sunder the bind in which it had ensnared her, Henriette uses a *corbeille* to bring her husband near death (he suffers a stroke and dies shortly thereafter) and turns the tables on her greedy family, ultimately winning the Mathéus fortune for herself.

Henriette's *corbeille* may have failed to seduce her, but its detailed description helps to clarify both its position of power in the ritual of the marriage transaction and its signifying power in a woman's transition from *demoiselle* to *femme mariée*. Prior to marriage, young girls from good families were typically dressed simply and primarily in white, no doubt signifying virginity—the unstated prerequisite of marriageablity. As Baronne Staffe admonishes, even as late as 1891, "Au dehors, ni même à la maison, elle ne porte jamais de vêtements singuliers ou excentriques et répudie toute couleur voyante qui 'tire l'œil'" (outside, and even at home, she never wears singular or eccentric clothing and eschews bright colors that "catch the eye").[12] In short, a young lady must not be too fashionable. This sartorial simplicity played an important strategic function in the marriage dance as well, for a girl who displayed too great a taste for opulence might not find a husband willing to support her expensive habits. Material worlds were thus intimately linked with the abstract worlds of women's social and legal status, for, once married, *la femme mariée* suddenly had access to luxury garments befitting and signaling her married status. In an 1850s fashion plate picturing a first communion, the *demoiselle*, dressed in white, gazes adoringly at a woman who must be her mother, central to the fashion plate (Figure 6). The *femme mariée* is resplendent compared to her monochromatic children (her son is dressed in black, typical of masculine costume of the nineteenth century). Her shawl, her laces, her flowers, and her gloves all bespeak her married status; and the fashion plate is clearly more interested in displaying the appropriate attire for the respectable mother at such an occasion than for her daughter, who recedes into the background, although it is *her* spiritual coming of age we are meant to witness. But a first communion was in a way a rehearsal for marriage, and the daughter's rapt gaze perhaps betrays rather more aptly her anticipation of her own entry into the world of color and luxury accessories than her spiritual awakening before God.

In a cautionary tale sure to impose moderation on a generation of young female readers imagined by Marie Emery in 1869 for *Le Journal des demoiselles*, one poor motherless girl, Juliette, entrusts the counseling of her fiancé on the matter of her *corbeille* to an older female friend, Madame Hortense Benoît. Edmond is prepared to include his mother's diamonds, the gems most closely linked to family wealth and its

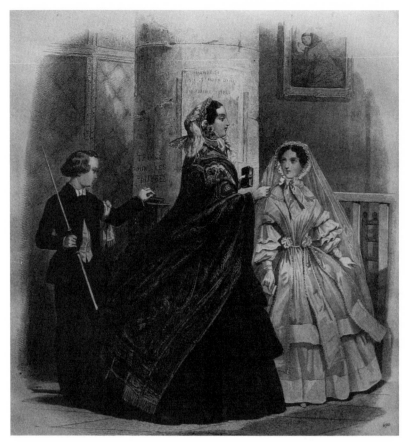

Figure 6. *Le Moniteur des dames et des demoiselles*, Maciet Collection, Bibliothèque des arts décoratifs.

transmission and most highly prized for their unchanging value and, as
such, customary jewels in the *corbeille*. No doubt with the best of intentions, Hortense makes the following supplemental suggestions to the
fiancé's offer in the fictional Juliette's *corbeille*:

> Les diamants ne servent d'ailleurs que pour les toilettes du soir, &
> toutes les femmes, les nouvelles mariées surtout, aiment à posséder
> quelques bijoux de moindre valeur, tels que les broches, pendants
> d'oreilles en turquoise, en émeraudes, je vous recommanderai plus
> spécialement les premières, parce que notre chère Juliette est blonde. Il
> est inutile de parler de la montre & de sa chaîne, cela est élémentaire.
> On en pourrait presque dire autant du cachemire long des Indes; je ne

crois pas qu'il y ait aujourd'hui une seule corbeille de mariée où il ne se trouve, & Juliette y tient essentiellement. Les dentelles noires & blanches, si nécessaires pour garnir nos robes de bal, n'occupent néanmoins que le second rang dans la nomenclature que je dois vous faire. A mon avis cependant, on ne saurait composer une corbeille sans volants de Chantilly. Une robe de velours est d'un bon effet, mais Juliette se contenterait de quelques robes en étoffe de soie, pourvu qu'elles fussent de la plus belle qualité. Je rappelle seulement pour mémoire le coffret refermant les gants, les nécessaires en or & autres bagatelles, la bourse pour ce que l'on appelait autrefois les épingles. Mais vous trouvez peut-être cette liste un peu longue? (83)[13]

[Diamonds anyway are only used for evening attire, and all women, especially new wives, like to have some less valuable jewelry, like brooches, turquoise or emerald earrings; I recommend to you the first in particular, because our dear Juliette is blonde. It is pointless to talk about the watch and its chain, this is elementary. We could almost say as much about the long Indian cashmere shawl; I don't think there is a single *corbeille* these days that doesn't contain one, and Juliette really wants one. Black and white laces, so necessary for decorating our ball gowns, take second place in the classification I need to do for you. In my opinion though, you cannot compose a *corbeille* without Chantilly lace flounces. A velvet dress makes a good impression, but Juliette would be happy with several silk dresses, as long as they are of the best quality. Allow me to add the glove box, the gold cases, and other trinkets, the purse for what used to be called pins. But perhaps you find this list a little long?]

Indeed, Juliette's stunned suitor, Edmond de Norville, is dumbstruck by the list and comes to the immediate conclusion that the beautiful Juliette's penchant for luxury would squander their modest fortune. He calls off their engagement, and Juliette's father pronounces the moral to his heartsick daughter and by extension to all the *demoiselles* of the journal's wide readership at the story's end: "la corbeille a tué le mari. En voyant quelles étaient les exigences de la fiancée, il s'est justement effrayé de ce que deviendraient celles de la femme. Puisse la leçon être profitable, ma chère, elle vous coûte assez cher" (85) (the *corbeille* killed the husband. Seeing all the fiancée's demands, he was rightly frightened of what the wife's would be. Let the lesson be profitable, my dear; it costs you dearly).[14] For all its excess and despite the presumed moral injunction against such an opulent *corbeille*, however, Madame Benoît's list nonetheless gave the eagerly reading *demoiselles* fodder for fantasy. A young lady could imagine what she might attain as a *femme mariée*, even if she dare not demand it and indeed had to feign disinterest.

The *corbeille* announces a girl's entry into matrimony, and with the signing of the marriage contract legally concluding the marriage transaction, just as she may now finally "toucher à sa dot" she may also "plonge[r] ses mains dans le fouillis, des bijoux, des dentelles, des éventails, des plumes offerts par le fiancé" (Bricard 130) (receive her dowry . . . plunge her hands into the jumble, of jewels, laces, fans, feathers offered by the fiancé). The *corbeille*'s contents were displayed publicly on the evening of the signing of the marriage contract, visible to envious young ladies and to their desperate sniping mothers: "les jeunes filles s'extasient, les femmes critiquent et tâtent, quand on ne les regarde pas" (Bricard 313) (the girls go into raptures, the women criticize and feel, when no one is watching them). By conferring social status, the *corbeille* became a tool in the struggle for position that characterized nineteenth-century social interactions. Newly permitted to display these luxuries, the married lady could now enter *le monde* as a suitably adorned *femme comme il faut*.

That the *corbeille* was offered on the day the contract was signed and that any deficiency in its contents could lead to the dissolution of the contract reinforce, however, its participation in the essentially financial transaction that marriage exemplified (Bricard 131). Baronne Staffe, writing with horror in 1891 about the proposed conversion of the *corbeille* into a more pragmatic coin, was ever so pleased that "la vieille mode a prévalu" (32) (the old ways prevailed). But the baronne's displeasure notwithstanding, it would not have been a simple conversion, for the *corbeille* is more easily understood through the concept of *trésor*, as we have seen, than through crude money, linked rather to the notion of *fortune*.[15] The luxurious objects constituting the *corbeille*'s treasure connoted more than their mere monetary value, their quality of *fortune*; they also embodied other forms of capital, such as respectability, virtue, elite origins, and, of course, good taste. These are what constitute a real *trésor*.

It is not difficult to see the *corbeille* as a residual trace of the practice of bridewealth, one of three forms of marriage transactions classified by anthropologists and ethnologists.[16] Bridewealth, or the payment of goods or money to the family of the bride by the family of the groom, was a practice associated with earlier, less complex European societies and with horticulturally based societies. Historian Diane Owen-Hughes explains that in early Germanic societies, such as that of the

Franks, the groom or his family began to pay the brideprice to the bride
herself in the form of gifts, and that later still, the Greco-Roman practice of dowry began to reassert itself.[17] Bricard perceives the inclusion
in the *corbeille* of "une bourse de louis d'or" (a purse of gold coins) as
a "lointain souvenir de l'époque où les Francs achetaient leurs femmes
et *payaient une dot!*" (a distant memory of the time when the Franks
bought their wives and *paid a dowry!*). But surely the entire *corbeille*,
and not just the purse of gold coins (which had to be newly minted and
virginal, meant for giving alms on the bride's wedding day), refers indirectly to the outmoded practice and to the underlying financial exchange that marriage rituals both concealed and revealed.[18]

TRÉSOR AND FORTUNE

Balzac's 1835 novella *Le Contrat de mariage* turns precisely on the interplay of *trésor* and *fortune*, gendered concepts that parallel symbolic and literal capital. While *trésor*, as I have been discussing, is a concept associated with the feminine and with the idealized packaging of
the abstractions of virtue and respectability in the luxurious contents
of the *corbeille*, *fortune* is more closely associated with the masculine
worlds of property and hard cash, which include the dowry that the
wife brings to her husband. Private female domesticity (another aspect of her characterization as *trésor*) balances male capital building
in the public sphere, and the female *trésor* of the fashionably adorned
wife pays homage to her husband's prowess in the market—his capacity to accumulate *fortune*. Balzac's novella plays with and even muddles
these conventions, however, mixing up *trésor* and *fortune*, exposing the
transactional nature of human relations and especially the falseness of
marriage rituals. By distorting and even reversing the gendered concepts of *trésor* and *fortune*, his text reveals fissures in the hierarchies of
gender and class that nineteenth-century French society was struggling
to maintain.

In raising the subject of the *corbeille* during the marriage contract
negotiations of her daughter, only to dismiss it in a moment of fake disinterest, the text's cunning female protagonist Madame Évangélista effectively converts *trésor* to *fortune* and gets her love-struck son-in-law
unwittingly to pay for both dowry and all that would have been contained in a *corbeille*. Like the hapless Juliette of the *Journal des demoiselles* cited earlier, Balzac's Natalie Évangélista also lacks suitors because of her penchant for excessive luxury. But she is unlike Juliette in

every other way, it turns out, and soon, with her mother's help, finds
the means to a wealthy husband even without possessing a *dot*. *Le Contrat de mariage*, set in the aristocratic circles of 1820s Bordeaux, aims,
the author tells us, to "retracer la grande comédie qui précède toute vie
conjugale" (retrace the great comedy that precedes all conjugal life).[19]

The novella develops in excruciating detail the financial labyrinth of
the marriage contract between the naive and sentimental Paul de Manerville and Natalie Évangélista, guided by her conniving mother. A
wealthy count, Paul returns to his native Bordeaux from Paris to marry
and settle. He immediately falls for the glamorous Natalie Évangélista,
the daughter of a successful Spanish merchant and his widow, descended from the illustrious Spanish aristocratic family of Casa-Réale. The
marriage contract ensues, and after three days of complex negotiations
that constitute the body of the novella, the couple is married and moves
back to Paris. Paul soon falls into debt due to the extravagant desires of
his wife, who remains financially protected by clauses in the contract
separating their possessions. Without a dowry, he is unable to use the
capital he should have received from his wife to increase his own fortune. Confusing *fortune* and *trésor*, Paul spends his own fortune to create a treasure, which is not actually his, as it turns out, since Natalie
never performs her wifely role. In order to preserve for herself the fortune that should go to Paul's heirs, Natalie refuses sexual relations with
her husband, thus forestalling any competition (from children). Intent
finally on rebuilding his fortune, Paul winds up banished from Paris on
a ship bound for India, where he learns of his wife's infidelity and his
mother-in-law's elaborate scheming.

Le Contrat de mariage circles around the *corbeille* and all it represents but in the end obviates it, thus signaling that something is quite
wrong in the march to marriage that Paul has undertaken. All those
luxury objects that should, by custom and propriety, be offered by
the groom in the *corbeille de mariage* are problematic in one way or
another in this work, indicating, along with the absence of the *corbeille* itself, an underlying and fatal problem with the marriage. The
novella details the precarious drafting of the contract, the revelation
of Natalie's squandered dowry, the creation of a *majorat* (or entail),
and the elevation of Natalie herself as *trésor* enough by her calculat-
ing mother. By referring throughout both directly and obliquely to
the distortion and even repudiation of the *corbeille*, Balzac's text reveals this object's centrality to the cultural construction of marriage
in nineteenth-century France.[20]

Madame Évangélista, a widow living in great luxury with her daughter, Natalie, has spent her daughter's share of her late husband's fortune and so cannot offer a dowry without ruining herself, a fact revealed during the contract negotiations. The solution that Mathias, Paul de Manerville's cautious family lawyer, devises is the creation of a *majorat*, or entail, so that the Manerville fortune and estate would be preserved intact for future male heirs.[21] Realizing that she is in a precarious position during these negotiations since she has no dowry to offer and her daughter is well known to have extravagant tastes, Madame Évangélista makes every effort to shield Paul from these facts and performs her role as naive aristocratic lady magisterially. Feigning a largesse and practicality that actually conceal her deep narcissism and prodigality, she absolves her future son-in-law from the expense of the *corbeille*, insisting:

> Il ne faut donc ni corbeille, ni joyaux, ni trousseau. Natalie a tout à profusion. Réservez plutôt l'argent que vous auriez mis à des cadeaux de noces, pour vous assurer à jamais un petit luxe intérieur. Je ne sais rien de plus sottement bourgeois que de dépenser cent mille francs à une corbeille de laquelle il ne subsiste rien un jour qu'un vieux coffre en satin blanc. Au contraire, cinq mille francs par an attribués à la toilette évitent mille soucis à une jeune femme, et lui restent pendant toute sa vie. D'ailleurs l'argent d'une corbeille sera nécessaire à l'arrangement de votre hôtel à Paris. (186)

> [You are not to give either *corbeille*, or jewels, or trousseau. Natalie has everything in profusion. Lay by the money you would otherwise put into wedding presents. I know nothing more stupidly bourgeois and commonplace than to spend a hundred thousand francs on a *corbeille*, of which nothing will be left in the end but an old trunk covered in white satin, when five thousand a year given to a young woman saves her much anxiety and lasts her lifetime. Besides, the money for a *corbeille* is needed to decorate your house in Paris. (translation modified)]

By forgoing a *corbeille* for her daughter, Madame Évangélista may seem generous; but, on the contrary, her gesture proves instead to be deeply motivated by her own financial interests. For if the dowry is really non-existent, a fact that emerges during the contract negotiations and is recounted to Paul by his trusty *notaire* ("il n'y a pas un sou de dot" [there isn't a penny for a dowry]), then technically, a *corbeille*, traditionally equal in value to a small percentage of the dowry, could hardly be required (162). In spite of the *corbeille*'s apparent absence, however, cash-

mere shawls, exquisite laces, fans, and diamonds—all items traditionally included in the *corbeille*—have particular significance in Balzac's
novella, as we shall see.

Natalie does in fact already have everything in profusion, but her
possessing them proves deeply problematic. For it is at least in part because of her ostentatious display as a *jeune fille* that at the ripe age of
nineteen, "nulle proposition de mariage n'était parvenue à l'oreille de
sa mère" (128) (no marriage offers had reached her mother's ear). As her
mother's spoiled only daughter, Natalie had been permitted the luxurious *toilette* of a *femme mariée*, and this had in fact ruined her chances
of finding a husband, even as her mother had hoped to inspire only
the most wealthy suitors for her daughter's hand: "Habituée à satis-
faire ses caprices de jeunes filles, mademoiselle Évangélista portait des
cachemires, avait des bijoux et vivait au milieu d'un luxe qui effrayait
les speculateurs" (128) (Accustomed to gratify her fancies, Mademoiselle Évangélista wore cashmeres and jewels, and lived in a style of luxury which alarmed all speculative suitors). Her *toilette* is as luxurious
as that of a married lady, which gives rise to the critiques of Borde-
lais society: "'Qui donc serait assez hardi . . . pour épouser une jeune
fille à laquelle sa mère donnait mille francs par mois pour sa toilette,
qui a ses chevaux, sa femme de chambre, et porte des dentelles?" (129)
(Who would be bold enough . . . to marry a girl whose mother gives her
a thousand francs a month for her *toilette*, who has horses and a maid
of her own, and wears laces?).

Louis Verardi's 1850s publication *Manuel du bon ton et de la politesse
française* offers the following clauses regarding appropriate *toilettes* for
young ladies:

> 31. La toilette d'une demoiselle sera toujours plus modeste que celle
> d'une femme mariée, parce que la vraie manière de se choisir un mari
> est de paraître *avoir les goûts simples.*

> 32. J'ai connu dix maris que leurs femmes ont ruiné par leur luxe, et
> qui cependant ne les avaient épousées que parce qu'*elles avaient les
> goûts simples.*

> 33. Pour qu'une demoiselle *ait les goûts simples*, il faut qu'elle ait hor-
> reur des cachemires et des riches fourrures, et le plus profond dédain
> pour les bijoux de prix et les diamants . . . jusqu'à ce qu'elle ait trouvé
> un bon mari.

> 34. Si elles font autrement, dit Mme Celnart, elles passent pour avoir
> un amour *effréné* du luxe, et elles se privent *du plaisir* de recevoir ces
> parures de la main d'un *époux.*

[31. The *toilette* of a young lady will always be more modest than that of a married woman, because the true way to choose a husband is to seem to have simple tastes.

32. I have known ten husbands whose wives ruined them by their luxury, even though they had married them because they had simple tastes.

33. For a young lady to have simple tastes, she must despise cashmeres and rich furs, and [have] the profoundest disdain for expensive jewels and diamonds . . . until she finds a good husband.

34. If they do otherwise, Mme Celnart says, they seem to have an excessive love of luxury, and they deprive themselves of the pleasure of receiving these *parures* from the hand of a husband.][22]

And Baronne Staffe, although writing at the end of the century, distills a century's worth of conventional wisdom when she writes: "Pour la fête du contrat, la fiancée ne se pare d'aucun des bijoux qui viennent de lui être donnés. Ils ne lui servent qu'après le mariage. Elle s'habille d'une simple et jolie toilette claire, sa dernière robe neuve de jeune fille" (34) (For the contract party, the fiancée does not adorn herself with any of the jewels she has just been given. They only serve her after the wedding. She dresses in a simple and pretty light-colored outfit, the last new dress of a maiden). Tinged as they are with satire, Vernardi's admonitions may sound less serious than Baronne Staffe's, but the longevity of the advice and its representation in a variety of conduct manuals as well as in fiction confirm the degree to which Natalie commits a social faux pas with her luxurious display.

Natalie disobeys these social rules of dress, and at her contract ball she stands out, blatantly ignoring the code of propriety: "aucune toilette, aucune femme, rien ne serait comparable à la beauté de Natalie, qui parée de dentelles et de satin, coquettement coiffée de ses cheveux retombant en mille boucles sur son cou, ressemblait à une fleur enveloppée de son feuillage" (198) (No bridal *toilette* was ever comparable with that of Natalie, whose beauty, decked with laces and satin, her hair coquettishly falling in a myriad of curls about her throat, resembled that of a flower encased in its foliage). Decidedly, Natalie already possesses the goods that a *corbeille* would afford her—notably the married lady's cashmere shawl and piles of laces—and, as we have seen, such a flouting of the norms can have serious social repercussions, just as they are discreet signals of unseemliness. The lawyer Mathias's remark during the contract negotiations, "si vous avez mangé de si bon appétit quand vous étiez fille, vous dévorerez donc quand vous serez femme" (159) (if you have eaten so heartily as a girl, you will devour when you

are married), resonates with the terrible lesson Juliette would learn for-
ty years later through her misadventure in the *Journal des demoiselles*
cited above.

This disruption of the traditional code of behavior regarding the *corbeille* and its contents, signaled in particular here by the cashmere, is
perhaps explained by Natalie's mother's Spanish and Créole origins—at
least that is what Madame Évangélista would have Paul believe.[23] More
important, however, Natalie's luxurious display has led directly to her
difficulty in finding a husband. The subsequent renunciation of the *corbeille* at the moment of the contract—which, as we have seen, normally
go hand in hand and are exchanged in a transactional way, the one's *trésor* quality compensating for the other's function to protect *fortune*—
points to a fundamental disruption of marriage customs and thus of
female roles. There is clearly something wrong with the contract, and
the marriage, it turns out, will be a tragic farce. "Ce mariage me semble
indécent" (227) (This marriage seems indecent), remark the gossips of
Bordeaux after the midnight marriage by torchlight. There are many
indications throughout the novella that while it seemed at first to be a
mariage d'inclination, it was fated to devolve into a *mariage de raison*.[24]
The narrator at several points refers to the evil omens that pursue the
couple, for example, the superstitions surrounding midnight torch-lit
ceremonies. But even before the mass, we learn that on the night of
the contract signing, Natalie "jouait avec l'écran en plumes indiennes
que lui avait offert Paul" (199) (Natalie played with a screen of pea-
cock's feathers given to her by Paul), a fan unlike the traditional *éventail brisé* or *plié* that was the staple of the *corbeille*. This fan perhaps retains too much of its oriental provenance and, Balzac tells us, augurs ill
for the couple as it is "d'après les croyances superstitieuses de quelques
pays ... pour l'amour un présage aussi sinistre que celui des ciseaux ou
de tout autre instrument tranchant donné, qui sans doute rappelle les
Parques de la mythologie" (199) (a gift which is to love, according to
superstitious belief in certain countries, as dangerous an omen as the
gift of scissors or other cutting instruments, which recall, no doubt, the
Parces of antiquity). Not only has Paul offered the wrong kind of fan,
but he has also offered it outside of the context of propriety—which is
the *corbeille*.

In the end, Madame Évangélista swindles Paul de Manerville out
of his fortune, and what she is after for the sake of her daughter far ex-
ceeds the expense Paul would have laid out for a *corbeille*. She accom-
plishes this with the help of a luxury item traditionally included in the

corbeille—diamonds—and her manipulation of this customary gift of the groom allows her ultimately to prevail in what she views as a combat with her future son-in-law.[25] In what has been termed "la comédie des diamants," Madame Évangélista ends up exchanging one type of diamond for another and manages to keep them all, even as she pretends to give them.[26] Madame Évangélista offers her diamonds as something of an afterthought as the lawyers are haggling over the nonexistent dowry. She is in possession of many fine jewels, among them newer diamonds (from Brazil, we learn), of inferior quality but more easily liquidated as cash, and old family treasures, such as the *Discreto* diamond, of Indian origins, which will accrue value over time.[27]

The two sets of diamonds symbolically illustrate the distinction introduced above and explored throughout Balzac's novella between *fortune* and *trésor*. The *Discreto*, Madame Évangélista explains, is a family heirloom "qui porte le surnom de Philippe II, et dont fut orné sa main royale, une pierre historique qui pendant dix ans le duc d'Albe a caressée sur le pommeau de son épée" (222) (a diamond which bears the name of Philip the Second and once adorned his royal hand, an historic stone which the Duke of Alba touched for ten years in the hilt of his sword). After the first day of contract negotiations, the widow has the value of all her jewels estimated by the jeweler Elie Magus, who explains to her privately the differences in value, quality, and provenance between the two sets of diamonds. Asian diamonds like the *Discreto* were considered to be of much higher quality than Brazilian diamonds; and given that the *Discreto* also bears the cultural value of aristocracy, since it was a gift from the duke and has been handed down over generations, the *Discreto* clearly carries more value than the set that Madame Évangélista will offer Paul. The "new" Brazilian diamonds are included under the marriage contract simply because these are the only ones the lawyers know about, and they are destined for sale to make the dowry payment—they thus constitute *fortune*. The *Discreto*, of much greater value but more difficult to convert immediately to cash, remains on the bosom of Madame Évangélista as her family *trésor*.[28]

But she will soon opt for *fortune* and manages to have it both ways, to her daughter's benefit and to Paul's detriment. After disclosing the absence of dowry, submitting to Maître Mathias's creation of a *majorat*, which would prevent the husband's fortune from passing to his wife, and realizing she has lost, Madame Évangélista enlists her daughter and schemes to gain possession of Paul's fortune for herself and Natalie after the wedding so that their luxurious lifestyle can remain unchanged.[29] In a maneuver whose groundwork she had already laid during the contract negotiations with her protestations of the value of *trésor* (representing Natalie) as superior to the financial crudeness of *fortune*, Natalie's mother will ultimately secure Paul's fortune for her daughter. Throughout the course of the negotiations, which Madame Évangélista had deplored as deeply offensive, she had set up the opposition of *fortune* and *trésor*, letting it be known that she valued more highly the financially incalculable *trésor* to the bookkeeping of *fortune*:

> J'ignorais ce qu'était un mariage en France, je suis Espagnole et créole. J'ignorais qu'avant de marier ma fille il fallût savoir le nombre de jours que Dieu m'accorderait encore, que ma fille souffrirait de ma vie, que j'ai tort de vivre et tort d'avoir vécu. Quand mon mari m'épousa, je n'avais que mon nom et ma personne. Mon seul nom valait pour lui des trésors auprès desquels pâlissaient les siens. Quelle fortune égale un grand nom? Ma dot était la beauté, la vertu, le bonheur, la naissance, l'éducation. L'argent donnerait-il ces trésors? (167)

> [I was ignorant of what the process of marriage is in France; I am a Spaniard and a Creole. I did not know that in order to marry my daughter it was necessary to reckon up the days which God may still grant me; that my child would suffer because I live; that I do harm by living, and by having lived! When my husband married me I had nothing but my name and my person. My name alone was a fortune to him, which dwarfed his own. What wealth can equal that of a great name? My dowry was beauty, virtue, happiness, birth, education. Can money give those treasures?]

She is being disingenuous, of course, and the opposition between *fortune* and *trésor* she repeatedly cites in hopes of avoiding payment of a dowry for her daughter's hand serves her well later when she lures Paul into an exchange in which he, or rather Natalie, will get the *trésor* (figured by the *Discreto)* and she, Madame Évangélista, the *fortune* (figured by the Brazilian diamonds), which in fact is what she wanted all along and what she truly values. With its royal pedigree, the *Discreto* signals aristocracy—it is equivalent to the great name so touted by Madame Évangélista as incalculable treasure since it emblematizes aristocracy, and she claims to care only for it. But the Brazilian diamonds, worth more in terms of liquidity, are what she ultimately desires because they offer financial power that even aristocratic pedigree cannot procure.

Mme Évangélista hands over the Brazilian diamonds after the contract is signed, and Paul promptly gives them to Natalie in a sort of parody of a *corbeille* gift. Mathias instructs him to sell them during the honeymoon, but the day following the contract's signing, Madame Évangélista approaches Paul with a trade. She wishes him to have the family heirloom instead, the *Discreto*, a diamond so valuable by its pedigree, a *trésor*, that he wouldn't think of selling it but will want rather to have it reset for Natalie and matched with other jewels purchased at his own cost:

> ... échangeons-les contre les joyaux que je vous livre pour accomplir mes engagements envers ma fille; vous y gagnerez, mais qu'est-ce que cela me fait! Je ne suis pas intéressée. Ainsi, Paul, avec vos économies vous vous amuserez à composer pour Natalie un diadème ou des épis, diamant à diamant. Au lieu d'avoir ces parures de fantaisie, ces brimborions qui ne sont à la mode que parmi les petites gens, votre femme aura de magnifiques diamants avec lesquels elle aura de véritables jouissances. Vendre pour vendre, ne vaut-il pas mieux se défaire de ces antiquailles, et garder dans la famille ces belles pierreries? (222)

> [Let us exchange them for the jewels I am giving you in order to fulfill my obligations toward my daughter. You will gain by the transaction, but what of that? I am not selfish. Instead of those mere fancy jewels, with the money you will have saved this way, Paul, you can enjoy designing for Natalie a tiara or a crown, stone by stone. Your wife will have fine diamonds that will bring her indescribable pleasure. Isn't it better that I should sell these bourgeois ornaments, which will surely go out of fashion, and that you should keep in the family these priceless stones?]

Paul accepts this ruinous swindle as a generous and thoughtful gesture from his mother-in-law, trading the Brazilian diamonds for the *Discreto*, which he gives his wife; and over the course of the next five years, as the spiteful Madame Évangélista had gleefully hoped, he spends what is left of his private fortune completing the treasure of his wife's jewels. In essence, Madame Évangélista makes *him* pay for both dowry and *corbeille*, in effect collapsing them together as precious *trésor* rather than converting them to necessarily expendable *fortune*. And Madame Évangélista, in (re)possession of the easily liquidated Brazilian diamonds, promptly sells them and acquires a head for business, economizing and amassing a fortune of her own as she profits from the downward spiral of Paul's investments and buys up his lost properties without his knowing it.

Now bankrupt, but with his wife financially protected through the legal machinations of the contract, in the novella's brutal conclusion

Paul explains his financial ruin to old Mathias on a stopover in Bordeaux before setting sail for India to make his fortune anew. Asked how he could possibly have fallen into such deep debt, Paul recites a script that was written unbeknownst to him by his mother-in-law:

> J'ai d'abord voulu compléter à ma femme la parure qui se trouvait commencée avec le collier de perles agrafé par le *Discreto*, un diamant de famille, et par les boucles d'oreilles de sa mère. J'ai payé cent mille francs une couronne d'épis. Nous voici à onze cent mille francs. Je me trouve devoir la fortune de ma femme, qui s'élève aux trois cent cinquante-six mille francs de sa dot. (232)

> [I wanted, in the first place, to complete for my wife that set of jewels of which she had the pearl necklace clasped by the family diamond, the 'Discreto,' and her mother's earrings. I paid a hundred thousand francs for a coronet of diamond wheat-ears. There's eleven hundred thousand. And now I find I owe the fortune of my wife, which amounts to three hundred and sixty-six thousand francs of her dowry.]

En route to India, Paul learns of his mother-in-law's deception and, worse still, of his wife's infidelity and illegitimate pregnancy. Both fortune and treasure lost to him, he travels to India to reconstitute his fortune, perhaps by importing luxury goods, like the *cachemires de l'Inde* that could end up as *trésor* in a lucky girl's *corbeille de mariage*. Although we never again hear from Paul de Manerville after his departure for Calcutta in 1827, it is tantalizing to imagine him there, contributing ironically from the Orient to the feminine economy of Paris.[30] For India was the exotic place of origin of both *cachemires* and diamonds, two of the most constant *trésors* to be found in the *corbeille*.

Balzac's short novel, focused almost exclusively around the extended scenes of the drafting of the marriage contract, plays with the conventions surrounding marriage, exposing the often dissimulated crude realities of negotiation. The contract documents those realities, and it is of note that the *demoiselle* and her intended do not seem to pay attention to the contract: it is more seemly for them to leave all this to parents and lawyers. Bricard explains: "Il est recommandé au jeune homme d'affecter la plus grande indifférence pendant que le notaire lit le contrat" (311). (It is recommended that the fiancé affect the greatest indifference while the lawyer reads the contract). If the contract negotiates the division and conservation of *fortune*, the *corbeille* is concerned with a less concrete notion of *trésor* linked to conceptions of virtue and idealized femininity. The *corbeille*, as the beautiful and luxurious offering exchanged in effect for dowry, is the contract's counterpart, its idealized equivalent, which helps to mask the financial transaction behind a splendid veil. The items it contains, as we shall see in the chapters that follow, contribute to the idealization of respectable women as *trésor* even as these items are also complex cultural artifacts that may potentially disrupt the very system of respectability that they help to maintain.

PERFORMING RESPECTABILITY

The *corbeille de mariage*, as we have seen, functioned in nineteenth-century French culture to mark the shift from *jeune fille* to *femme mariée* and thus to define both the costumes and the customs of propriety. It served as a reward to an obedient and virtuous daughter and a symbol of how and for what she was valued. Emblematic of the conventions of marriage, it was the beautified double of the cruder contract, which openly enumerated details of the financial transaction of marriage. Most important, the *corbeille* signified, through its structuring and displaying of the garments of propriety, the performance of respectable femininity. At the same time, the display of exotic fabrics and luxury objects designed for seduction visually depicts the unmentionable erotic subtext of the transition to womanhood. The *corbeille* captured the theatrical moment of becoming a *femme comme il faut*: it was both treasure chest filled with the costumes of the starring role and altar of respectability upon which *la jeune fille* was required to throw herself.

The concept of respectability gained importance in France in the early nineteenth century, and, like its earlier counterpart in England, it was closely linked to the theme of gentility conventionally associated with class origins. For women, respectability was inseparable from "domestic femininity," which demanded certain behaviors and practices. Historian Woodruff Smith traces the origins of respectability in England through an evolving set of contexts, among them gentility, luxury, virtue, and the gendered spheres of masculinity and femininity.[31] Unlike earlier forms of individual status, however, respectability "was constructed on a profoundly different basis of assumptions. . . . A person was respectable if he or she *acted* respectable" (205). Thus, respectability as a form of status could be performed, contesting earlier notions of status by birth and necessitating the props and accoutrements of that performance. The acquisition of those props and accoutrements was lubricated by the consumer boom of the late eighteenth and nineteenth centuries, for respectability, as Smith maintains, was "probably the primary factor defining consumption in Western economies" and was therefore "a substantial part of the general phenomenon of modernity" (24). Consumption of luxury goods was not excluded from the context of respectability, especially as oriental luxury goods could be appropriated and domesticated to the purposes of constructing the respectable image of a comfortable home (211). As the repository of the costumes of feminine respectability, the *corbeille de mariage* contained the objects that best incarnated the ideal feminine in this new context. Fans, shawls, laces, and gloves both connote modest behavior because they cover and protect female flesh and suggest sensual pleasure through their softness, their dainty craftsmanship, their quality of molding and leaving partially visible that same female flesh.

The importance of the *corbeille de mariage* in nineteenth-century France lies in its power to domesticate exotic goods and appropriate them for the social theater of Paris, which offers a central role to the feminine ideal of respectability. From oriental harem to Parisian wardrobe, the mythology of the object expands and adapts to the demands of a society seeking visible markers of its power and limits. The frontispiece engraving from Jouy's *Hermite de la Chaussée d'Antin* cited earlier provides a graphic pendant to what Mallarmé (alias Marguerite de Ponty) would envision sixty years later, when the "oriental folds" of a cashmere shawl slipped from the shoulders of a woman to envelop an overstuffed *corbeille*. The engraving illustrating Jouy's story entitled "L'Histoire d'un schall" included in the collection from 1815 pictures a large wooden structure, surrounded by luxury goods—shawls, feather fans, jewels—resting against a backdrop of palm trees and other exotic flora, as if attesting to the exotic provenance of the luxury contents (Figure 7).[32] Floating in a kind of bubble, a graceful, bare-breasted, dark-skinned, turbaned woman seems to dance erotically as she waves her cashmere shawl. This vision transfixes a horrified European man (the narrator of Jouy's "Histoire"), who is being led away by a native. The woman seems to incarnate Western fantasies of oriental women as highly eroticized just as it includes readable references to Western femininity as well. The engraving shows her wearing the sheer white muslin gown imported from India, first introduced to France by Marie-Antoinette and later popularized in the First Empire, thus linking her to images of Western femininity, but fully exposing her dark breasts, reminding the viewer of her otherness.[33] On her opposite side, a wooden structure, which appears to be a miniature replica of the object below the bubble, is engulfed in smoke. The woman, it turns out, however, is a young Indian widow, about to be immolated on the funeral pyre of her sixty-year-old husband, and she offers her shawl to the European, who brings it back to France to become fashion's favorite. Jouy's readers can have it both ways: the image alone feeds Western fantasies of the erotic exotic, and the story that accompanies the image explains that this woman is none other than respectability incarnate—a faithful wife.

Jouy's story of the shawl's many adventures ends in the nineteenth century, when, after having been originally conceived and expertly crafted as the prized gift of the mogul of Bengal to his only child-producing wife (and thus his one true wife), it finds its way into the *corbeille de noces* of "la fille d'un ancien employé à la régie," only to be eventually "coupé en morceaux . . . pour en faire des gilets" at the end of the tale (316–17) (the daughter of a former employee of the company . . . cut into pieces . . . to make waistcoats out of them).[34] The fantasy bubble of the exotic, eroticized, and hyperbolically faithful wife offering her shawl as she dances to her death sits atop an object that by visual analogy conjures the *corbeille de mariage*, as it seems to spill forth luxury goods. Ironically, this object is mirrored as the funeral pyre in the smaller image. The link between pyre and *corbeille* is implicit, but legible. Both imply a requisite obedience and fidelity from the wife: while the Indian widow must prove her fidelity by self-immolation, the Western bride promises hers by accepting the gift of her intended; and the objects contained in the *corbeille* thus achieve moral significance through their association with marriage. Jouy tells us that the Indian wife for whom the shawl was originally made was the one (of many in the oriental harem) who produced an heir and who was thus legitimate. Her loyalty and her legitimacy earn her respectability, honored by the gift of the treasured shawl.

The oriental wife's metropolitan foil, Balzac's Natalie Évangélista learns through her mother's spiteful tutelage to avoid maternity and thus undo the penalty of the *majorat*. Just as before she was married she illegitimately seized the prerogatives of the *femme mariée*, after her marriage, she represents and reproduces illegitimacy, subverting the cultural ideal of the feminine through her manipulation of sartorial and social customs. The *corbeille* was the very index of French feminine respectability through its connotation of marriage and its literal function as repository for the costumes of the *femme mariée*. Disingenuously eschewed by Natalie's mother, only to reappear in a monstrously

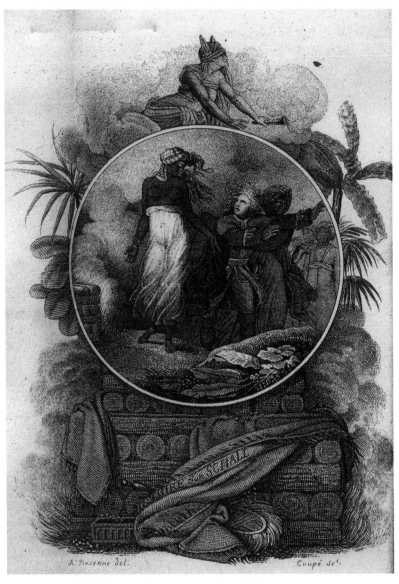

Figure 7. "L'Histoire d'un schall," *L'Hermite de la Chaussée d'Antin*, 1815, Bibliothèque nationale de France.

distorted form in Balzac's text, the *corbeille* as emblem in Jouy's work unites in a single paradoxical image the complex strains of bourgeois femininity.

CONCLUSION

In the engraving, both woman and shawl embody marital fidelity, even as they both contribute to an erotic staging of female martyrdom. As Jouy's text suggests, it is when the shawl enters the French fashion system that it begins to shed its aura of respectabilty and is eventually reduced to raw commodity. By sanctifying the sartorial signs of feminine virtue, however, through their inclusion in the *corbeille de mariage*, the fashion system, speaking primarily through the fashion press, repackages the exotic for a domestic consuming public. The feminine material world of fashion and accessories that the *corbeille* refers to concretizes the more abstract worlds of women's legal and social status in nineteenth-century France.

The *corbeille de mariage* wielded the power to broker a marriage and contributed crucially to the theater of bourgeois femininity, but it also embodied the tension between the erotic and the respectable. The moralizing impulse behind the associations of the *corbeille* treasures with respectable femininity is ironized in Gyp's dialogue entitled "La Corbeille de mariage" from her 1888 collection *Pauvres petites femmes*.[35] Here the author personifies the objects from the *corbeille*, while the mute *mariée* (bride) looks on and is advised by "la voix du bien" and "la voix du mal." Good and evil seem to have more to do with fashion's do's and don't's than with what constitutes respectable behavior in nineteenth-century France, and Gyp is capitalizing on the moral associations of these accessories to comment on the female condition. That the *mariée* is classified as a "personnage muet" (mute character) and remains silent throughout this short comic piece is perhaps commentary enough. But by giving voice to the objects themselves—lace, diamonds, cashmere shawls, undergarments, among other objects— the text animates those key accessories that have so much to instruct about nineteenth-century conceptions of the feminine. The *Cachemires* speak: "Nous sommes les cachemires, aujourd'hui méconnus, mais néanmoins on n'ose nous supprimer, et notre place est toujours marquée dans toutes les corbeilles"(6) (We are the cashmeres, unrecognized today, but nonetheless no one dares get rid of us, and we always have a place in all *corbeilles).*

Without exception, and even well after it was no longer considered a stylish accessory, one item remained constant in the *corbeilles de mariage*, and thus in the material fantasies, of young ladies: *le cachemire*. Dangling from the fingers of Jouy's Indian martyr, it eventually passes to the shoulders of Mallarmé's imagined beauty, from whose body it slips to surround the *corbeille* itself in the fashion writer's suggestive text. In the following chapter, I will examine in detail this most prized accessory, which made its début in the fashion landscape with the century's beginning and was to become much more than a fashion trend. Charged at once with moral and erotic imperatives, it became, rather, the very garment of luxurious respectability.

CHAPTER THREE

"Cashmere Fever"

Virtue and the Domestication of the Exotic

Après des années d'espoir, de désirs, de craintes, d'impatience, je le tiens,
le voilà . . . je le tiens. quelle finesse de tissu! quelles couleurs! quel éclat!
quels dessins! mon beau cachemire, nous ne nous quitterons plus!

"Monologue du cachemire"

A satirical piece published in *La Silhouette* in 1830 entitled "Monologue du cachemire" depicts a young girl nearly swooning with rapture as she receives a long-coveted cashmere shawl from her lover, who is stationed in the new French colony of Algeria (Figure 8). A military metaphor is evoked and sustained throughout the piece.

The soldier Édouard defeats any potential romantic rivals with his heroic gift of this luxury garment, and whether it was procured from "quelque Circassienne dont il aurait enfoncé le sérail" (some Caucasian woman whose harem he penetrated) or from "quelque *colonel* turc dont il aura coupé la tête" (some Turkish colonel whose head he chopped off) is of little matter, for "c'est un cachemire!" (it's a cashmere!), the monologist raves, and "cela excuse tout!" (that excuses everything!).[1] More crucial still, on the social battlefield, the anonymous musing *demoiselle*, newly armed with her cashmere, will crush her own fierce competitors:

> Oui je veux m'en parer aujourd'hui, à l'instant même; je ne retard-
> erai pas mon triomphe d'une minute. Zoé, Clothilde, Paméla, vont en
> étouffer de dépit. Elles se croient plus jolies, plus aimables, plus adroites
> que moi. Allons, mesdemoiselles, s'il en est ainsi, avec tant de beauté,
> d'amabilité, d'adresse, essayez; ayez un cachemire, il est temps, ou bien,
> si vous n'êtes pas assez habiles pour l'obtenir, contentez-vous du meri-
> nos et de la bourre de soie. (12)

> [Yes, I want to wear it today, at this very instant; I will not delay my tri-
> umph for one minute. Zoe, Clothilde, Pamela will suffocate with envy.
> They think themselves prettier, friendlier, cleverer than I. Let's go,

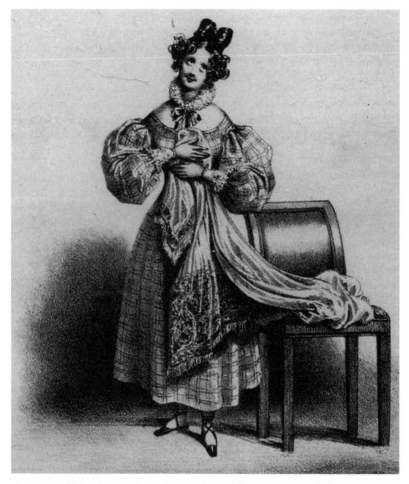

Figure 8. "Monologue du cachemire," *La Silhouette: journal des caricatures, beaux-arts, dessins, mœurs, théatres, etc.*, The Pierpont Morgan Library, New York. Bequest; Gordon N. Ray; 1987. PML 140321.

girls, if it is so, with so much beauty, likability, and skill, you try; have a cashmere, it's time, or, if you are not clever enough to get one, you'll have to be happy with merino wool and rough silk.]

The girl is well aware of the hierarchy of fabrics. Cashmere trumps lesser wools and silks: she is now unstoppable. The cashmere's association with the *corbeille de mariage* proves Édouard's worthiness as a suitor, but it also goes on to guarantee the young lady's value as a commodity in the marriage market. The gift of the cashmere spells out her married future, just as merino wool and rough silk, considered common and unrefined fabrics, indicate both lower economic status and unwelcome variations on the unmarried condition to which she happily consigns her competitors.[2] In the privacy of this parodic monologue (the subtitle of the publication is *Journal des caricatures*), we learn that she has been dreaming of her cashmere since birth ("j'y songeais dès le berceau"), just as other *demoiselles* dream of having a husband. She had tried her luck and suffered through seducing several eligible bachelors—a clerk, a lawyer, a doctor—but only the soldier Édouard, at the propitious colonial moment and place, was able to procure the long-coveted luxury item.[3] The monologue makes fun of the cult of fashionable appearances that endows a garment with the power to bestow abstract moral qualities, such as respectability, and slyly suggests that the "respectability" conferred by such a garment can be taken off and put on at will.

Appearing in 1830, the year of the French conquest of Algeria as well as of the advent of Louis-Philippe to the French throne, the monologue deftly convenes the discourses of French colonialism, particularly in Algeria, French social practices of courtship and marriage, and feminine status anxiety, which covers for broader social anxieties. The intersection of these discourses occurs at the most fashionable of sites: the oriental luxury garment par excellence, the *cachemire*, whose power is in full view in the monologue. Its appeal supersedes that of merely one man, as the monologue amply demonstrates. "Depuis six semaines qu'il m'a quittée; le temps commençait à me paraître long. Je n'aime pas la solitude, et l'absence, l'ennui, les occasions.... Mais ce cachemire qui vient de lui, c'est presque lui-même, c'est une société.... Oh! mon cher Édouard! mon beau cachemire!... je crois que j'en deviendrai folle" (12–13) (For six weeks now since he has been gone, time was beginning to go slowly. I don't like solitude, and the absence, the boredom, the opportunities.... But this cashmere that comes from him, it is almost him, it's company.... Oh! my dear Edward! My beautiful cashmere!... I think I will go mad for it). More potent than the lover himself, even usurping him as lover, both signifying his love and guaranteeing her fidelity, the *cachemire* sensually compensates for the girl's loneliness.

The shawl's exoticism conjures at first erotic, then valorous fantasies, both of which exist in relation to the context of French colonialism. Her fantasy of Édouard's capture of her cashmere imitates fantasies of colonial exploits: she imagines first his penetration into the feminized and oriental space of the harem, which contains the prized white harem girl (the *Circassienne*), her own double, and then the gory decapitation of an Oriental himself. The monologue exemplifies the phantasmic construction of the Orient in nineteenth-century France.[4] The young Parisienne revels in a double fantasy born of colonialism flaunting masculine power: the harem-ravaging scene bleeds into battlefield heroism, and the conquest of the erotic, sensual, and private space of the oriental woman is doubled by the public conquest of the barbarian. Erotic and military conquests both become vehicles of male power, and the *cachemire* is the spoils of that double conquest, bringing multiple pleasures back home. The colonial context thus serves as a signifier of masculine power, and that power defines female position.

When the symbol of conquest comes home to France, it is taken up by the fashion system and apparently seamlessly incorporated into a domestic economy. As recipient of those spoils, however, the Parisienne participates in the colonial exploit, especially when she wields social power of her own and functions as a screen on which to project male success and female virtue. The garment is quickly converted from exotic signifier to domestic currency, as its new proprietress prepares to leverage it against her rivals in the Parisian social scene. At the same time, however, she doubles her exotic counterpart, taking on the mantle of objectified colony herself. Even in ancient Eastern cultures, gifts of fine garments like *cachemires* "were intended to establish a hierarchical relationship between the giver and the recipient, whose acceptance acknowledged submission."[5] Fashion makes that submission palatable, even desirable, as the objectification, like the object, can lead to power. For the monologue also clearly illustrates the construction of detailed socializations, as women come to signal class and learn to manipulate the signs of power.

Finally, the *cachemire* is completely assimilated to Édouard himself, even to the point of effacing him altogether, as the girl rapturously declares that she has fallen madly in love with it ("j'en deviendrai folle"). In a mock marriage vow, personifying the *cachemire* and conflating it with the absent Édouard, she cries "Oh mon cher Édouard! Mon beau cachemire! Que je vais t'admirer, te choyer, te chérir!" (Oh my dear Edward! My beautiful cashmere! How I will admire you, pamper you, cherish you!). The cashmere is thus the site of multiple and interrelated pleasures: erotic, material, and social. She has become a happy victim of "cashmere fever."

"Cashmere fever" was in full swing by 1830, but its onset in France can be traced to an earlier colonial moment: the First Empire. In the opening "Convolute" of *The Arcades Project*, taking for his subject "Arcades, Magasins de Nouveautés, and Sales Clerks," Walter Benjamin identifies the cashmere shawl as the essential hot commodity of the early to mid-nineteenth century. Quoting an 1854 volume entitled *Paris chez soi*, Benjamin offers the following synopsis of the life span of the shawl:

> In 1798 and 1799, the Egyptian campaign lent frightful importance
> to the fashion for shawls. Some generals in the expeditionary army,
> taking advantage of the proximity of India, sent home shawls . . . of
> cashmere to their wives and lady friends. . . . From then on, the disease
> that might be called cashmere fever took on significant proportions. It
> began to spread during the Consulate, grew greater under the Empire,
> became gigantic during the Restoration, reached colossal size under
> the July Monarchy, and has finally assumed Sphinx-like dimensions
> since the February Revolution of 1848.[6]

Benjamin's source conflates two favorite nineteenth-century discourses in his brief chronology—that of malady (disease, fever, spread) and that of the exotic (Egypt, India, Sphinx-like)—linking the two through the concept of size (gigantic, colossal, etc.). The expanding "epidemic," we should note, was mirrored literally in the expanding size of cashmere shawls themselves. The "epidemic" refers to the ever increasing skirt and crinoline size of the mid-nineteenth century and thus participates in a satirical critique of the crinoline popular in the 1850s and 1860s, when skirts reached their most voluminous circumference. According to Benjamin's bemused speaker, the cashmere shawl, oriental signifier and unparalleled Parisian must-have accessory, unlike most other shorter-lived fashion trends, possessed an ever expanding appeal that serves as a metaphor for social mobility as it was grafted onto women in nineteenth-century France.

What this feverish acquisition of cashmere shawls indicates about French society and its consumption habits in the nineteenth century, the cultural impact of the object itself, both the oriental and French versions, and the oblique relationship of Western women to colonialism that lurks beneath the surface of the story of cashmere in France constitute the subject of this chapter. In the "Monologue du cachemire," the shawl is a sign for female eroticism inasmuch as it represents the spoils of colonialism, an emblem of male power. The fantasy of Édouard's "penetration" into the harem, taking the shawl, and giving it to his fiancée suggests the Parisian woman is colonized by transfer, by her willingness to be claimed by male power, now in a more socially delicate form appropriate to her social aspirations—marriage conferring respectability. The whole process renders colonization itself, whether domestic or oriental, erotic—and that serves to make an unequal gender economy more palatable to the subjected. At the same time, the monologue illustrates a curious transfer of power: as the cashmere moves from masculine to feminine hands, from the supersensual Orient to the domestic space of Paris, it becomes a sign of social superiority and a vehicle for social mobility.

In the pages that follow, I trace the rise of the exotic cashmere shawl as principal sign of female status and respectability in France during the first half of the nineteenth century. I first explore the colonial context of the introduction of the *cachemire* into cultural practice in nineteenth-century France through a historical discussion of its cultural valence. I then turn to two primary literary texts that rely heavily on what I call a cashmere plot: first, Balzac's 1846 *La Cousine Bette* and, second, Flaubert's 1869 *L'Éducation sentimentale*. These readings bring the circulating cashmere shawl into focus as a central leitmotif in the production both of the novels' plots and the conflicts over feminine virtue governing each. I conclude by considering the further domestication of the shawl as it loses its luxury appeal by the turn of the century. These novels, although squarely set in Paris and offering complex portrayals of distinctly Parisian society, offer a view into the structures of power elucidated and maintained by colonialism. The *cachemire* is the circulating object that draws out a series of analogies that sometimes look more like oppositions—between colonized place and Western woman, between the socially marginal woman and her respectable counterpart, between exotic fashionable object and the adorned woman herself.

By investigating the trajectory of cashmere shawls in Balzac's *La Cousine Bette* and Flaubert's *L'Éducation sentimentale*, I propose that the story of the *cachemire* as fashion trend expresses social and cultural concerns—namely, the interrelated anxieties over authenticity and social mobility—that preoccupied the nineteenth-century imaginary, and that these concerns were bound up in the colonial context as the fantasy of the supersensual Orient dovetailed with the fantasy of the domestic and idealized feminine. By reevaluating the exploitation of and economic and moral values surrounding cashmere and by considering the ways in which certain exotic objects were assimilated into the service of sexual propriety and bourgeois values, this chapter explores the impact of colonialism on France's fashion economy, which, as we shall see, worked in concert with its moral economy.

Two general trends inform the question of women and imperialism and the latter's corollary, orientalism: representations and analyses first of Western women *in* the Orient, exploring, travel writing, colonizing, and, second, of oriental women as objects of otherness.[7] Less frequent is discussion of how "the oriental," that by-product of colonialism, permeated the everyday lives of Western women and what this assimilation and consumption meant culturally.[8] Part of colonialism's staying power with the metropole lay in the colonizing culture's assumption of oriental goods into its own signifying systems—the goods became domesticated, that is, converted into an appealing and consumable form of domination over Western women and their bodies. These objects only retained their power inasmuch as they continued to refer to the exotic/erotic and were acquired at great expense. Desire was introduced and then reproduced through the collision and collusion of imperial and marketing projects. Feeding the female consumer's desire for the exotic became itself a reinforcement of empire, while at the same time, it threatened to corrupt bourgeois femininity. In her essay in *Western Women and Imperialism*, Nupur Chaudhuri presents the tantalizing argument that Anglo-Indian women helped make cashmere shawls and curry cultural mainstays of the bourgeois Victorian woman's household. However, her analysis stops short of (and indeed calls for) a real consideration of what happened to the oriental object once it was incorporated into the everyday lives of Western women. Furthermore, and inversely, what happened to the Western woman as she appropriated the aura of the oriental object? Did she become more virtuous (more French) or more dangerous (more oriental)? Before turning to the novels to deepen the analysis of these questions, let us explore the historical and cultural context of cashmere itself in nineteenth-century France.

CASHMERE IN CONTEXT

An expensive, handwoven textile brought to France from the East through Napoléon's campaigns, the cashmere shawl was to become a cultural fetish evoking sensual fantasies of a constructed Orient before falling out of fashion in the latter half of the century. Cashmeres were available in France as early as the seventeenth century, when explorers traveled to India and Persia at the behest of French kings.[9] But it was around 1800 that the cashmere shawl began to be imported to Europe systematically. Frank Ames, in his history of the Kashmir shawl, describes the first point of contact between fashion and empire: "When

Napoléon returned from Egypt, the generals and officers who had served under him brought back mementoes of the Orient. Among these were Kashmir shawls which they wore wrapped around their waists as belts, and which had been plundered from the Mamelukes, the soldiers of the Egyptian army."[10] From its origin as a war souvenir, emblematic of male power, the shawl, back in Paris, was quickly transformed into fashion's *dernier cri*, in part for its beauty but also for its functionality in the new, simpler fashions of the First Empire, which necessitated warm coverings for exposed *décolletages* and gauzily clad limbs (135) (Figure 9). An erotic vestimentary sign because of its great expense, its power to evoke the exotic East, and the eroticized notion of male conquest, and because of its tactile delicate softness replicating female skin, the cashmere shawl permitted fashionable ladies to dress scantily in public and still remain decorously covered.

The shawl thus possessed the dual and paradoxical capacity of representing both feminine virtue *and* female seduction. In the first sense, the shawl illustrates the metropolitan appropriation of a colonial object as a French fashion accessory used to indicate status and respectability. Through its revaluing and participation in the European fashion economy, becoming, for example, the centerpiece of the *corbeille de mariage*, the shawl simultaneously began to reflect, even to construct, a moral economy. It is in this sense that we can say that the *cachemire* in European hands and circulating through European markets, both visibly commercial and less visibly so in its associations with marriage through mandatory inclusion in the *corbeille*, facilitated a domestication of the exotic. By *domestication* I mean at once the importation of the object itself into France, its incorporation into the specifically feminine fashion system, and, as a result, its value shift into what we might call a domestic feminine fantasy.[11] One fantasy was exchanged for another: the supersensual object connoting the erotics of the East was converted into the symbol of female virtue, but not without retaining some traces of its erotic allure.

For as a cultural sign of the Orient, this luxury garment was linked to the erotic through its very exoticism. As Woodruff Smith argues, "Exotic imports served as tokens of the excitement supposedly available in the lands they came from. Thus the pleasant feeling of soft fabrics . . . was desirable . . . because it suggested images of Eastern lands where sexual activity supposedly took place with more variety and style than in Europe, and amid a profusion of soft textiles."[12] The *cachemire*, as the monologue above suggests, projected deep as-

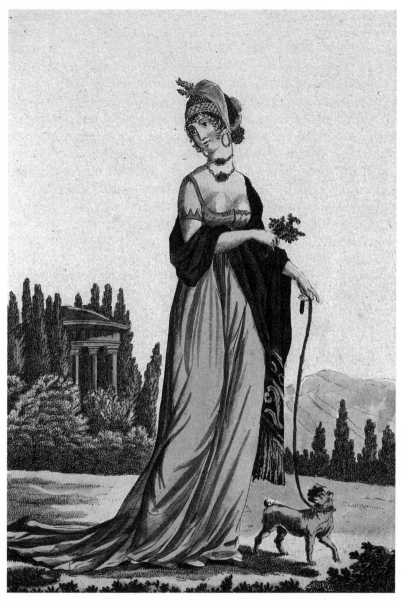

Figure 9. "Triple aigrette de diamants," *Costumes de France, 1795–1815*, Bibliothèque nationale de France.

sociations with sensuality and feminine eroticism. Both hiding and
revealing, richly textured and blanket-like, thus suggesting intimate
spaces, the *cachemire* epitomized Western fantasies of feminized oriental splendor.[13] The garment that was once synonymous with the
masculine, public domain of the military, its appropriation indicating conquest and power, shifted as it moved into the feminized, private, and domestic sphere of fashion but remained powerful nonetheless. The *cachemire* now facilitated conquest of a marriageable lady,
who would in turn sport the signs of her husband's economic conquest. The two fantasies discussed earlier in relation to the "Monologue du cachemire"—penetration of the harem and social/economic
conquest, both presented through the military metaphor—converge
domestically and are virtually simultaneous.

The *cachemire*'s rise to premier status symbol of the mid-nineteenth
century was set in motion by the trend setting and exorbitant spending
of Empress Joséphine, who reputedly never asked the price of a shawl
(Ames 135).[14] Following Joséphine, every fashionable lady required a
shawl to complete her wardrobe and signal her standing among the social elite of early nineteenth-century Paris. Napoléon included seven-
teen Kashmiri shawls in the *corbeille de noces* of Marie-Louise, his second wife, as if reiterating his imperial conquests in his own very public
domestic sphere (Maskiell 39). From the imperial court on down, wom-
en as consumers were thus implicated in the imperial project even as
they attended balls and operas draped in exotic splendor.

Not only did the appropriation of the exotic *cachemire* set in motion
a complex fantasy exchange between harem girl and domestic wife, but
the cashmere also functioned socially as symbolic capital because of the
wealth it represented. The *cachemire* was a marker of economic status
and one's proper use of it a marker of class, but it could also be translated into literal capital. As an illustration of the cash value of a cashmere
shawl, an 1806 inventory of Empress Joséphine's possessions "evaluated
her 45 shawls at 36,000 francs, a Rubens at 1,500 and a Leonardo *Virgin and Child* at 1,000."[15] Of course, there were gradations of value even
among the French imitations, which were perfected over the course of
the century; but the genuine Kashmiri shawl was always the most highly valued, followed by the "Parisian" shawl, and finally the "provincial"
shawl.[16] An article on the "Exposition des Produits de l'Industrie de
1839" written for the *Journal des demoiselles* by fashion correspondent
Alida de Savignac reveals at once the great fashion for and the hierarchy among shawls:

Malgré la mode des mantelets, les fabriques de châles n'ont point
suspendu leurs efforts pour égaler les châles de cachemire; on peut
même dire que l'un de nos fabricans [sic] a surpassé tout ce que l'Inde
et la Perse peuvent offrir de plus merveilleux. Figurez-vous un châle
d'une grandeur extraordinaire, et sur ce châle sont représentés des
jardins, des pagodes, des processions de personnages divers. Ce sont
des prêtres, des musiciens, des soldats, des caravanes, tout cela se dé-
tachant assez nettement, et aussi facile à distinguer que s'il s'agissait
d'une gravure. Il est impossible de pousser plus loin l'audace de la composition, l'éclat et l'harmonie des couleurs, que ne l'a fait M. Gaussen
dans l'exécution de ce châle prodigieux. A côté de ces merveilles, aux-
quelles les têtes couronnées peuvent seules mettre un prix, les fabricans de Paris ont exposé de fort beaux châles *tapis*, dont la chaîne et la
trame sont en pure laine cachemire. La fabrique de Lyon offre aux fortunes médiocres des châles indous, dont la chaîne est en bourre de soie.
Enfin, Nîmes est parvenu à tisser des cachemires très jolis et d'un prix
si modéré, que cela semble un rêve. (188–89)

[In spite of the fashion for mantelets, shawl manufacturers have not
stopped their efforts to equal cashmere shawls; one could even say that
one of our manufacturers surpassed everything magnificent that India
and Persia could offer. Imagine a shawl of extraordinary size, and on
this shawl are depicted gardens, pagodas, and processions of various
people. These are priests, musicians, soldiers, caravans, all of it clearly
delineated and as easy to distinguish as if it were an engraving. It is impossible to take too far the audacity of the composition, the effect and
harmony of the colors that M. Gaussen has produced in the execution
of this prodigious shawl. Next to these wonders, which only royalty
could afford, the Parisian manufacturers have displayed some beautiful
"carpet" shawls, in which the warp and the weft are in pure cashmere
wool. The Lyon manufacturers offer Indian shawls for average fortunes
whose weave is in rough silk. Finally, Nîmes has managed to weave
very pretty cashmeres at such a reasonable price that it seems to be a
dream.]

Mme de Savignac's description of the prodigious Gaussen shawl rivals
passages from Flaubert's *Bouvard et Pécuchet*. It contains an excess of
oriental referents, belying its inauthenticity, its "trying too hard," but
her narrative nonetheless attests to the great power of the cashmere
shawl to inflame the desires of a wide range of shoppers. That "indous"
shawls could possibly emerge from Lyon or that French manufacturers could produce shawls more oriental than Persian manufacturers
is, of course, absurd, but such claims demonstrate the selling power

of the Orient, just as they confirm that the Orient is in fact a Western invention.

Most potent in terms of its symbolic signifying value, the prized *cachemire* was morally charged—linked not only to social and economic status but also to feminine virtue, the corollary to masculine honor and a notion seemingly at odds with the erotic fantasy of the Orient. Occasionally a trousseau item, a *cachemire* was sometimes handed down from mother to daughter, but more traditionally in France it was purchased at great expense before her wedding by her fiancé and placed in her *corbeille de mariage*. As Isabelle Bricard explains in *Saintes ou pouliches*, and as I elaborated in the previous chapter, the promise of a well-stocked *corbeille* could exert more influence than parental authority in deciding girls to accept a husband, and the *châle de cachemire* held a place of honor amid the many luxuries contained in the *corbeille*. If, for example, the *corbeille* contained "des cachemires en nombre insuffisant" (311) (an insufficient number of cashmeres), the marriage contract could be broken. The *corbeille* itself, a repository of (mostly) oriental luxuries, was "[d]ésignée au début du siècle sous le nom de *sultan*" (designated by the term *sultan* at the beginning of the century), thus further emphasizing the association of luxury goods and the Orient and hinting at the erotic (because exotic) nature of the transactions at hand and to come.

The *cachemire*, both the fashionable fabric and the fantasized space to which it referred, was the subject of several vaudeville plays in the early part of the century, attesting to the popular obsession with the garment and its symbolic powers.[17] The conflation of potential husband and *cachemire* mocked in the monologue was already a trope of the vaudeville stage of the First Empire. In the 1811 *Le Cachemire, ou l'étrenne à la mode*, two sisters vie for the affections of the same man (also named Édouard). When their father sends home a *cachemire* from afar, charging his wife with the choice of which daughter to give it to, she devises a way of determining the girls' true feelings by having each choose between the *cachemire* and her heart's desire. Adèle, the elder, chooses Édouard, while Aglaé, the younger, more fashionable one, declares that nothing could please as much as a *cachemire* ("Y a-t-il quelque chose au monde qui puisse plaire autant qu'un Cachemire?" [15]). Adèle is then promptly rewarded for her dutiful behavior with not only a husband but one who bestows on her a *cachemire* of her own, as is the custom. For while these luxuries are deemed necessities by the flighty Aglaé ("demandez à toutes les femmes si ce n'est pas un objet nécessaire au bonheur" [15]), Adèle (the older and wiser) qualifies their necessity in relation only to marriage: "Si nécessaire, qu'il est d'usage d'en faire mention dans les contrats de mariage" (15) (So necessary, that it is normal to mention them in marriage contracts). Aglaé, like her later incarnation, the anonymous heroine of the monologue, nonetheless relishes the prospect of attracting everyone's attention in society when she wears her *cachemire*, conflating it with, and perhaps preferring it to, her nonexistent fiancé. The play clearly makes Aglaé the loser, and uses the *cachemire* to express the social reward system for the proper prioritization of a young girl—her remaining within the structure of marriage—just as it also makes the *cachemire*'s inappropriate predominance over a young girl's heart the occasion for a critique of misplaced values and the possible specter of spinsterhood.

The *cachemire* was instrumental, then, in the construction of the etiquette surrounding marriage and indeed signified marriage and respectability just as it simultaneously conjured fantasies of Arabian nights. "Comme le précise la presse féminine, le châle est le surtout de demi-saison que, seules, les femmes mariées ont le droit de porter" (Lévi-Strauss 100) (As the feminine press specifies, the shawl is the cover-up for fall and spring, which only married ladies have the right to wear). In short, as fashion journals and novels alike make explicit, the *cachemire* was an accessory reserved for married or marriageable women. As Philippe Perrot reminds us, "Unmarried nineteenth-century French women, no matter how wealthy, were discouraged from wearing Kashmiri shawls, for to do so would 'lead people to believe that they are possessed of an unbridled love of luxury and deprive themselves of the pleasure of receiving such finery from a husband'" (100).[18] Inappropriate women's appropriation of it signals at once their desire to be respectable and, more generally, the sartorial imposture of the lower class as the upper class.[19] In a court transcript recorded in 1867 in the case of "M. X*** contre Mlle Z*** pour un cachemire des Indes," the lawyer for the merchant trying to recover a shawl that had not been fully paid for reminds the court of the breach of decorum Mlle Z*** has committed by assuming the right to wear a shawl as an unmarried woman: "Qu'il me soit permis de vous rappeler que, depuis longtemps, le droit de porter un cachemire des Indes est regardé comme un privilège dont jouissaient seules les femmes mariées" (May I remind you that for a long time the right to wear an Indian cashmere has been regarded as a privilege enjoyed only by married ladies).[20] To the many targets of the *Silhouette*'s 1830 monologue that opened this chapter, the idealized and innocent *demoiselle* is no exception: for this young lady's etiquette-defying public display of her new cashmere, as well as her having "shopped around" to locate its procurer, reveals her erotic experience. While she is clearly a caricature, and the monologue exposes the sham of her manipulation of fashionable appearances to lay claim to abstract moral qualities such as respectability, those appearances were nonetheless powerful enough to inspire feverish consumption of Indian *cachemires* and equally feverish attempts by French textile manufacturers to imitate them.

For its erotic, social, economic, and moral signifying power, then, the cashmere shawl emerged as an important marker of distinction, that quality of uniqueness that the dominant social group cultivates in order to maintain its place in the hierarchy, as we saw above. The authentic cashmere shawl was coveted by all but difficult to obtain, thus ensuring and augmenting its cultural value. As the fortunate *demoiselle* of the "Monologue du cachemire" fully realized, not only was the shawl valuable in and of itself, beautifully confected as it was of a precious foreign textile and vibrant with color and pattern, it also exerted the social power of conferring value, of signifying at once desirability and respectability. The *cachemire's* authority of distinction eventually gave way to imitation, however, as fashion typically, and paradoxically, illustrates, and imitation French cashmeres became readily available, no longer serving as a clear class marker.[21]

In his historical study of the shawl, John Irwin recounts the rise of the European shawl industry, the eventual success of which would depend on mass production, which caused the ultimate decline in the value of the cashmere shawl as a luxury item reserved for the elite. Irwin tells us that in 1801, "M. Guillaume Louis Ternaux, a well-known shawl manufacturer, obtained the semi-official support of the French Government to sponsor a trip to Tibet to acquire a flock of goats. . . . By the time he reached France most of the goats had died; the rest suffered severely from a scab disease. . . . Initial results . . . were disappointing."[22] Eventually though, the shawl was successfully imitated, and Ternaux's name became synonymous with the most common imitation shawl on the market.

Typologies and gradations of cashmeres emerged that resembled the classifications of women we saw in some of the physiological texts analyzed in Chapter 1. The problem of authenticating a cashmere shawl was commonplace enough that in 1846, the weekly journal *L'Illustration* offered a full-page caricature of the authentication process (Figure 10). The image tells the true story of two rival French manufacturers as they struggle for dominance of the French market for cashmeres. In the classic tale of modern capitalism, domestic cashmeres could be mass produced at lower cost than imported handwoven ones. The "bureau de la vérification des cachemires" (office for the verification of cashmere shawls) opened to offer a legitimate authority to determine the authenticity of cashmeres. Ultimately, the image tells us, the only way truly to know one's cashmere is authentic is to carry the genuine Kashmiri goat on one's back.

In her article on the history of the cashmere shawl in France, Monique Lévi-Strauss describes the social necessity for such a bureau to exist precisely for the purpose of verifying the authenticity and thus the value of the cashmere. Authenticity carried high stakes, both for the manufacturers, whose literal profit hinged on it, and for consumers, who made symbolic profit in the form of social ascendancy. In the literary texts I will now turn to, the parallels between the luxury garment and its best consumers become apparent. For as the century progressed, the overdetermined cashmere shawl began to circulate, focusing the desires of the dying aristocracy, the rising bourgeoisie, and the Parisian *demi-monde* alike. Like the cashmeres they desired, the women who wore them were also subject to scrutiny, and great pains were taken, as we saw in the first chapter, to distinguish legitimate, authentic ladies from those who would pretend to be so.

CLASSING WOMEN AND *CACHEMIRES*

Similar to Balzac's *Ferragus* discussed earler, both *La Cousine Bette* and *L'Éducation sentimentale* are built around a recurrent pairing of female characters of diverging classes (wives and mistresses, *femmes comme il faut* and *comme il en faut*), and both novels are consequently driven by a dynamics of opposition, imitation, and exchange between these two apparent poles. In Balzac's novel, against the virtuous and socially superior Hulot women (Adeline and Hortense—mother and daughter) is pitted a series of foils. The rapacious bourgeoise Valérie Marneffe (a courtesan in disguise), several figures from the Parisian *demi-monde*, and the vengeful Bette (Adeline's cousin), who passes freely among these social realms, serve as rivals to the Hulot *femmes comme il faut*. In Flaubert's novel, we also find a complex set of rivalries: Marie Arnoux, the virtuous married bourgeois lady, is alternately opposed to Madame Dambreuse, the nouveau-riche wife of a former aristocrat, and Rosanette Bron, the low-level courtesan involved with both Jacques Arnoux,

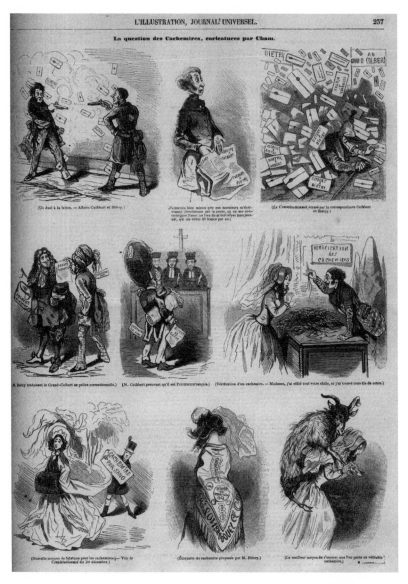

Figure 10. "La question des Cachemires, caricatures par Cham," *L'Illustration*, 1846, Vassar College Library, Poughkeepsie, N.Y. Reprinted with permission of the Famille Baschet.

Madame Arnoux's husband, and Frédéric Moreau, Madame Arnoux's besotted admirer.

Balzac's Bette and Flaubert's Rosanette are both loose variations on the working-class *grisette*—Bette because she works in the industry of *passementerie*, embroidering uniforms for the army and the national guard, and Rosanette because she began her social climb within the Parisian *demi-monde* to the rank of *lorette* as a silk weaver. She also claims to have been a shopgirl, which further links her to the social class of the *grisette*. Like Frédéric, we know little more of her history than that she has ascended the ranks of the Parisian *demi-monde* out of squalor. Perhaps more salient, Rosanette's origins in the Lyon silk-weaving industry mark her as emanating from the dangerous working class.[23] As for Bette, had she been pretty, she probably would have been a true *grisette*.

That both women are linked to the activity of weaving and sewing merits mention. Bette's line of business, Balzac tells us, is gold and silver embroidery, and it "comprenait les épaulettes, les dragonnes, les aiguillettes, enfin cette immense quantité de choses brillantes qui scintillaient sur les riches uniformes de l'armée française et sur les habits civils" (included epaulettes, sword-knots, aiguillettes; in short the immense mass of glittering ornaments that sparkled on the rich uniforms of the French army and civil officials).[24] Bette's involvement and indeed her great skill in this world (she is considered the finest workwoman in Pons's shop) place her in a position of control over the social "language" of the world to which she only marginally belongs. As Sarah Maza argues, since uniforms and costume more broadly are the essential social markers of this world, Bette's mastery of this important social sign system suggests that she exercises a degree of power within that realm. Bette embroiders the very vestimentary signs that guarantee masculine power—the military, its hierarchy, and the protection of civil order. It is Bette who orchestrates Valérie Marneffe's infiltration of the Hulot marriages primarily through a manipulation of fashion in the careful disguising of the courtesan as a proper lady. Equally significant, if not as evident, is Rosanette's connection to the textile business. The daughter of silk weavers, she was sold into prostitution by her mother at the age of fifteen. Her early tie to textiles and to the production of luxury goods ironically prepares her ascension to the position of consumer (and consumed). While less diabolical than Bette, Flaubert's Rosanette occupies a similar space, figuring both social and sartorial imposture.

Both novels also involve complex, if oblique, political plots. While Balzac's novel is less overtly political than Flaubert's, critics have pointed out that both novels may be read as political allegories.[25] *La Cousine Bette* exposes the social degradation that results from the corruption and materialism of the July Monarchy, and *L'Éducation sentimentale* recounts the violent birth of the Second Empire through the blind eyes of a self-interested protagonist. Both novels present important commentaries on the dramatic shifts in social hierarchies that were occurring in mid-nineteenth-century Paris through their panoramic views of society, which stage the disquieting indeterminacy of social position in an emerging modern world. At stake in the conflicts of both novels is social (in)stability, brought into focus through narratives around the paired (and gendered) values of virtue and honor and the paired (and gendered) spaces of the domestic and the political. In both novels, it is the ornamental, the oriental—indeed, the feminine—cashmere shawl that serves to weave these narrative threads together.

SOCIAL AND SARTORIAL IMPOSTURE IN
LA COUSINE BETTE

The feminized plots of marriage, seduction, and commodification that constitute the heart of Balzac's novel are constructed and played out around exotic objects. *La Cousine Bette*'s explicit Orient is Algeria, but its implicit Orient is in fact Paris itself—the money to pay for decadent Parisian luxuries comes from swindling the army and the French government in Algeria. Balzac's Algeria is not merely a historicizing *effet de réel*, a parody and extension of Napoléon's 1798 *expédition d'Egypte*, but also a colonial setting whose seemingly tangential presence in the novel erupts at key moments in the heart of Paris to expose local scandals. Likewise, key exotic objects figure in the text at moments when women perturb the bounds of propriety. French masculine honor explodes as extortion in Algeria, just as its double, feminine virtue, is imploding in Paris. Paris in the end becomes the much-fantasized Orient, complete with its emasculated men, its harem girls, its excessive luxury. I am interested here in considering how the Orient works on women in this novel and how these women in turn use exotic objects to reinforce, contest, or pastiche stereotypes about respectable femininity. If "the Orient" is a woman of loose morals, an easy leap to the courtesans of Paris—exemplified in Balzac's novel by the representation of Valérie as Delilah—why, then, do "oriental" objects enter France's fashion economy as signifiers of *virtue*? Through the common trope of conflating Orient and woman, Balzac uses those signifiers in this novel to represent the feminine threat. Might we say that assimilated exotic fashion accessories are de-domesticated and reoriented in a novel that uses them to signal breaches in feminine respectability? In *La Cousine Bette*, the circulating "oriental" *cachemire* both domesticates the barbarian Bette and "orientalizes," that is, subverts, the structure of feminine respectability on which Parisian society relies to be intelligible.

Published in 1846 and set during the July Monarchy, Balzac's *La Cousine Bette* explicitly takes up the analysis of a society in flux through the prism of a single family that has complex relations with elements from all social levels. An Alsatian peasant, Bette was brought to Paris during the First Empire to accompany her more fortunate and beautiful cousin Adeline, who, many years before, had married the Baron Hulot, a wealthy and titled soldier of Napoléon's army. When the novel begins, in 1838, Napoléon is already long gone, the baron's former imperial splendor is faded and most of his fortune squandered on courtesans, and Adeline's daughter, Hortense, in spite of her stunning beauty, is dowry-less and thus cannot find a husband. Her *cachemire* will have to be provided by her mother, since a *cachemire*-stuffed *corbeille* comes only in exchange for a resplendent *dot*. Bette is driven to deceive and destroy her family by a single passion—which she has been cultivating since childhood with the aim of exacting revenge against her kinder cousin by reversing their social positions. Both the broader social context of the novel (the portrayal of a decaying empire society and the rise of an entrepreneurial bourgeois class) and the individual circumstances that generate the novel's plot (Bette's envy of Adeline, which motivates her to conspire to ruin the family financially, morally, and even physically) find a symbolic representation in the yellow cashmere shawl that circulates throughout the novel.

To Bette, Adeline's cashmere shawl, a wedding gift from the baron, which has since made its way into her daughter Hortense's trousseau, represents everything the "poor relation" has been denied, materially and emotionally. From the outset of the novel, "ce précieux tissu" (this precious cloth) is the one object for which Bette is willing to compromise her secrets. The young and eligible Hortense promises her mother's *cachemire* on the condition that Bette prove that she has a lover. Bette's desire to one-up Adeline is set into motion as she divulges information that will eventually—and ironically—lead to Hortense's marriage with the mysterious lover Bette herself has been hiding. The shawl, and what it represents, is more valuable than Wenceslas, the young, handsome, and impoverished artist whom Bette has been keeping for herself.

> La cousine Bette, en proie depuis son arrivée à Paris à l'admiration
> des cachemires, avait été fascinée par l'idée de posséder ce cachemire
> jaune donné par le baron à sa femme, en 1808, et qui, selon l'usage de
> quelques familles, avait passé de la mère à la fille en 1830.
>   Depuis dix ans, le châle s'était bien usé; mais ce précieux tissu, tou-
> jours serré dans une boîte de santal, semblait comme le mobilier de la
> baronne, toujours neuf à la vieille fille. (91)

> [Cousin Betty, who, since her first arrival in Paris, had been bitten by
> a mania for shawls, was bewitched by the idea of owning the yellow
> cashmere given to his wife by the Baron in 1808, and handed down
> from mother to daughter after the manner of some families in 1830.
> The shawl had been a good deal worn ten years ago; but the costly ob-
> ject, now always kept in its sandal-wood box, seemed to the old maid
> ever new, like the drawing-room furniture. (41)]

Bette's fascination is linked to an uncharacteristic fashion lust but,
more important, it is tied to her desire for power and her recognition
of the shawl's value in the vestimentary language that is the currency
of the social world to which she aspires. *Possession* is the key term here,
as it is "l'idée de posséder" that drives Bette to relinquish her own most
treasured possession, her secret attachment to the Polish sculptor, in
exchange for another, more material possession—the shawl. On the social and familial margins, she is the quintessential "have-not" rivaling
the Hulot "haves," and she thus represents on the invisible political level of the text the "perceived" indeterminate social threat posed by the
urban underclass.[26] Possession of the shawl potentially demarginalizes
Bette, as we shall see.

    Adeline's yellow cashmere shawl is a polyvalent sign. First, it sig-
nifies imperial luxury, now faded, but still glorious to Bette. That the
shawl, a cultural sign of the Orient, may also hint at a residual trace of
imperialist fantasies resurrected in 1840s France is affirmed by an important colonial subtext in this novel. This plot, which risks the honor
of the Hulot family, involves the conspiracy by several government officials to defraud the French government in one of its burgeoning and ex-
ploitative enterprises in Algeria, the new colony. The Algerian debacle
is the public social scandal compromising the concept of honor that is
duplicated on the private level of family, both with Hulot's unredeemed
philandering (he promises the cook that she will become the next bar-
oness once his wife dies in the final pages of the novel) and with Adeline Hulot's eventual capitulation to the craven Crevel's propositions
(in the end she offers herself to Crevel to save her family). The blemishes

to public honor and private virtue are interwoven through the theme of fraud. Bette is deeply implicated in this deceit, defrauding her cousins of both wealth and honor by luring the baron into the embrace of a prostitute in respectable woman's clothing. The shawl is linked to Bette's "imperialist" fantasy of conquest, and Bette's acquisition of it symbolically figures the masking of social identity that will allow her nearly to vanquish the family.[27]

Second, in the textual economy of La Cousine Bette, the shawl represents marital bliss, as it was a gift from the baron to his wife when they were first married and has now become their daughter's trousseau treasure. One aspect of Bette's social lust is certainly to shed her spinster status. The shawl is still "new" ("toujours neuf") to the "old" maid ("la vieille fille"), thus suggesting that by its acquisition, Bette will appear more marriageable. Bette is in fact endlessly characterized as an old maid, as opposed to her beautiful cousin who, although a peasant, defied all odds by marrying into the aristocracy, albeit the hybrid aristocracy created by Napoléon. The cashmere shawl for Bette is clearly an emblem of social ascendancy, indeed, to return to Bourdieu's idiom, one of distinction bound up in the respectability of marriage.

Finally, and related to its social symbolism, the shawl is a sign of fashionability, for, in spite of its being the worse for wear, it is still chic, and possessing it may well afford Bette access into worlds from which she has heretofore been excluded. It is thus a sort of social skeleton key. And Bette's eventual acquisition of the shawl marks her rise to power in the novel and her entry into fashionability, just as its loss marks Adeline and Hortense's downfall.

Described as a spider in the center of her web (224/167), the vengeful seamstress sets out to take or to destroy what is Adeline's, and after some time, she succeeds in sabotaging Hortense's marriage, luring both Wenceslas and Baron Hulot into erotic relations with her protégée and instrument, Valérie, channeling what is left of the Hulot fortune into her own (and Valérie's) pocket and convincing her unsuspecting cousin that she, Bette, should be married to the baron's older brother, Maréchal Hulot, a man of uncompromising honor. In her moment of glory, "Ainsi restaurée, toujours en cachemire jaune, Bette eût été méconnaissable à qui l'eût revue après ces trois années" (211) (Thus furbished up, and wearing the yellow cashmere shawl, Lisbeth would have been unrecognizable by anyone who had not seen her for three years [155]). The exchange of the shawl in the opening scene of the novel was but the first step, then, in a series of orchestrated maneuvers that Bet-

te had hoped would ultimately lead to the reversal of status and fortunes of these two rival cousins, Bette's social and moral opposites. The
centrality of the shawl in this scene (which parallels Crevel's proposi-
tioning of Adeline Hulot in exchange for her daughter's dowry) and its
punctuation of the novel at key moments express the essential theme of
social imposture in *La Cousine Bette*, just as its initial exchange models the various forms of circulation so vital to this novel's representation of an emerging economy of commodities and mass production.
The shawl's fabled exotic provenance and its subsequent domestication
into the marriage market of the Hulot women potentially reconstruct
Bette as a marriageable lady when she acquires it. At the same time,
however, that Hortense would *sell* her precious trousseau treasure and
subsequently *purchase* her husband with her "jolie bourse algérienne"
indicates the potential perturbation in the moral economy that the
feminized oriental object can facilitate.

CIRCULATION AND SUBSTITUTION IN
L'ÉDUCATION SENTIMENTALE

Like Balzac, Flaubert uses a shawl simultaneously to structure his novel
and to indicate the blurring of social boundaries that is one of its central themes. The two novels present strikingly similar structures in this
regard: both contain liminal shawl scenes that offer keys to reading,
and both novels reintroduce the shawl plot at their midpoints to mark
the climactic moment of social and sartorial imposture on which their
plots hinge.

The cashmere shawl is key to Flaubert's novel, the majority of which
is also set in 1840s Paris. When in the opening scene of *L'Éducation sentimentale* Frédéric Moreau rescues Marie Arnoux's "châle à bandes vio-
lettes" from falling into the muddy waters of the Seine, he is performing what fashion history reveals to be a heroic gesture indeed, given the
enormous popularity and value of the *cachemire* in nineteenth-century
France.[28] In fact, the *Journal des dames et des modes* recounts a more
daring, real-life feat of fashion valor when in 1833 "a young man who
dived into the Seine to save a drowning woman, deposited her on shore,
then swam back to the middle of the river to rescue her Cashmere
shawl" (Werther 8). Like the personified shawl of the fashion magazine, Marie Arnoux's shawl is invested with untold value. For Frédéric,
before even speaking to his unknown beloved, her shawl becomes the
repository for his fantasies of intimacy: "Elle avait dû, bien des fois, au

milieu de la mer, durant les soirs humides, en envelopper sa taille, s'en couvrir les pieds, dormir dedans!" (*L'Éducation sentimentale* 24) (How many times, out at sea, on damp evenings, she must have wrapped it around her body, covered her feet with it, or slept in it!).[29]

Madame Arnoux's *cachemire* is metonymic, inspiring Frédéric's erotic fantasies as well as his act of bravado. It is also a source of textual inspiration, for no sooner has Frédéric saved the shawl from destruction than it is resurrected a second time, indirectly, in the harpist's "romance orientale où il était question de poignards, de fleurs et d'étoiles" (24) (eastern romance, all about daggers, flowers and stars [19]). The shawl, then, is established from the outset as the fetish object for Frédéric's sexual fantasies about Madame Arnoux, and it is symbolically linked to the textual representation of the Orient, obsessively related in the nineteenth-century French male imagination to the hyperfeminized, supereroticized space of the harem. Frédéric assumes the as-yet unidentified Marie Arnoux with her splendid "peau brune" (brown skin) to be Andalusian or perhaps Creole. Her exoticism is qualified, however, by the sudden appearance of her *négresse*, whose presence quickly repatriates her as French and whitens her up without completely erasing the erotic/exotic residue left by the first impression. In fact, that first impression lingers, trailing its sensual exoticism in the dirty Seine, and it is that fantasy that Frédéric recovers when he catches Madame Arnoux's shawl before it disappears into the river. The shawl both embodies and animates the fantasy on which much of the novel's action will turn.

L'Éducation sentimentale offers a second pivotal shawl scene, and since Flaubert's novel places the Revolution of 1848 at its invisible center, the shawl plot may be read as a metaphor in domestic miniature for the wider social upheavals of the novel. As in *La Cousine Bette*, in *L'Éducation sentimentale*, the detail of the shawl serves to interweave the gendered spaces of private and public, domestic and political.

Jacques Arnoux, a middle-class dealer in art reproductions, among a series of other kitsch objects all related to the emerging industries of mass production in nineteenth-century France, is torn between his wife, Marie, and his mistress, Rosanette.[30] Rosanette nags him relentlessly for a *cachemire*, desiring it for its value in the wardrobe of a coquette as well as for the status it confers on its bearer—status of wealth and of propriety, as we have seen. An extremely costly gift, for Arnoux to offer it would signify his financial commitment to the courtesan. In fact, the *cachemire* is equivalent in Rosanette's mind to Arnoux's investment profits, which he had also promised her, a comparison that designates the shawl as a form of currency: "Il lui avait promis un quart de ses bénéfices dans les fameuses mines de kaolin: aucun bénéfice ne se montrait, pas plus que le cachemire dont il la leurrait depuis six mois" (188) (He had promised her a quarter of his profits from the famous kaolin mines: no profit was showing, no more than the cashmere shawl with which he had been teasing her for the past six months [150]). Arnoux finally does give Rosanette the *cachemire*, and this object is then further invested with textual significance as it now becomes both the vital plot link between Marie Arnoux and Rosanette and the sign of illicit lust in the text.

After Arnoux's gift, Madame Arnoux goes "chez le Persan" to have her own shawl repaired and is mistaken by the shopkeeper for the "other" Madame Arnoux, to whom a similar shawl had been recently expedited. The receipt for Rosanette's *cachemire* confirms Madame Arnoux's worst suspicions about her husband's infidelity. Aghast, she retreats with the evidence, only to confront her husband with his infidelity in the presence of her admirer, Frédéric, who himself is soon to enter the triangle when he also becomes Rosanette's lover. The cashmere shawl, then, is the vehicle of substitution, or exchange—mistress for wife, *femme comme il en faut* for *femme comme il faut*. Beneath the ubiquitous "cashmere fever" of nineteenth-century France clearly lies the commodification of women. Rosanette can be bought with a shawl, and the fateful moment of confusion, indeed substitution, occurs in the commercial space of a shop showcasing exotic feminine accessories.

The shawl plot overlays several layers of transaction, but nowhere in the novel is the conflation of woman and object more apparent than in the symbolic death scene of Madame Arnoux at the "vente aux enchères" (auction) toward the end of the novel, historically situated on December 1, 1851, the eve of the coup of Louis-Napoléon. Much has been written about the importance of this scene as the final stage in Frédéric's *éducation*, the metaphorical denuding of the ideal of modesty, and, in particular, the crass purchase of the famous *coffret* by Madame Dambreuse, now Frédéric's fiancée, which had alternately belonged both to Marie Arnoux and to Rosanette.[31] It should come as no surprise that in the advertisement for the auction, the following items once belonging to Marie Arnoux are now up for sale: "batterie de cuisine, linge de corps et de table, chemises, dentelles, jupons, pantalons, cachemires français et de l'Inde, piano d'Érard, deux bahuts de chêne Renaissance, miroir de Venise, poteries de Chine et du Japon" (498) ("'kitchen utensils, personal and table linen, chemises, laces, petticoats, drawers, French and Indian cashmeres, an Erard piano, a pair of Renaissance oak chests, Venetian mirrors, Chinese and Japanese porcelain'" [403]). Interspersed with items of the most personal intimacy (*linge de corps, chemises*, etc.) and those reflecting high resale value because of their pedigree and provenance (*piano d'Érard, miroir de Venise*, etc.), Madame Arnoux's *cachemires* bridge the gap between intimate garment and collectible object. The authentic cashmeres (*de l'Inde*) and their reproductions (*français*) represent the poles in the cashmere hierarchy, and their commingling on the auction block subtly suggests the social chaos this novel portrays. But the mention of the *cachemires* also recalls the earlier scene of the discovered bill of sale disclosing Arnoux's infidelity and linking through substitution of Marie Arnoux and Rosanette, just as it anticipates the convergence of Rosanette and Madame Dambreuse through the circulating *coffret*.[32]

In this scene of bald commerce, we find present all three principal female protagonists (Marie only metonymically), and it is here that Flaubert revives the opposition announced by Balzac in his early texts in a new confrontation between Rosanette and Madame Dambreuse. Rosanette arrives for the sale gussied up "en gilet de satin blanc à boutons de perles, avec une robe de falbalas, étroitement gantée, l'air vainqueur" (wearing a white satin jacket with pearl buttons, a flounced dress, tight gloves, and a triumphant expression); Madame Dambreuse "l'avait reconnue; et, pendant une minute, elles se considérèrent de haut en bas, scrupuleusement, afin de découvrir le défaut, la tare,—l'une enviant peut-être la jeunesse de l'autre, et celle-ci dépitée par l'extrême bon ton, la simplicité aristocratique de sa rivale" (502-3) (had recognized her; and for a full minute, they looked each other up and down, with scrupulous attention, in search of some flaw or blemish—the one perhaps envying the other's youth, while the latter was annoyed at her rival's good taste and aristocratic simplicity [407]). The overt opposition between the two women is written as one of style: Rosanette plays *la femme comme il en faut* to Madame Dambreuse's *femme comme il faut*. Madame Dambreuse may well project aristocracy, but she is also an imposter of sorts and every bit the golddigger that is Rosanette. She is, we learn, "tout simplement, une demoiselle Boutron, la fille d'un préfet" (267) (quite simply, a Boutron girl, the daughter of a prefect [214]). Neither emerges victorious in the end, as Frédéric dumps them both, leaving them to their catfight and making them equals in rejection. Most significant, however, is that Madame Arnoux, the icon of respectability, is reduced to her material accessories and that "ses reliques" (her relics) (including her *cachemires*) have entered the public sphere of commerce for purchase by the likes of Rosanette and Madame Dambreuse.

Both *La Cousine Bette* and *L'Éducation sentimentale* reveal the power of costume and material possessions to stage social belonging. And in their satirical representation of the frenzied acquisition of the accoutrements of social standing, both novels make a searing critique of the obsessive materialism that shadows the dramatic social and political upheavals of the day. The *cachemire*, luxury oriental import, served both to reinforce standards of feminine virtue, especially inasmuch as it signified marriage and marriageability, and to corrupt female respectability, as it was equally associated with Western fantasies of erotic harems and allowed women a form of social and economic transgression.

CONCLUSION

In February 1870 on the Paris vaudeville stage, playwright Eugène Labiche presented a comedy in one act entitled *Le Cachemire X.B.T.* The play is set entirely within the confines of a Parisian boutique called "Le Castor Laborieux" (The Busy Beaver), specializing in the commerce of cashmere.[33] Labiche's lightweight comedy stages several layers of social and domestic strife through a scene of commercial success gone awry. The two merchants Rotranger and Lobligeois are mocked by their shopworkers, cuckolded by their wives, and at each other's throats over the failure of their business, each blaming the other for the flagging sales of the once luxury item, the *cachemire*. The ugliest shawl in the shop becomes the centerpiece of the swirling disputes of the play. Because no one will purchase the shawl, the shopgirl acquires it, only for it to be sold under her nose to a rare customer, a young dandy lawyer who claims to be searching for a birthday present for his mother but who seems rather more interested in seducing the shopkeeper's flirty wife. After paying an outrageous sum for a phony "cachemire des Indes," the young lawyer shortly returns, prodded by his horrified mother, and threatens a lawsuit for having been defrauded: "c'est un cachemire d'Amiens que vous m'avez livré.... Je ne pense pas que le département de la Somme fasse partie de l'Indoustan" (452) (it's a cashmere from Amiens you have delivered me.... I don't believe that the department of the Somme is part of Hindustan). One commercial transaction begets another, however ("les affaires sont les affaires! [business is business!]), and all is made square when the shopkeeper's lubricious wife exchanges kisses for the bill of sale.

Labiche's play reiterates what we recognize as a common nineteenth-century plot involving a cuckolded husband and the purchase of a woman with a luxury garment. But by staging his play in a shop, he also makes plainly explicit the connection between sexual commerce and business transactions, the link between lust and *luxe* that was perhaps only implicit in earlier texts. Furthermore, his 1870 production dramatizes the cultural dénouement of one of the great luxury items of the nineteenth century. Once the staple only of the proper Parisian lady's wardrobe, the *cachemire* was now within the grasp of every common shopgirl. No longer unique, imported, handwoven garments signifying social distinction, by the 1870s cashmere shawls had fully entered mass production in France and were thus both infinitely reproducible and affordable. The sinking business of the Busy Beaver really has little to do with the commercial ineptitude of the bumbling buffoons behind the counter. It has, rather, everything to do with the social intersection that transpires in the public/private space of the shop. For here, lowly shopgirl, petit bourgeois, rising bourgeois professional, and his *maman* with her "grande dame" affectations meet, interact, and exchange both money and kisses, effecting a leveling out of social distinction repeatedly represented in the symbolic drama of the cashmere shawl.

As mass production and distribution made the imitation of cashmere shawls possible in France, and as more and more women were able to afford them, the *cachemire* lost its luster. The anxiety over social "authenticity," which no doubt masks nineteenth-century anxieties over political legitimacy following the collapse of the old regime, is pointedly illustrated in the debates that raged in fashion journals over the authenticity of a lady's *cachemire*. Balzac's virtuous aristocratic heroines are threatened with replacement by *demi-mondaines* and spurious bourgeoises, a scenario that enacts the fragililty of categories such as distinction; in *L'Éducation sentimentale*, Madame Arnoux's relationship of substitutability with Rosanette demonstrates a latent reversibility of the respectable Parisienne and the *demi-mondaine*; and finally, in Proust's fin de siècle in the character of Odette de Crécy, courtesan becomes wife, *la femme comme il en faut* becomes *la femme comme il faut*, reinventing Balzac's metaphor of Paris as the *grande courtisane* and bracketing the pronoun (en) of his witticism. Odette, Rosanette, and Bette are all necessarily "othered" in these texts—like the *cachemires* they covet, procure, or symbolically double, the socially marginal woman signifies the decadent eroticism of the exotic Orient, and the erotic trace just barely lingering in the garment of respectability that lines the *corbeille* still threatens to overwhelm its domestic counterfantasy of idealized virtue.

By the time we reach Proust, the *cachemire* has indeed entirely lost its value. In the first volume of the *Recherche*, cashmere goes underground. Relegated to indoor status, it no longer serves its important social function and is worn by Marcel's father to soothe his aching head: "il était encore devant nous, grand, dans sa robe de nuit blanche sous le cachemire de l'Inde violet et rose qu'il nouait autour de sa tête depuis qu'il avait des névralgies" (he was still in front of us, a tall figure in his white nightshirt, crowned with the pink and violet cashmere scarf which he used to wrap around his head since he had begun to suffer from neuralgia).[34] And *Le Temps retrouvé* finishes the job, designating the once hot commodity "le cachemire d'autrefois," a sign of outmoded fashion, which has now been replaced by "le satin et la mousseline de soie" (the cashmere of former days by satin and chiffon).[35] By the end of the *Recherche*, Odette de Crécy (Mme de Forcheville) has been reformed as aristocratic—very few characters remember her dubious origins. But perhaps more surprising than Odette's rise to high society is the ascendancy of the ultimate *bourgeoise*, Madame Verdurin. For the triumph of Madame Verdurin reverses Balzac's original exclusion of the *bourgeoise* from the categories of *femmes* he had laid out in his *études*. Balzac had judged that

> Quant à la bourgeoise, il est impossible de la confondre avec la femme comme il faut; elle la fait admirablement ressortir, elle explique le charme que vous a jeté votre inconnue. La bourgeoise est affairée, sort par tous les temps, trotte, va, vient, regarde, ne sait pas si elle entrera, si elle n'entrera pas dans un magasin . . . la bourgeoise entend très bien les pléonasmes de toilette. (*Autre étude*, 69–70)

> [As to the *bourgeoise*, the citizen womankind, she cannot possibly be mistaken for the lady; she is an admirable foil to her, she accounts for the spell cast over you by the Unknown. She is bustling, and goes out in all weather, trots about, comes, goes, gazes, does not know whether she will or will not go into a shop . . . she is accomplished in the redundancies of dress. (38)]

No one in Proust's universe is more verbose than Madame Verdurin, either in real speech or in the metaphorical language of clothes. Proust replaces one elaborate system of distinction with another, however, for the crucial subtext of his intensely private yet equally intensely social novel is surely that taste, snobbery, and the shifting patterns of distinction of a dying world emerge on the other side of a century intact but with a new wardrobe—a new set of distinctions.

In this chapter, I have examined the apparent opposition and potential reversibility of social poles within two landmark French novels of the mid-nineteenth century by focusing on a single overdetermined object. The circulation of the cashmere shawl in Balzac's and Flaubert's novels presents a pointed commentary on nineteenth-century views on social decline. Studying its circulation both focuses that social commentary and provides a vital key to reading the structures and themes of the novels themselves. The shifting cultural dynamics of opposition, imitation, and exchange reveal themselves in these novels in a quintessentially modern way—through the code of consumer culture, which in turn recites a chapter in the social history of the nineteenth century. The cashmere shawl and its social history should be read as an allegory within the realm of fashion for the shifting social landscape of nineteenth-century Paris. The hierarchy among shawls and the concern over a shawl's authenticity or its quality as a reproduction mirror the social hierarchy among women in nineteenth-century France and women's interest in establishing their status among the "legitimate," that is, the respectable, class. But the rise and fall of such a cultural artifact also offers important insights into the actualization of feminine identities in modern French society. For while social and political anxieties clearly underlie the story of cashmere, perhaps more significant still is the threat presented to the discerning *male* by the sartorial imposture of "inappropriate" women that the changing status of cashmere permits. The cashmere shawl is a vital accessory in the wardrobe of a lady of distinction, but it is the proper lady herself, the *femme comme il faut*, who serves as the necessary accessory for the socially successful man. And as Swann painfully illustrates, social marginalization awaits the man who cannot discern or who willingly ignores the distinction inherent in Balzac's little pronoun.

Finally, associations between colony and metropole come into clearer focus as exotic objects are assimilated to the fashion economy of France, reaffirming, among other things, the commercial underpinnings of French colonialism and the implication of Western women in the colonial project. More important perhaps, this fashion economy is tightly tied to a moral economy constructing and maintaining a Western ideology of the feminine. Like the Orient itself, these objects and their social circulation reveal the peculiar role of the feminine in nineteenth-century society: as screens on which to project masculine power and status, women must function ornamentally; and the fashion accessories with which they adorn themselves, very often of oriental provenance, hyperbolically reinforce this role and thus support the imperial project both literally and figuratively. At the same time, perhaps still possessing the decadent aura of their origins, these objects can also serve to subvert the ideology of the feminine they supposedly support. And by looking at exotic objects assimilated to Western notions of female respectability, we can begin to relocate some of the work of colonialism in the drawing rooms and boudoirs of Paris.

CHAPTER FOUR

Mademoiselle Ombrelle

Shielding the Fair Sex

*Dans cette œuvre d'art qui s'appelle la toilette d'une
femme, l'ombrelle joue le rôle du clair-obscur.*

OCTAVE UZANNE

As Emma Rouault enters the foreground in the opening sequences
of *Madame Bovary* and makes her play for the country doctor, she is
enveloped in the soft glow, the special effect, of an "ombrelle, de soie
gorge-de-pigeon, que traversait le soleil, [et qui] éclairait de reflets
mobiles la peau blanche de sa figure" (parasol, made of marbled silk,
[which] as the sun came shining through it, spread shifting colors over
the whiteness of her face).[1] The spell of illusion is cast in the *clair-obscur*
of the *ombrelle*'s visual trick: Charles is smitten by Emma's picture of
idealized femininity, with its promise of submission, fidelity, and un-
tarnished beauty. Her whiteness, emblematic of her desirability and
beauty within nineteenth-century aesthetic standards, is both guaranteed and enhanced by this requisite outdoor fashion accessory. Several
chapters and a wedding later, however, Emma's *ombrelle* is closed, and
as she wanders through the countryside for only the reader to see, her
ombrelle comes to figure the very crystallization of her discontent: "ses
idées peu à peu se fixaient et, assise sur le gazon, qu'elle fouillait à petit
coups avec le bout de son ombrelle, Emma se répétait:—Pourquoi, mon
Dieu, me suis-je mariée?" (73) (Then her ideas gradually came together,
and sitting on the grass, poking at it with the point of her sunshade,
Emma kept saying to herself:—Oh, why, dear God, did I marry him?
[34]). Her own illusions of romance, in which the feminine ideal stars
in the leading role, are laid bare in the harsh light of banal lived experience, untempered by special effects; and the *ombrelle*, stripped here of
its fashion-use value, signals instead Emma's slippage from the norma-

tive role prescribed to women in nineteenth-century France as it punctuates her plaintive lament on marriage.

This chapter focuses on the role of the *ombrelle* in the production and perturbation of idealized bourgeois femininity. In particular, here I wish to develop an analysis of the *ombrelle* as a highly gendered guarantor of respectability, indicating, above all, leisure and its presuppositions. In the fashion plates of the nineteenth century from the First Empire to the fin de siècle, the most visible and ubiquitous accessory for outdoor activities associated with leisure was the *ombrelle*. Because this accessory was ostensibly used to protect tender female skin against sun, not rain, the cultural imperatives of leisure and domesticity defining bourgeois femininity were implicit in the object's function to ensure and valorize whiteness. The *ombrelle*, a "dôme portatif de taffetas" (portable taffeta dome), married domesticity and leisure by reproducing on a small, symbolic scale the private, domestic interior of its carrier in the public great outdoors (Figure 11).[2]

The development of leisure as a concept and the expansion of a leisure class have been well documented by contemporary historians such as Bonnie Smith in her influential study of nineteenth-century bourgeois women in northern France, *Ladies of the Leisure Class*, and by early economists such as Thorstein Veblen, whose 1899 *Theory of the Leisure Class* offers still-pertinent observations on the relationship of women to luxury. With the rise of capitalism and the shift from their role as laborers to curators of domesticity, Smith argues, bourgeois women's responsibility as the signposts of family status and propriety became increasingly heavy.[3] As Veblen convincingly argues, status was predicated on wealth and leisure, but it was also linked to the domestic space, morally idealized and removed as it was from the brutal world of masculine industry, which, of course, subsidized domesticity's idealization (Smith).[4] Both leisure and domesticity privileged whiteness as a key sign of participation in their linked value systems, which were constructed simultaneously on a marked separation from work—both manual, organizing women by class and race, and industrial-financial, organizing them by gender.

The *ombrelle*, by its shape and construction, as we shall see in the analyses I set forth below, incarnated the feminine itself. Like the fashion doll and later the fashion mannequin, the *ombrelle* figured woman in an inanimate fashion accessory, performing the double act of dehumanizing and fetishizing her, just as it represented and sought to maintain iconic femininity, predicated on a domestic ideology of vir-

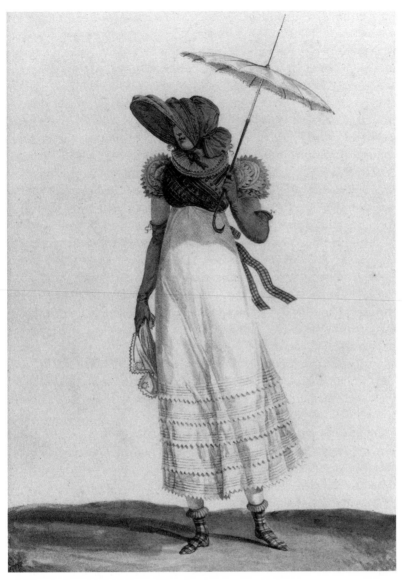

Figure 11. "La Merveilleuse," Bibliothèque nationale de France.

tue, purity, and submission. Because the *ombrelle* was to become the embodiment of the feminine, no accessory could have been more overtly gendered. From the early classification of the elite *ombrelle-marquise*, to fashion writer Octave Uzanne's characterization of the "frêle ombrelle," to the early twentieth-century acculturating children's fable "Mademoiselle Ombrelle," this accessory was distinctly female. Indeed, its official definition asserts as much. The dainty *ombrelle* is defined in nineteenth-century dictionaries in relation to its predecessor, the parasol. It was a "petit parasol dont se servent les dames" (a small parasol used by ladies).[5] The word *ombrelle* in fact seems to have entered the French lexicon in the 1800s, although the parasol had been widely used for centuries. The dictionary entry is telling in its delimiting of this form of small parasol for use uniquely by "les dames" (ladies), thus indicating that the object was restricted in terms of both gender and class.

That the *ombrelle* was hyperbolically feminized, as we shall see primarily through a series of images from nineteenth-century popular visual culture, risks obscuring that it was also classed and raced. Like the other feminine fashion accessories examined in this book, the *ombrelle* was a class marker. It was extremely popular, especially from the mid-nineteenth century on, figuring among the "indispensable accessories" of a proper lady; it thus expressed and bolstered gender and class norms.[6] Indeed, a wide range of *ombrelles* existed to serve the female social gamut. The tiny silken *marquise* emblematized wealth and leisure as it was designed for carriage use, while less elaborate models manufactured from less luxurious elements were widely available for purchase by a middle-class clientele. At both ends of the bourgeois social spectrum, however, the *ombrelle* clearly presupposed leisure, as it had to be carried in a free hand and as its primary function was to protect its bearer from the elements and complete a *toilette*, hardly the concerns of working-class women. Unlike the other accessories examined in this book, the *ombrelle* was explicitly linked to whiteness by virtue of its marking feminine bourgeois separation from work, and it thus helped to naturalize fair skin as one of the foremost standards of feminine beauty.[7] Functionally, the *ombrelle* served as a sunscreen to protect this powerful component of the nineteenth-century Western beauty aesthetic, which epitomized leisure and class and which also developed in contemporary ideologies of race as a moral indicator.[8]

In the *ombrelle*, then, as index of leisure par excellence, ideologies of class, gender, aesthetics, and race converge. Fashion writing and imagery illustrative of the *ombrelle*, together with the details surrounding its construction and use, mark this accessory as a key component of what has been termed the "fair sex ideology," especially widespread in eighteenth- and nineteenth-century North America but having its origins in Western Europe.[9] French historian Elsa Dorlin explains that early European anthropologists and naturalists considered "le blanc" to be "la couleur primitive de l'homme" (the original color of man), suggesting that all other colors/races were degenerate forms of the original and thus opening the door to the blending of two notions of purity: racial and moral.[10] This ideology, springing from the conflation of eighteenth-century physiognomic theories of the equation of beauty and morality with ideas of racial hierarchies, helped to shape nineteenth-century concepts of womanhood.[11] In his comprehensive study on whiteness in the Western tradition, cultural critic Richard Dyer argues that "the moral and aesthetic resonance of whiteness can and often has been mobilised in relation to white-skinned people" and illustrates this mobilization in representations of whiteness that emphasize "purity, cleanliness, virginity" (70). Dyer continues, "In Western tradition, white is beautiful because it is the colour of virtue. This remarkable equation relates to a particular definition of goodness. All lists of the moral connotations of white as symbol in Western culture are the same: purity, spirituality, transcendence, cleanliness, virtue, simplicity, chastity" (72). Dyer cites entries from the *Oxford English Dictionary*, but the *Dictionnaire de l'Académie française* of 1835 yields similar associations of *blanc/che* with innocence, virtue, and cleanliness.[12] As guarantor of whiteness, the *ombrelle* participated in Western ideologies of race and morality and was thus an integral component of the nineteenth-century formula for ideal femininity.

In the following pages, I present the *ombrelle* through a three-part structure, organized overall through the concept of leisure, in which gender, class, and race all participate as central factors. I suggest that the *ombrelle* is a strongly gendered female accessory as it simultaneously visually replicates ideal femininity, reproduces in miniature the protected, feminized domestic space, and functions to naturalize standards of feminine beauty. I demonstrate this primarily through an analysis of visual materials from both the female-oriented fashion press and the male-oriented popular, satirical press. But the *ombrelle* is also a class marker whose circulation between classes both produces social anxiety and potentially undermines the very normative femininity it incarnates. It contributes to idealized femininity through its marking of elite status, especially through certain models of *ombrelles*, as we shall see. The second movement of this chapter demonstrates this problem by juxtaposing two literary texts, from both elite and popular culture. Episodes from Flaubert's 1869 novel *L'Éducation sentimentale* and the Trouvé brothers' 1861 vaudeville play "Une ombrelle compromise par un parapluie" (An *ombrelle* compromised by an umbrella) take up the problematics and implications surrounding the *ombrelle*'s class slippage. Finally, the *ombrelle* works to ensure a racialized hierarchy. It is no surprise that the *ombrelle* reaches its fashionable peak during the Second Empire, when French colonialism was expanding exponentially and thus introducing new racial elements into domestic culture. The *ombrelle* guarantees whiteness and refers to the ethos of leisure, thereby reinforcing the racial order. The final movement of this chapter, then, analyzes two texts separated by nearly fifty years: Balzac's 1836 *Le Lys dans la vallée*, which helps to elucidate the connection between complexion, virtue, and the feminine fashion accessory, and Zola's 1880 *Nana*, which reconsiders Nana's perturbation of normative white femininity through the lens of the *ombrelle* and its relation to the prostitute's parodic enactment of leisure. These analyses, taken together, aim to make visible the hidden rhetorics of class and race bound up with one of the most persistent fashion emblems of womanhood in nineteenth-century France, the *ombrelle*.

LA FRÊLE OMBRELLE

Fin-de-siècle fashion writer, historian, and bibliophile Octave Uzanne offers a clear entry point to a discussion of the gendering of the *ombrelle* and the ways in which this fashion accessory operated in and on nineteenth-century French culture. In his 1883 *L'Ombrelle, le gant, et le manchon*, Uzanne produces an explicitly gendered personification of the *ombrelle* in his attempt to link this object with an idealized femininity predicated on an elite and nostalgic model. Like the fashion illustrations I will consider in this section, Uzanne's text expresses an assimilation of woman to accessory. This assimilation, accomplished through a hyperfeminization of the object, produces a personification of the *ombrelle*, just as it also produces a reification of the woman who wields it.

Uzanne presents his treatise as a sequel to his study of the fan, a "book for the boudoir," as he calls it. Both books were illustrated by artist Paul Avril, best known perhaps for his "sapphic" illustrations (Figure 12). Avril's erotically charged illustrations complement Uzanne's thesis that the *ombrelle* is like woman herself, dainty and delicate, and that it serves to protect femininity, to shield the fair sex. The playful eroticism of the illustrations, however, also points to the eroticization of the *ombrelle* as weapon, both feminized as seductive shield when opened, which perhaps suggests the missing skirts of the naked nymphs, and masculinized as phallic sword when closed, which may suggest any number of uses, from Emma Bovary's expressive instrument to Avril's cherub's plaything.

In his opening remark about the *ombrelle* cited in the epigraph to this chapter, Uzanne tells us that "[d]ans cette œuvre d'art qui s'appelle la toilette d'une femme, l'ombrelle joue le rôle du clair-obscur" (63) (in this work of art that is a woman's *toilette*, the *ombrelle* plays the role of *clair-obscur*). Comparing women's fashion to high art by embedding its terminology into his phrase, Uzanne suggests both a gendered relationship between art and fashion and a visual facticity produced by the *ombrelle* in particular. Properly deployed, the *ombrelle* produces an effect of light and shadow, a flattering frame and tool of idealization for its female subject that hinges on the contrast of transparency and opacity, visibility and invisibility, virtue and seduction. Constitutive, then, of a key fantasy of the nineteenth-century feminine, the *ombrelle* also has old associations with (oriental) royalty and by the nineteenth century is clearly linked to status and leisure and, thus, respectability.

Uzanne places the *ombrelle* in the category of "les parures protectrices de [l']être délicat" (finery protective of the delicate sex), thereby inscribing its function within a discourse of female respectability that speaks to her preciousness and her weakness in relation to male strength. And through the use of the adjective "délicat," he implicitly refers to fairness of complexion, whose protection is also embedded in the *ombrelle*'s function.[13] *Ombrelles* were strictly feminine, while *parapluies*, much larger, were masculine objects, serving a purely utilitarian end and signaling ignominiously both the absence of carriage and the bourgeois concern for protecting one's garments.[14] Maurice Gardot, a contributor to the *Journal des demoiselles* writing in 1883, muses on the classed and gendered associations with the *parapluie*: "Riflard [a *parapluie*] en 1830, il personnifia longtemps et presque exclusivement le bourgeois tranquille, épicier retiré des affaires, rentier du Marais, n'ayant plus que deux ambitions: pêcher une friture et . . . la manger" (317) (*Riflard* in 1830, for a long time it personified almost exclusively the dull bourgeois, the grocer retired from business, the stockholder of the Marais, having no more than two ambitions: fishing for his fried

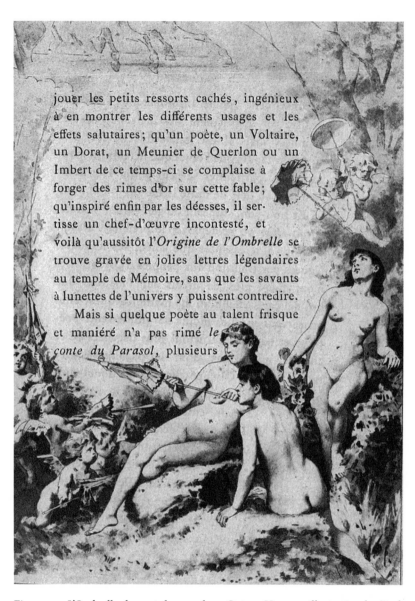

jouer les petits ressorts cachés, ingénieux à en montrer les différents usages et les effets salutaires; qu'un poète, un Voltaire, un Dorat, un Meunier de Querlon ou un Imbert de ce temps-ci se complaise à forger des rimes d'or sur cette fable; qu'inspiré enfin par les déesses, il sertisse un chef-d'œuvre incontesté, et voilà qu'aussitôt l'*Origine de l'Ombrelle* se trouve gravée en jolies lettres légendaires au temple de Mémoire, sans que les savants à lunettes de l'univers y puissent contredire.

Mais si quelque poète au talent frisque et maniéré n'a pas rimé *le conte du Parasol,* plusieurs

Figure 12. *L'Ombrelle, le gant, le manchon,* Octave Uzanne, illustration by Paul Avril, 1883, Vassar College Library, Poughkeepsie, N.Y.

supper and . . . eating it).[15] The pedestrian *parapluie* was thus historically associated with the petit bourgeois whose sole interests were pragmatic (eating, keeping dry) and not symbolic (signifying up in a social
class system). Not so for the *ombrelle*, which was pure surplus and a
sign of social status. Baronne Staffe illustrates this gendered distinction
between raw utility and genteel ornament in a chapter on "les visites"
in her 1889 conduct manual *Usages du monde*: "Les visiteurs laissent,
dans l'antichambre ou le vestibule les parapluies, les cache-poussière,
les doubles chaussures, etc., dont ils peuvent s'être munis contre les in-
tempéries. Les femmes gardent leur ombrelle ou leur en-cas, leur boa,
leur manchon pour entrer dans un salon" (104) (Visitors leave in the
foyer or the vestibule umbrellas, dusters, galoshes, etc., that they can
don in inclement weather. Women keep their *ombrelle*, or their *en-cas*,
their boa, their muff, when they enter the drawing room).[16] Unlike the
purely utilitarian and masculinized *parapluie*, which had to wait in the
foyer, the *ombrelle* accompanied the lady into the social space of the salon and participated in the conduct of the visit. Its objective to complete
the *toilette* of a lady, to signify propriety and status, was more valuable
than its ostensible use value as sunshade. Gardot remarks on the super-
fluity of the *ombrelle* given the Parisian climate: "Le soleil est, en effet,
si pâle et si rare que l'on se demande presque s'il ne s'est pas refroidi"
(317) (The sun, in fact, is so pale and rare that we have to wonder almost
if it hasn't been frozen). It hardly seems necessary, Gardot contends, to
protect one's complexion under such inclement skies, but this superflu-
ity only begs the question of the object's deeper cultural significance.

Gray Parisian skies notwithstanding, *ombrelles* were de rigueur for
outdoor promenades and came into fashion seasonally, just as certain
fabrics and colors did. Countless fashion plates from the First Empire
to the fin de siècle depict women engaged in typical outdoor leisure activities and toting the requisite *ombrelle*. An account of the latest fashions (and clearly a plug for the *ombrelle* shop of Mottet) in the anonymous "Bulletin des modes" column in the fashion journal *La Mode* in
March 1847 expressly justifies the feminizing and elite classing of this
accessory:

> chez M. MOTTET . . . nous avons tenu en nos mains et vraiment admi-
> ré des ombrelles destinées au printemps, dont la forme est si coquette
> et l'étoffe si fraîche, dont la petite canne d'ivoire est si artistique-
> ment fouillée, qu'elles nous ont paru tout-à-fait dignes d'être appelées
> ombrelles duchesses, ombrelles Maintenon, et ombrelles Victoria.
> M. Mottet nous a montré encore un parasol de campagne, servant en

même temps de paraverse sans être pour cela d'une ampleur exa-
gérée et d'un poids incommode. Cet industriel a compris que dans les
longues excursions champêtres faites souvent en plein soleil, une ombrelle trop lourde eût été une sorte de supplice et de contre-sens (524).

[At Mottet's . . . we held in our hands and really admired the new
spring models of *ombrelle*, whose shape is so coquettish and whose
material so fresh, whose little ivory handle is so artistically turned, that
they seemed completely worthy of being called *ombrelles duchesses,
ombrelles Maintenon,* and *ombrelles Victoria.* M. Mottet also showed us
a country parasol that could serve as well as a windscreen, but without,
for all that, being of an exaggerated size or of an ungainly weight. This
manufacturer has understood that for long country excursions, often
made under a full sun, an *ombrelle* that is too heavy would be a torture
and counterproductive.]

Mottet's clients engage in precisely the kinds of leisure activities
deemed appropriate for elite and upwardly mobile bourgeois ladies in
nineteenth-century France. The crucial accoutrement for strolling under the sun, the *ombrelle* had to be usable—not too large or cumber-
some, thus presupposing the delicacy of its owner, and stylish—that
is, combining shapely coquetry, fresh fashionable fabrics, and artistic
details, all of which contributed to a classed and elegant look. A description from the issue of *Journal des dames et des modes* of April 1837
explicitly links delicacy and elegance, stating the express purpose of
the tiny *ombrelle-marquise*—to protect the face: "En attendant le soleil,
Verdier fabrique de charmantes ombrelles garnies en or. Les ombrelles
de calèche, dites *marquises* préserveront cette année toutes les figures
frêles et élégantes du hâle de l'été, si toutefois il y a un été" (163) (As
we await the sun, Verdier is making charming *ombrelles* trimmed with
gold. Carriage *ombrelles*, called *marquises*, will protect all the fragile
and elegant faces this year from the tanning effects of summer, if there
ever is a summer). As both excerpts indicate, as an extension of herself,
the *ombrelle* was assimilated to the woman who carried it and marked
both social status and its attending feminine aesthetic, which married
beauty with leisure and delicacy.

This personification process was widespread: adjectives used in the
fashion press to describe *ombrelles*, such as *charmantes, coquettes, jolies, élégantes, fraîches,* clearly feminize the accessory; and, it should
be noted, these objects were with great frequency colored white. Along
with fashion discourse, literary figures too promoted the symbolic
nexus of whiteness and purity, a connection I will explore in more de-

tail below.[17] Another important trend in *ombrelles* was to match them to dresses, particularly in the latter part of the century, further emphasizing this parallelism between woman and object: the *ombrelle* was "dressed" according to the fabric and color scheme of the dress the lady was wearing and often concealed lacy or silken linings visible on the *ombrelle* when open. Indeed, one anonymous fashion writer for the *Journal des demoiselles* describes the vogue of matching dresses with *ombrelles* and even proclaims the tastefulness of matching *ombrelles* and *gants*, also meant to protect from the sun, further crystallizing their related function in the maintenance of a racialized beauty ideal. In describing a *"costume de cachemire gris perle,"* the fashion writer elaborates on a complete outfit, each detail of which is nuanced in shades of gray, down to the "gants & ombrelle gris perle, car il est de bon goût de les assortir aux toilettes" (pearl gray gloves and *ombrelle*, since it is in good taste to match one's *toilettes*).[18] Similarly, a fashion plate from an 1883 number of *La Mode illustrée* picturing two women dressed in outdoor wear designed and most probably designated for the typical leisure activities of elite and bourgeois women—visiting, walking, and the races—illustrates the fashion of matching *ombrelles* in color and fabric to dresses (Figure 13). One *ombrelle* is opened to protect the lady's face from the sun, its blue silk trim matching the fabric of her dress and hat; the other, closed, is fabricated from a rose silk that matches the bonnet and printed flowers on the bearer's dress. This *ombrelle* is garnished with a tied ribbon that repeats the bonnet ribbon tied around this lady's throat, reinforcing the parallelism between woman and accessory. Like fashion descriptions, illustrated plates tout the value of symmetry in color and fabric in the production of tasteful and appropriate dress, inscribing metonymic links between accessory and dressed woman. Often, toward the end of the century, as suggested earlier, "like the frothy underwear hidden under the plain skirts, many plain parasols when opened revealed elaborate linings," again reproducing the parallel relationship of woman and accessory.[19] Like so many women's fashions that carried with them the moral and social values of respectable femininity they presumably served to safeguard, the *ombrelle* was also a potent instrument in the erotic play of feminine seduction, concealing and revealing the sensuality that was ostensibly prohibited for respectable women.

The silks and laces used to confect and ornament *ombrelles* were part of the treasure trove of the *corbeille de mariage*. By the 1860s, *ombrelles* were also widely available ready-made at all price ranges, especially af-

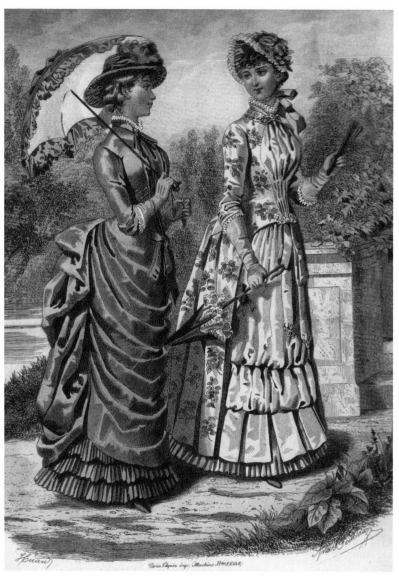

Figure 13.   Plate 24, *La Mode illustrée*, 1883, private collection.

ter the advent of the department store, which as Zola's 1883 novel *Au Bonheur des Dames* documents, led to the near extinction of the artisanal fabrication of fashion accessories like the *ombrelle*. His novel pits every small local fashion boutique and craftsman against the monolithic department store. The neighborhood's final holdout, Bourras, the *ombrelle* and *parapluie* maker who carves his own handles and sews his own laces onto the frame, in the end succumbs, crushed by the volume of product and clientele that his rival Mouret can command. In one of the great scenes of consumption in this novel, Zola describes a magnificent display of *ombrelles* at the Bonheur, designed to mesmerize customers by defamiliarizing the object from its usual outdoor setting:

> C'était l'exposition des ombrelles. Toutes ouvertes, arrondies comme des boucliers, elles couvraient le hall, de la baie vitrée du plafond à la cimaise de chêne verni. Autour des arcades des étages supérieurs, elles dessinaient des festons; le long des colonnes, elles descendaient en guirlandes; sur les balustrades des galeries, jusque sur les rampes des escaliers, elles filaient en lignes serrées; et, partout rangées symétriquement, bariolant les murs de rouge, de vert et de jaune, elles semblaient de grandes lanternes vénitiennes, allumées pour quelque fête colossale. Dans les angles, il y avait des motifs compliqués, des étoiles faites d'ombrelles à trente-neuf sous, dont les teintes claires, bleu pâle, blanc crème, rose tendre, brûlaient avec une douceur de veilleuse; tandis que, au-dessus, d'immenses parasols japonais, où des grues couleur d'or volaient dans un ciel de pourpre, flambaient avec des reflets d'incendie.

> [It was the display of parasols. Wide open and rounded like shields, they covered the hall from the glazed ceiling to the varnished oak mouldings. They formed festoons around the arcades of the upper storeys; they hung down in garlands along the pillars; they ran in close lines along the balustrades of the galleries, and even on the banisters of the staircases; symmetrically arranged everywhere, speckling the walls with red, green, and yellow, they seemed like great Venetian lanterns, lit for some colossal entertainment. In the corners there were complicated patterns, stars made of parasols at ninety-five centimes, and their light shades—pale blue, creamy white, soft pink—were burning with the gentleness of a night-light; while above, huge Japanese sunshades covered with golden cranes flying across a purple sky were blazing with glints of fire].[20]

The crowds of *ombrelles* both mimic and invite into the department store the masses of female consumers of every social rank and economic means. Zola's crowds are feminized and multiplied in his excessive

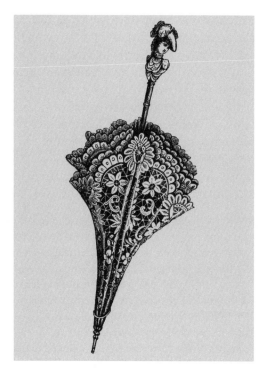

Figure 14. "Poignet d'ombrelle." Reprinted with permission from Dover Publications.

display of the fashion accessory that most clearly embodies the feminine. Open like shields, Mouret's *ombrelles* both reveal their feminized hidden interiors and present an army of irresistible merchandise, the front line in Mouret's offensive against the woman consumer. But Zola's equivalence of *ombrelle* and woman in this novel merely illustrates the assimilation, propagated by both the fashion press and the manufacturers of *ombrelles*, between woman and her accessory. One *ombrelle* from 1884, for example, even displays a carved lady's head as its handle (*poignet*), exemplifying the metaphorical relationship between accessory and woman (Figure 14). And if its handle could reproduce a lady's head, when opened, the *ombrelle* mimicked in its shape the voluminous skirts of the mid-nineteenth century. Introduced in the 1840s, the crinoline was frequently illustrated and ridiculed in satirical journals just as it was being widely promoted in ladies' fashion journals.[21] The doubling of woman and *ombrelle* recurs visually in caricatures as well as in the fashion plates, as in the Daumier sketch in Figure 15, which paints

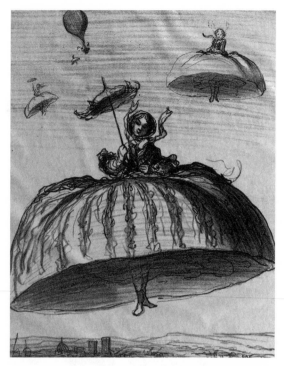

Figure 15.   "Manière d'utiliser les jupons nouvellement
mise à la mode," Daumier, 1856, Bibliothèque nationale
de France.

a Parisian sky raining women. Her hat ribbons fluttering, the principal
female figure looks demurely downward, her complexion protected by
her tiny *ombrelle* and her fall broken by her parachute-like skirt, under
which the viewer has a rare full view of lacy petticoats, undergarments,
legs encased in stockings, and, naturally, tiny booted feet. The analogy of form between skirt and *ombrelle* is amusingly on display in the
drawing, but the caricature, while it seems to ridicule the excess and
frivolity of women's fashions, also mirrors in many ways the structures
of the fashion plate.

    Like many other ladies' fashion accessories in nineteenth-century
France, the *ombrelle* refers nostalgically to the eighteenth-century era
of high fashion and decorative excess known as the Pompadour period
(1721–64). In fact, the most popular model for the *ombrelle* in the mid-
nineteenth century was called a *marquise*, after the marquise de Pompadour herself, the paragon of eighteenth-century feminine coquetry.

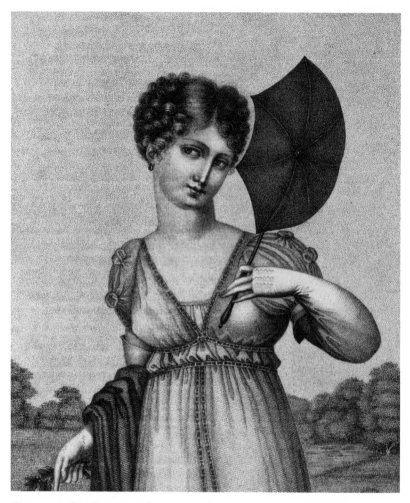

Figure 16.   "La Coquetterie," *Costumes de France, 1795–1815*, Bibliothèque nationale de France.

Costume historian Annie Sagalow asserts that the *ombrelle-marquise*
was particularly important during the Second Empire but that it was
already in evidence as early as 1802 (Figure 16): "Dès 1839, R. M. Cazal, l'un des plus importants fabricants d'ombrelles et de parapluies du
XIXe siècle, expliquait dans un brevet, le mécanisme spécial qui dif-
férencie, entre autres, l'ombrelle-marquise des ombrelles fabriquées
précédémment: une charnière, au sommet du mât, permet d'incliner
en écran pare-soleil la couverture de l'ombrelle" (28). (By 1839, R. M.

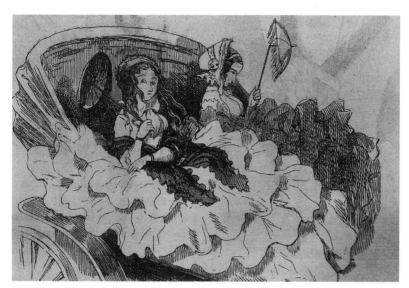

Figure 17. "Le Bois de Boulogne: Habituées," *Petit Journal pour rire*, Émile Marcelin, 1856, private collection.

Cazal, one of the most important *ombrelle* and umbrella makers of the nineteenth century, was explaining in a patent the special mechanism that differentiates, among other things, the *ombrelle-marquise* from *ombrelles* made earlier: a hinge, at the top of the rod, permits one to tilt the cover of the *ombrelle* as a sunscreen). Because the *marquise* operated with a hinge in the stem, this distinct *ombrelle* could be bent in order to protect the face directly. It was specifically designed for carriage use, thus marking its bearer as socially superior. The illustrator Émile Marcelin depicts the *habituées*, or the regulars, of the Bois de Boulogne riding in carriages and screening their faces with their tiny *ombrelles-marquises* in his series of caricatures of the life of the Bois de Boulogne (Figure 17). This illustration, from *Le Petit Journal pour rire* of 1856, demonstrates that the *ombrelle* is as much social tool as skin protector, as it allows for control over who sees what (or whom). And again, the fringed ornamentation of the *marquise* echoes the flouncy frou-frou of the ladies' skirts, which spill out of the carriage in an excess of cloth. Taken together with the other signs of wealth and class apparent in the drawing, the *marquises* signify midcentury snobbery.

Finally, to return to Uzanne's text where I began this analysis of the visual and discursive gendering of the *ombrelle*, the fashion writer fantasizes about the *ombrelle*'s signifying value during the idealized eighteenth century (ever his historical point of reference for all things respectably fashionable), which he hopes to re-create in his fin-de-siècle reading public. In the following passage, he produces a multipronged commentary at once on the accessory and on its proprietress, as if the two were indistinct:

> Comme tous les objets de la parure entre la main des femmes, l'ombrelle au siècle dernier, devient presque, comme l'éventail, un léger et gracieux hochet qui sert à ponctuer une expression, à arrondir un geste, à armer une attitude, à peindre la rêverie lorsque, conduite par une jolie main indolente, la pointe trace de vagues dessins sur le sable. Au souffle brûlant des déclarations amoureuses, souvent la frêle Ombrelle s'échappe des mains d'une belle en signe d'armistice et comme un aveu d'abandon (41).

> [Like all accessories in the hands of women, the *ombrelle* in the last century became practically, like the fan, a light and graceful toy which served to accentuate an expression, fill out a gesture, defend an attitude, depict a dream, when, wielded by a pretty indolent hand, its point traces vague drawings in the sand. At the ardent breath of declarations of love, the *frêle Ombrelle* often falls from the hands of a *belle* as a sign of both armistice and an avowal of abandon.]

Only distantly related to the practical, masculine, and functional umbrella, as we have seen, the decorative *ombrelle*, in the hands of a woman, is converted to plaything, arm of seduction, cosmetic enhancer, and extension of the female body. It figures female expressions, gestures, and feelings and even serves female art production (let us not forget that Uzanne has likened the ladies' *toilette* to *une œuvre d'art*) as it mimics, albeit aimlessly, the artist's pencil drawing in the sand (cf. *Madame Bovary*). Most important, as Uzanne demonstrates in his "frêle Ombrelle," which is assimilated to the "belle" herself through rhyme and personified though Uzanne's capitalization, the *ombrelle* doubles the swooning woman. It may well protect this delicate creature from the burning rays of the sun, but, hyperbolically feminized, according to Uzanne, the *ombrelle* is frailty itself against burning declarations of love, just like the lady who carries it. Female capitulation in the face of male ardor is also encoded in the delicacy proclaimed by the *ombrelle*'s importance for the *frêle femelle*. The weaker sex must maintain her delicacy as it symbolizes a series of cultural values on which a certain conceptualization of the nation depends, and she must also willingly faint before male desire.

The gendering of the *ombrelle* is visible in print and picture throughout the nineteenth century, and, as I have suggested, its classing was difficult to disengage from this gendering. In the next section, I consider the object as class sign in greater depth and demonstrate how the anxiety over class assignment is both expressed and worked out in the *ombrelle*.

CLASSING THE *MARQUISE*: FROM VAUDEVILLE TO FLAUBERT

Both the classing and the gendering of the *ombrelle* are quite visible in an 1861 vaudeville play entitled *"Une Ombrelle compromise par un parapluie"* (Figure 18), written by Messieurs Arsène and Eugène Trouvé, which figures its protagonists precisely through these two accessories and unfolds a convoluted jealousy plot resolved only through the correct reassignment of the objects to their rightful, and appropriate, owners.[22] The play takes up the topical issue of the new law requiring that one check personal items on entering museums. In this one-act play, Madame Pépin, the coat check attendant at the entry to a horticultural exhibit, complains about the thrift of the fashionable exhibition-goers: "Voyez-donc cette belle dame . . . elle est mise comme une duchesse et met sa marquise dans sa poche, plutôt que de donner deux sous" (1) (Have a look at that beautiful lady . . . she is dressed like a duchess and puts her *marquise* in her pocket, rather than pay two cents). But when an anonymous "dame" enters, accompanied by a young man, Jules, who seems to have been stalking the lady from the omnibus, Madame Pépin is relieved to be charged with the brand new *ombrelle* "charmante, d'un goût parfait" (charming, in perfect taste) of a real lady. The *ombrelle* indeed figures this respectable lady, who takes great pains to ensure that Madame Pépin check the young man's *canne* "séparément," as the *dame* emphatically insists they are *not* together, notwithstanding young Jules's continued attentions and their entering the exhibit together.

In a classically burlesque series of events, turning on the recognition and misattribution of an *ombrelle*, bourgeois jealousy erupts, only to be righted at the last possible moment, when both objects and people return to their proper places.[23] For in the meantime, Godichon, the lady's husband, happens to be lunching and imbibing in the next-door café, unaware that his wife is visiting the exhibit. Bored, he begins to peruse the contents of the adjacent coat check, amusing himself with a drunken social critique of the exhibition-goers based on their accoutrements. His monologue is worth quoting at length, for it serves both to

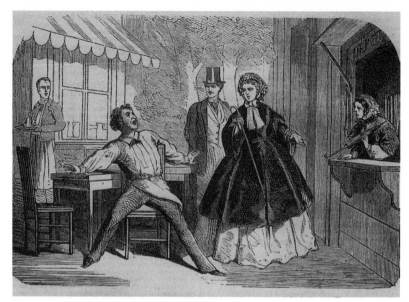

Figure 18. *Une Ombrelle compromise par un parapluie*, University of Florida George
A. Smathers Libraries, Special & Area Studies Collection, Rare Book Collection.

develop further the gendered and classed characteristics of the accessories and to expose the moment of recognition at which the jealousy
plot takes off:

> Voyons si la société est choisie . . . Peuh! voici des cannes bien vul-
> gaires . . . des ombrelles bien rapées . . . Cette branche en houx n'est pas
> mal . . . un certain air aristocratique! . . . cette petite ombrelle . . . nous
> avons bien la mine, mademoiselle, d'arriver en droite ligne du quartier
> Bréda . . . Regardez ces deux vieux rotins de chaque côté de cet en-tout-
> cas pudique . . . la chaste Suzanne entre les deux vieillards . . . la canne
> d'un étudiant . . . celle d'un septuagénaire, la pomme brillante, le bout
> tordu . . . Voilà une ombrelle . . . (Il regarde attentivement.) qui ressemble
> à celle de ma femme . . . c'est étonnant! . . . Si je n'étais pas sûr . . . mais
> c'est incroyable! . . . C'est elle! . . . je la reconnais à cette tache qu'elle y fit
> en assaisonnant la salade, un certain jour . . . Elle est ici? . . . Je ne puis
> le croire! . . . Et ce parapluie formidable qui y est attaché! . . . Ma tête
> s'égare! Elle a voulu sortir seule . . . Il me passe une foule de choses dés-
> agréables devant les yeux! Si j'étais . . . et le bec de ce grédin de parapluie
> tourné vers celui de mon épouse! . . . Il me prend une folle envie . . . de le
> pourfendre . . . de l'ouvrir . . . cet ignoble parapluie! . . . Et toi, ombrelle
> adultère . . . tiens! (Il lui allonge un coup de canne.) (3).

[Let's just see if this is high society . . . Bah! these are very vul-
gar canes . . . really worn-out parasols . . . This holly stick isn't
bad . . . a certain air of aristocracy! . . . this little parasol . . . you
seem, mademoiselle, to have come straight from the Bréda neighborhood . . . Look at these two old canes on either side of the prud-
ish "en-tout-cas" . . . chaste Suzannah between the old men . . . the
student's cane, . . . an old man's cane, its brilliant handle, its end
twisted . . . Here's a parasol . . . (he takes a closer look) that looks like
my wife's . . . how peculiar! . . . If I wasn't sure . . . but this is unbeliev-
able! . . . It *is* hers! . . . Here is the stain that she got on it while dressing a salad the other day . . . Is she here? . . . I can't believe it! . . . And
this fabulous umbrella attached to it! . . . I'm losing my mind! She
said she wanted to go out alone . . . I'm thinking of terrible things! If I
were . . . and what of the point of this despicable umbrella, facing my
wife's parasol! . . . I'm dying to . . . to slay . . . to open . . . this ignoble
umbrella! . . . And you, adulterous parasol, . . . take that! (He stretches
out to strike her with his cane.)]

The conflation of object and person is complete: the *parapluie*, emblematic of the usurping male, is an ignoble *grédin* (rascal), who stands in
much too close proximity to the adulterous *ombrelle*, who receives a
physical blow for her crime. The gendering of the object comes plainly into view through Godichon's revenge on the metaphoric *ombrelle*,
which is punished for adultery in the way husbands were legally permitted to punish their wives. The hyperfeminine *ombrelle* (albeit stained,
indicating perhaps its presumed moral blemish) is locked in the embrace of a large, formidable, need I say, phallic *parapluie*.

Godichon hatches an elaborate scheme to catch the objects' human
counterparts in the act, which is already being rehearsed by their accessories. But he is mercifully saved from his misguided jealous rage
when he discovers that the proprietors of the scandalous *parapluie* and
ombrelle are a grandfather and granddaughter, to whom Madame Godichon had given her stained *ombrelle* earlier in the day. Young girls
(fitted for corsets from a tender age) were never too young to learn
to be young ladies.[24] Godichon is so relieved to find his wife untaint-
ed by adultery ("[e]nfin je te retrouve . . . et pure!" [finally I've found
you . . . and pure!]) and in possession of a new *ombrelle* that he fails to
realize that his wife is still being pursued by the young man with the
canne, and that the *canne* and the *ombrelle* had indeed been exchanged
in the vestiary, an entanglement that should have given greater cause
for alarm than that of the *parapluie*. For *cannes* were typically the accessories of wealthy, aristocratic dandies, while *parapluies* were stolidly

bourgeois.[25] This one-act play revolves entirely around popular conceptions of propriety and their public demonstration through fashion accessories like the *ombrelle*. The *ombrelle*, figuring the woman who carries it, is also a social weapon, defending class and standing.

The *ombrelle* is thus associated with both gender and class norms, as the vaudeville play demonstrates and as Uzanne also emphasizes. Uzanne's descriptions work to shape fashion as expressive of a normative society, which, as he seems only half aware, has been mutating over the better part of the nineteenth century. Uzanne concludes his "history" of the *ombrelle* with a typical lament over its democratization: "L'Ombrelle se trouve aujourd'hui entre toutes les mains; en ce siècle utilitaire et pratique cela devait être. Il n'est point, à l'heure actuelle, de femme ou de fille du peuple qui n'ait son Ombrelle ou son *en-tout-cas* de satin" (61) (Today the *Ombrelle* is found in every hand; in our utilitarian and practical century it must be thus. At the present moment, there isn't a single woman or girl of the people who doesn't have her own *Ombrelle* or satin *en-tout-cas*). Uzanne decries the modern accessibility and, indeed, the bourgeoisification of this essentially elegant accessory and its collapse into utility with the *en-tout-cas*, a kind of woman's umbrella, a hybrid of *ombrelle* and *parapluie*. He thus resists the modernity of social mobility and fashion's role in it. And yet Uzanne nonetheless offers up his book for consumption by a bourgeois female readership hungry to be fashionable and thereby participates in the very commodification and democratization he claims so to despise. While Uzanne's fashion discourse does not express any apparent awareness of the paradox of its own position, nineteenth-century literary discourse is acutely aware of both the paradox and the slippage of fashion's role from a normalizing system upholding social hierarchies to an equalizing system in which those hierarchies are increasingly less visible.

Flaubert's *Éducation sentimentale* provides a compelling example of the disturbance of proper social assignment amid the cultural and political chaos of midcentury France. In an obscure but vital narrative surrounding Madame Arnoux's *ombrelle*, we can discern the threat modern fashion and thus modernity itself posed to both class and gender categories. If the Trouvé brothers' vaudeville play used the *ombrelle* to construct a jealousy plot revolving around tenuous gender and class relations, insinuating trouble in hierarchical paradise, Flaubert's monumental historical novel uses the *ombrelle* to upend class relations altogether.

It is worth remembering that when Frédéric Moreau first sees Marie

Arnoux aboard the *Ville-de-Montereau* in the novel's opening scene, he
falls for her metonyms—that is, her composite parts, most of them detailed elements of fashion: her "large chapeau de paille, avec des rubans
roses, . . . sa robe de mousseline claire, tachetée de petits pois, etc." (23)
(large straw hat with pink ribbons . . . her dress of light, dotted muslin, etc.). As Evelyne Woestelandt has written, fragile, airy *mousseline*
was new and popular in the nineteenth century and contributed significantly along with the multiplying feminine accessories of the period to the "jeu d'apparences" that produced "un fragile équilibre entre
avances et modestie, extravagance et mesure, anarchisme et respect de
l'ordre" that was central to the allure of bourgeois femininity (the game
of appearances . . . a fragile balance between seduction and modesty,
extravagance and measure, subversiveness and respect for order).[26] Madame Arnoux is fully accessorized: as we saw in Chapter 2, Frédéric's
pickup line is predicated on the "rescue" of her cashmere shawl, and
when he does approach her, "il se planta tout près de son ombrelle, posée contre le banc" (23) (he plopped down right near her *ombrelle*, set
against the bench).

The *ombrelle* plot develops as a narrative about the circulation and
equalization of women from opposite classes and, thus, opposite moral-
ities. Desperate to meet her again in Paris, Frédéric barges in at the Arnoux house one evening, to be admitted by Jacques Arnoux "non dans
le boudoir ou dans sa chambre, mais dans la salle à manger" (not in the
boudoir or in the bedroom, but in the dining room) where we (but presumably not the dense Frédéric) observe *two* glasses of champagne on
the table. Nervous at his unwelcome reception at Arnoux's house, Frédéric becomes clumsy and, bumping into a chair leg, "fit tomber une
ombrelle posée dessus; le manche d'ivoire se brisa" (91) (knocked over
an *ombrelle* set against [the chair]; the ivory handle broke). Naturally,
this *ombrelle* cannot belong to Madame Arnoux, who is away tending
her sick mother in Chartres and who would surely not leave her *ombrelle*, a daytime accessory, lying about in the dining room anyway; further evidence of its suspect ownership lies in Arnoux's "singulier sourire" when Frédéric nearly dies of chagrin "d'avoir brisé l'ombrelle de
Madame Arnoux" (91) (peculiar smile . . . for having broken Madame
Arnoux's *ombrelle*). Blind to all the obvious signs of Arnoux's infidelity,
Frédéric makes amends for what he perceives to be his "maladresse" by
purchasing a fashionable and expensive new *ombrelle* for his idol for her
birthday: "une marquise en soie gorge-pigeon, à petit manche d'ivoire
ciselé, et qui arrivait de Chine" (109) (a *marquise* in dove gray silk, with

a small carved ivory handle, which came from China). Woestelandt remarks that this description represents the most detailed of any accessory in *L'Éducation* ("Système de la mode," 252). While Madame Arnoux is most frequently dressed in somber colors, thus reflecting midcentury codes of bourgeois propriety—and distinguishing herself from the gaudy colors and loose morals of a Rosanette—here she acquires a shimmering dove-gray silk filter through which to be viewed and idealized.

The *ombrelle* bespeaks luxury, artisanry, and exoticism and evokes orientalist fantasies through its material components of silk and ivory, both traditionally associated with the Far East, and it thus also evokes erotic fantasies. For this freshly imported *ombrelle*, defined by its *clarté*, recalls Madame Arnoux the *inconnue* of Frédéric's initial idealizing vision of her in the scene of the *coup de foudre*. Likewise, less perceptibly, it links Madame Arnoux to her *demi-mondaine* rival, whose *ombrelle* Frédéric is unwittingly replacing.

The *ombrelle* plot, then, is inextricably linked to the infidelity plot, and the one elucidates the other for the reader. As Frédéric offers his gift to Madame Arnoux, she is pleased but perplexed when he replies, "Mais, c'est presque une dette! . . . j'ai été si fâché" (112) (Well it is practically a debt! . . . I was so upset). Arnoux cuts him off before he has a chance to explain his motivations for offering an *ombrelle* and thus to expose Arnoux's infidelity. But it is indeed at this same birthday party, set in the countryside near the Arnoux factory, that Madame Arnoux just a little later learns of Arnoux's affair with Rosanette when Arnoux himself carelessly wraps a bouquet of roses for her in a letter from Mlle Vatnaz, Rosanette's "secretary."

The circulating *ombrelles* of *L'Éducation sentimentale* point to the anxiety surrounding class assignment as it gets attached to femininity in the nineteenth century. The reversibility of class incorporates a threat to appropriate gender roles by confusing *bourgeoise* with *courtisane*, virtuous with venal. Class blurring is in fact also a gender problem because, as the *ombrelle* plot instructs, the flirty Rosanette can penetrate the private space of the superchaste *über*-matron Madame Arnoux, who is as susceptible to substitution, if as precious, as an *ombrelle* (or a *cachemire*, a pair of *pantoufles*). Not only is the *ombrelle* classed and gendered in nineteenth-century France, however, it is also raced, as we shall see. That the *ombrelle* guarantees whiteness only further contributes to this accessory's participation in maintaining clearly demarcated social and cultural borders.

L'OMBRELLE DE SOIE BLANCHE

In his *Code de la toilette* of 1829, Horace Raisson succinctly proclaims the normative female beauty ideal with respect to skin tone: "On discutera encore longtemps sur les mérites divers de la couleur brune ou blonde; mais on demeurera toujours d'accord sur ce point, que la peau la plus blanche est la plus belle!" (28). (We will continue to debate the various merits of brunettes and blonds; but we will always agree on one thing: that the whitest skin is the most beautiful!).[27] Cultural historian Philippe Perrot documents the prizing of *la blancheur du teint* among the *bourgeoises* of the nineteenth century in his *Le Travail des apparences*, citing medical evidence that supported the aristocratic aesthetic and moral judgment of "la blancheur du teint, signe de santé" (a white complexion, sign of health) in the perpetuation of the ethic of conspicuous leisure. Perrot quotes a Doctor Marrin, who writes prescriptively:

> Je me borne à rappeler . . . que l'air vif du littoral est mauvais pour les personnes sujettes au hâle, aux taches de rousseur et autres colorations *anormales* qui doivent au moins être protégées par une large ombrelle, un chapeau à bords rabattus, une voilette sérieuse, des gants longs. (145)

> [I limit myself to recalling that the strong air of the seashore is bad for people susceptible to tanning, freckles, and other *abnormal* colorings, who should at least be protected by a large *ombrelle*, a hat with turned-down edges, a serious veil, long gloves.][28]

Given the unanimity of opinion announced consistently over the course of the nineteenth century and the historical changes to urban social spaces, such as the transformation of the dark Paris streets into sunlit boulevards and the renovations of public spaces like the Bois de Boulogne in the latter half of the century, along with the rise of leisure, shopping, and tourism generally, it is no wonder that the *ombrelle*, the accessory most closely linked to preserving a white complexion, was so crucial to a lady's *toilette* in nineteenth-century France.[29]

The fashion press vigorously promoted this aesthetic, each year heralding the advent of spring with the arrival of new styles of *ombrelles*, which were essential to maintaining white skin. A description in the February 1847 number of the journal *La Mode* combines shameless promotion of a favored boutique with an evocation of the "dangers" of the sun in order to boost consumption: "Dans le soleil de mars, il y a souvent comme de la trahison cachée, et il y a danger à sortir sans ombrelle. Où nos lectrices pourraient-elles aller en choisir de plus légères et cependant de plus abritantes qu'au magasin du boulevard Poissonnière, no. 7?" ("Bulletin des Modes" 401) (Under the March sun, there is often a hidden treachery, and there is danger in going out without an *ombrelle*. Where might our readers go to choose the lightest-weight and yet the most protective of these if not to the shop at number 7, boulevard Poissonnière?). The potentially damaging effects of ultraviolet rays were hardly cause for alarm in the mid-nineteenth century, as they were as yet undiscovered, but the danger of darker skin was only too great and to be avoided at all costs. Ladies could purchase their protective shields from M. Mottet, "cet habile industriel" (this clever industrialist) of the boulevard Poissonnière, who managed at once to beautify and protect women by combining "le reflet de ses étoffes de manière à embellir la femme qui se défend des ardeurs du soleil sous ces petits dômes portatifs de taffetas" (the reflection of his fabrics in a way to beautify the woman who protects herself from the sun's ardor beneath these little portable taffeta domes).[30]

Moral purity indicated through whiteness is a master trope of Western culture, but it attained mammoth proportions during the nineteenth century. Status and wealth, signaled by white skin, marked separation from work, as Dyer explains:

> Color distinctions within whiteness have been understood in relation to labour. To work outside the home—literally out of doors but also away from the values of domesticity—is to be exposed to the elements, especially the sun and the wind, which darken white skin. In most hierarchical social systems, however much the toiler may be lauded in some traditions, the very dreariness and pain of their labour accords them lowly status: thus to be darker, though racially white, is to be inferior. Gender differentiation is crossed with that of class: lower-class women may be darker than upper-class men; to be a lady is to be as white as it gets. (57)

This signifying system extended also to clothing and accessories that indicated women's engagement with leisure activities, such as city promenades, shopping excursions, country outings, carriage rides, visits to exhibits and to the races, and, to a growing degree, travel.[31] The valuing of white skin was supported as well by a booming cosmetics industry in the nineteenth century, which offered a wide array of products, some of them quite deadly because of their toxic chemical components, for the whitening of complexion.[32] Kessler discusses the importance of makeup in the construction of what she calls the perfect "bourgeois *visage*," citing whiteness of skin as the requisite foundation upon which other delicate shades could be applied. Quoting Restif de la Bretonne, who in turn quotes Vandermonde, Kessler describes the ideal face in terms of natural elements: "now it gives bloom to lilies and roses; now one sees only the somber violet, or the dark fruit of the myrtle" (37).[33] Kessler argues that the imperative of a natural application of rice powder and other potions for beautification was paramount in the production of ideal feminine beauty, and that the visibility of the application, like the visibility of the seams in the clothing of Balzac's *femme comme il en faut*, was a clear sign of suspect morality. Crucially different from makeup, then, because it highlighted and shielded the coveted "naturalness" of white skin, the *ombrelle* announced the essential nature of the white complexion of its bearer and her engagement with leisure, even as it nonetheless participated in the construction of this *visage* and its attendant value system. The *ombrelle* thus marshals ideologies of race and class into the service of a feminized ideal of purity and domesticity.

Many French texts of the nineteenth century are inflected with this ideology. Arguably one of the most enduring and iconic literary characters of the nineteenth century, Chateaubriand's Indian princess Atala (1801), daughter of Spanish general Lopez and an Indian convert to Christianity, is described explicitly in terms of a conjunction of whiteness and virtue. First, as she frees the bound Chactas, she appears to him as "une grande figure blanche" (69) (a large white figure) rescuing him from death, and then, at her funeral, she emerges as allegorical Virginity in a scene replete with white symbolics linked to virtue that was to be replicated in master paintings and collectible dinner plates alike in the early nineteenth century:[34]

> Vers le soir, nous transportâmes ses précieux restes à une ouverture de la grotte, qui donnait vers le nord. L'ermite les avait roulés dans une pièce de lin d'Europe, filé par sa mère: c'était le seul bien qui lui restât de sa patrie, et depuis longtemps il le destinait à son propre tombeau. Atala était couchée sur un gazon de sensitives de montagnes; ses pieds, sa tête, ses épaules et une partie de son sein étaient découverts. On voyait dans ses cheveux une fleur de magnolia fanée. . . . Celle-là même que j'avais déposée sur le lit de la vierge, pour la rendre féconde. Ses lèvres, comme un bouton de rose cueilli depuis deux matins, semblaient languir et sourire. Dans ses joues d'une blancheur éclatante, on distinguait quelques veines bleues. Ses beaux yeux étaient fermés, ses pieds modestes étaient joints, et ses mains d'albâtre pressaient sur

son coeur un crucifix d'ébène; le scapulaire de ses voeux était passé à
son cou. Elle paraissait enchantée par l'Ange de la mélancolie, et par
le double sommeil de l'innocence et de la tombe. Je n'ai rien vu de
plus céleste. Quiconque eût ignoré que cette jeune fille avait joui de la
lumière, aurait pu la prendre pour la statue de la Virginité endormie.
(119–20)

[Toward evening, we took up the precious remains and brought them
to an opening of the grotto facing northward. The hermit had wrapped
them in a piece of European linen, which had been spun by his mother:
it was the only possession he still had of his native land, and he had
long intended it for his own tomb. Atala lay on a carpet of mountain
mimosa. Her feet, her head and shoulders, and part of her breast were
uncovered. In her hair was a withered magnolia blossom—the very
one I had laid on the maiden's bed to foster her fertility. Her lips, like a
rose bud picked two days before, seemed to languish and smile wanly.
In her dazzling white cheeks blue veins were visible. Her fine eyes were
closed and her modest feet together, while her alabaster hands pressed
to her heart an ebony cross. Suspended from her neck was the scapu-
lary of her vows. She seemed enchanted by the Angel of Melancholy
and by the twofold slumber of innocence and death. Never have I laid
eyes on anything more heavenly. Whoever was unaware that the maid
had once enjoyed the light of day might have taken her for a statue of
sleeping virginity. (72)]

As Naomi Schor has elegantly argued, Atala is allegorized as virginity in order to reframe femininity as pure and submissive in the wake
of the limited but threatening female empowerment witnessed by the
French Revolution. "By making the lifeless corpse of the young Indian maiden an allegory of Virginity," Schor contends, "Chateaubriand
successfully manages to capitalize on the legitimating power of feminine allegory, while voiding the feminine form of female corporeality
and desire and erasing from it the marks of racial difference" ("*Triste
Amérique*," 147).[35] His purifying move is a whitening on several levels.
From the mountain mimosa, the *mimosa pudica*, on which her shroud-
ed white body is lain to the white magnolia flower in her hair (emblematic of potential maternity, not sensuality); from her gleaming white
cheeks to her alabaster hands; from her modest feet to the celestial innocence of the virgin—Atala's chastity is staged through the repeated representation of her whiteness. Setting, physical attributes, and,
finally, moral characteristics are all linked through the master trope
of whiteness. If, as Schor proposes, *Atala* "founds . . . the tradition of
representing woman in nineteenth-century French fiction as sexually

stigmatized" (138), I would add that crucial to that representation is the symbolics of whiteness.

Central to this French genealogy, Balzac's *Le Lys dans la vallée* (1836) features the long-suffering and self-abnegating Madame de Mortsauf, a realist literary daughter of the allegorical Atala. Madame de Mortsauf, Henriette or Blanche (her nickname), is consistently dressed in white, the better to reinforce her lily-white virtue, and carries a white *ombrelle* as she walks through the countryside of the Indre with her platonic lover Félix.[36] If Atala inaugurates this image of the feminine that in Schor's account would have the "ideological effect[s]" of "putting into place . . . a cultural construction of femininity adequate to the reactionary sexual regime brought into being with the French Revolution" (137), Blanche de Mortsauf, as we shall see, consolidates this equation. The version of respectable womanhood she epitomizes, by definition white and virtuous, was signaled in part in the nineteenth century by the ownership and wielding of an *ombrelle*. Seemingly only a peripheral accessory of dress, the *ombrelle* was a powerful sign of essentialized femininity that carried with it the value systems of leisure and domesticity that defined the ideal elite and bourgeois woman of nineteenth-century France.

Le Lys dans la vallée's Blanche (Henriette) de Mortsauf carries an *ombrelle de soie blanche*, as if reinforcing in the accessory both its utility in preserving whiteness and the moral purity it proclaims for its human double.[37] In an important scene from this novel, in which Henriette/Blanche establishes the boundaries of chastity in her passionate relationship with Félix Vandenasse, her *ombrelle* produces a simulacrum of the sacrosanct domestic space that is threatened by the potential adulterous relationship. She opens her *ombrelle de soie blanche* as she, her lover Félix, and son Jacques gaze over the valley of the Indre, which has become the physical repository for the unfulfilled passions of the lovers. Henriette's *ombrelle* opens to cover and protect all three of them in a gesture that converts Félix from lover to son:

> elle me dit alors de cet air faussement impatienté, si gracieux, si coquet:—
> Allons, voyez donc un peu notre chère vallée? Elle se retourna, mit son
> ombrelle de soie blanche au-dessus de nos têtes, en collant Jacques sur
> elle; et le geste de tête par lequel elle me montra l'Indre, la toue, les prés,
> prouvait que depuis mon séjour et nos promenades elle s'était entendue
> avec ces horizons fumeux, avec leurs sinuosités vaporeuses. Elle savait
> maintenant ce que soupire le rossignol pendant les nuits, et ce que répète
> le chantre des marais en psalmodiant sa note plaintive. (172)

[. . . she said in her tone of affected impatience, so gracious and so insinuating—"Come, let us look at our favorite valley!"

She turned, holding her white silk parasol over our heads, and clasping Jacques closely to her side; the movement of her head by which she directed my attention to the Indre, to the punt, and the fields, showed me that since my visit and our walks together she had made herself familiar with those misty distances and hazy curves. Nature was the cloak that had sheltered her thoughts; she knew now what the nightingale sobs over at night, and what the marsh-bird repeats in its plaintive droning note. (143)]

Through the vehicle of the *ombrelle*, Henriette transforms a traditional gesture of coquetry into maternal instinct—this is precisely what defines her behavior and her character throughout the novel. Her equalizing of Jacques and Félix under the *ombrelle*'s white dome stresses the control to which she must submit her desire: this *ombrelle*'s special effect is to make lover equivalent to son and thus to give visible form to Henriette's demand that Félix be "rien que [m]on fils" (172) (nothing but my son) so that she can continue to see him and not suffer the guilt of a social and moral transgression even in thought. The *ombrelle* signifies the privileging of the feminized domestic space characterized by virtue, matrimony, and family and thus works here to produce a perception shift, to transform a cruel reality (unfulfillable passion for Félix) into a bearable fiction (Félix becomes a son of the family). The *blancheur* of the *ombrelle*'s silk, twice doubling the prized complexion of nineteenth-century female beauty ideals through white color and silken texture, functions usefully to refract the sun and thus to protect that precious and desirable white skin in the valley of the Indre, but it also clearly functions symbolically in this novel to cue the reader to the moral superiority of its bearer and to enforce the domestic imperative.[38]

For all its virtuous signifying power, however, the *ombrelle de soie blanche* cannot help but refer also to the sensual, and excessively white, female flesh that it is shielding. This flesh is described in stunning detail in the scene of the *coup de foudre* that inaugurates this tale of repressed passion, which results in Félix de Vandenasse's strangely indecorous and passionate embrace of Madame de Mortsauf's *dos*, provoked by the sight of her "blanches épaules" (white shoulders), which in turn refer to the "globes azurés" (blue-veined orbs) of her breasts. It is worth citing the passage at length to get at the nexus of whiteness, sensuality, and virtue that the *ombrelle*, it turns out, implies:

Mes yeux furent tout à coup frappés par de blanches épaules rebondies sur lesquelles j'aurais voulu pouvoir me rouler, des épaules légèrement rosées qui semblaient rougir comme si elles se trouvaient nues pour la première fois, de pudiques épaules qui avaient une âme, et dont la peau satinée éclatait à la lumière comme un tissu de soie. Ces épaules étaient partagées par une raie, le long de laquelle coula mon regard, plus hardi que ma main. Je me haussai tout palpitant pour voir le corsage et fus complétement fasciné par une gorge chastement couverte d'une gaze, mais dont les globes azurés et d'une rondeur parfaite étaient douillettement couchés dans des flots de dentelle. Les plus légers détails de cette tête furent des amorces qui réveillèrent en moi des jouissances infinies: le brillant des cheveux lissés au-dessus d'un cou velouté comme celui d'une petite fille, les lignes blanches que le peigne y avait dessinées et où mon imagination courut comme en de frais sentiers, tout me fit perdre l'esprit. Après m'être assuré que personne ne me voyait, je me plongeai dans ce dos comme un enfant qui se jette dans le sein de sa mère, et je baisai toutes ces épaules en roulant ma tête. (21–22)

[My eyes were suddenly fascinated by white rounded shoulders that made me long to bury my face in them, shoulders faintly pink, as if they were blushing to find themselves bare for the first time, bashful shoulders with a soul of their own and a satin skin shining in the light like a silken fabric. Between these shoulders ran a furrow which my eyes, bolder than my hand, glided into. My heart beat as I stood up to look over them, and I was entirely captivated by a bosom modestly covered with gauze, perfect in roundness, and bluely veined as it lay softly bedded in lace frills. The least details of the charming head were allurements stirring me to endless delight: the sheen of the hair knotted above a neck as peach-like as a little girl's, the white partings made by the comb along which my imagination played as in a new-made path— everything together turned my brain.

Looking round to make sure that no one saw me, I buried my face in that back as a baby hides in its mother's breast, and kissed those shoulders all over, rubbing my cheek against them. (17)]

Madame de Mortsauf's *épaules* not only figure her breasts but also her cheeks, as they seem capable of blushing. Her *épaules* are described in terms of clothing as well—*satinée, tissu de soie*—suggesting the delicacy of the skin and the special effect of sunlight as it passes over and through silk. The *flot de dentelles* seductively conceals Madame de Mortsauf's bosom, creating a link to the materials of the *ombrelle*'s construction. Woman and accessory are thus once more assimilated in Balzac's 1836 novel, perhaps best understood for its thematization of the married woman's repressed sensuality and the price of virtue.[39] It is through the white symbolics of this initial description that Madame de Mortsauf's fleshly sensuality is linked to her decorous maintenance of virtue, signaled by her repeated white *toilettes* and, as we have seen, her *ombrelle de soie blanche*.

Recalling the virginal whiteness of young ladies' dress before marriage, the ubiquitous white *ombrelle* was marketed to appeal to the moral standards of the era, which prized the whitest of linens, undergarments, *mouchoirs*, and *gants* as emblematic of cleanliness, elite status (because laundering was so expensive), and, above all, purity of character. The trope of whiteness and its link both to female beauty and to the paired ideologies of domesticity and leisure are central to Zola's 1880 novel of Second Empire Paris and the *demi-monde*, *Nana*, in which the eponymous heroine is from the novel's first set piece characterized by her dazzling white skin.[40] She has no talent for singing or acting, but she has "sacrédié . . . une peau, oh! une peau!" (damn her . . . a skin—oh, such a skin!).[41] "Si blanche et si grasse" (56) (so white and so plump) (23) are repeated epithets used to describe Nana throughout the novel; she eclipses the other stars, and in particular the small, dark Rose Mignon. In the finale of her début as *la Blonde Vénus*, she appears "nue avec une tranquille audace, certaine de la toute-puissance de sa chair. Une simple gaze l'enveloppait; ses épaules rondes, sa gorge d'amazone dont les pointes roses se tenaient levées et rigides comme des lances, ses larges hanches qui roulaient dans un balancement voluptueux, ses cuisses de blonde grasse, tout son corps se devinait, se voyait sous le tissu léger, d'une blancheur d'écume" (62–63) (She appeared in her nakedness with a calm audacity, confident in the all-powerfulness of her flesh. A slight gauze enveloped her; her round shoulders, her amazonian breasts, the rosy tips of which stood out straight and firm as lances, her broad hips swayed by the most voluptuous movements, her plump thighs, in fact, her whole body could be divined, nay seen, white as the foam, beneath the transparent covering [29]).

Nana's gleaming whiteness is indeed showcased in the opening chapter of the novel, and the whiteness of her flesh, enhanced by clouds of *poudre de riz* as she makes up for the stage, as well as her recurring white *toilettes* with the obligatory *ombrelle*, all point to a hyperbolic whiteness characterizing this figure.[42] But as Sander Gilman has argued in his influential study of racial and gender stereotypes in the nineteenth century, Nana's whiteness actually masks her blackness, her otherness, her venality.[43] As a prostitute, Zola's Nana, modeled on Manet's 1877 painting, which was in turn modeled on Zola's first figuring of Nana in his novel of the same year, *L'Assommoir*, is morally and sexually equivalent to a black woman—that is, impure and erotically promiscuous according to the prevailing racist stereotype of the time (102).[44] Like her white stage powder, which Manet captures her applying in the painting and to which Zola likewise refers, Nana's *ombrelle* serves to whiten her, both through its value as a signifier of white respectability and as a literal protection of skin from the darkening effects of the sun. Like her *maquillage* too, her *ombrelle* can only serve as a prop for the social theater and cannot express any essentialized notions of Nana's femininity, as it did in the case of Henriette de Mortsauf. For Zola's self-conscious and even parodic use of this accessory in the hands of Nana exposes rather the prostitute's affront to the idealized feminine. This text uncovers the theatricality of femininity, or as Janet Beizer contends, discussing Nana's social makeover in the second half of the novel, "Reality is once more shown to be an extension of representation, a re-presentation of a representation" (181).[45] As Kessler has elucidated in her analysis of Baudelaire, *maquillage* is a visible tool in the construction of a "bourgeois *visage*," and its overuse exposes the artifice of that construction (38, 49). The *ombrelle*, on the contrary, is not visibly a constructive tool but rather, as we have seen, serves to protect the whiteness already there. That Nana is repeatedly illustrated concocting her whiteness with powder and then using her *ombrelle* as a weapon rather than a protective device doubly underscores the performative nature of her actions. At the same time, Nana's disruptive use of the *ombrelle* nonetheless works to reinforce this accessory's place in the production of respectable femininity.

Nana's staging of her misbegotten respectability naturally takes place out of doors. The working girl's sudden access to leisure activities, thanks to the wealth of the besotted Muffat, Steiner, and a string of other admirers, leads her first to a country outing and then to the races at Longchamp, two *topoi* of upper-class leisure as conspicuous consumption. Nana's leisure activities are clearly parodies, and her/Zola's use of the hyperfeminized *ombrelle* reveals multiple degrees of slippage in the normative definition of the feminine on the levels of race, class, and gender. Nana wreaks havoc with her *ombrelle*—the accessorial embodiment of femininity.

When Nana first arrives at the country house, purchased by one of her lovers, she brings with her the appropriate accoutrement of feminine bourgeois leisure: an *ombrelle de soie blanche*. She then misuses her *ombrelle* as a *parapluie* in the driving rain, soiling its whiteness and blackening it as she tramps through the garden and explores her new domain on the evening of her arrival. This scene, as Therese Dolan has indicated, points to Nana as the contaminating social element, showing up respectable society by appropriating and besmirching its symbols. In the garden under the pouring rain

> Elle ouvrit son ombrelle de soie blanche, courut dans les allées. . . . La femme de chambre ne bougeait pas. Il fallait vraiment que madame fût enragée. Maintenant l'eau tombait à torrents, la petite ombrelle de soie blanche était déjà toute noire; et elle ne couvrait pas madame, dont la jupe ruisselait. Cela ne la dérangeait guère. Elle visitait sous l'averse le potager et le fruitier, s'arrêtant à chaque arbre, se penchant sur chaque planche de légumes. . . . Et Nana, qui s'était accroupie dans la boue, lâcha son ombrelle, recevant l'ondée. (197–98)

> [She opened her white silk parasol, and ran along the paths. . . . But the maid did not stir. Madame must really be mad. It was now pouring in torrents. The little white silk parasol already looked quite black, and did not cover madame, whose skirt was sopping. But this did not worry her. In spite of the rain she inspected both the kitchen and fruit gardens, stopping at each tree, and leaning over each bed of vegetables. . . . And Nana, who had stooped down in the mud, let go of her parasol, and received the full force of the shower (165)].

Nana's misuse of the lady's fashion accessory undoes the gendering and classing that the *ombrelle* usually enacts. As discussed above, the *parapluie*'s inherent masculinity and its unrefined associations make it an unsuitable accessory for a lady. When the courtesan trashes her delicate white *ombrelle* by using it as raingear and dragging it through the mud of the garden in the evening, she deflates the accessory's signifying power to produce female respectability. The *ombrelle*'s transformation anticipates Nana's own demise from smallpox (veiled syphilis) at the novel's end, when her excessively white flesh is reduced to a rotting black mass: "d'un aspect grisâtre de boue, elles [les pustules] semblaient déjà une moisissure de la terre, sur cette bouillie informe" (524) ("with the greyish aspect of mud, they already seemed like a mouldiness of the earth on that shapeless pulp" [449]).[46] But more interesting to me, Nana's conversion of *ombrelle* to *parapluie* declasses and defeminizes her. Nana's most disturbing threat resides in her upending of gender norms: as we know from the novel, she reduces the powerful men around her to sycophantic parasites and subverts the heterosexual economy through her liaison with the prostitute Satin.[47] Her appropriation of the accessorial sign of elite respectable femininity and her subversive use of it in a parody of the leisurely country retreat signal her affront to social and gender norms.

Likewise, in the second of such episodes of parodied elite leisure, the scene of the races at Longchamp brings Nana into direct contact with the social world from which she has been ostensibly ostracized; and here too Nana's disruptive use of her *ombrelle* proclaims her subversion of a sign system intended to maintain gendered and classed norms. Much has been written about this scene, detailing the racecourse stand's strict spatial economy that replicates the social hierarchy of the day, the entrance of the many different types of carriages, each of which reflects a nuance of social caste, and, of course, the bestiality of Nana as she doubles the filly who was named for her and who triumphs at the race, just as Nana the prostitute breaches the social barrier and emerges triumphant in elite drawing rooms after the Longchamp scene.[48] I wish to explore what happens to Nana's *ombrelle*, however, and ask what it can tell us about Nana's perturbation of normative femininity, constructed, as we have seen, through a social and racialized ideal connoting domesticity and leisure.

Outfitted in a *toilette* of white and blue satin, mimicking the colors of the Virgin Mary but apparently honoring one of her lover's stable colors, at Longchamp Nana carries this time an "ombrelle de soie bleue" to match her dress (358). Seemingly nothing more than an accessorial detail of her costume, the *ombrelle* in fact comes to figure a complex series of rivalries—sexual, social, and professional—on which are founded the broader subversions of order that Nana's character represents. Nana attends the races with the Hugon brothers, whom she ultimately ruins. As she asks Philippe to hold her *ombrelle* for her to free up her hands so that she can use her binoculars to scrutinize her upperclass lovers and rivals, Georges (Zizi, as she calls him), the younger of the two, seizes it rapturously, as if it were Nana herself. "Georges d'un mouvement brusque, avait devancé son frère, ravi de porter l'ombrelle de soie bleue à frange d'argent" (358) (But George, with a quick movement, forestalled his brother, and was quite delighted at holding the blue silk parasol, with silver fringe [330]). For Georges, holding her precious accessory is tantamount to possessing the desired woman herself, but in fact, it is he who is possessed by the woman and placed in the female position in the gender binary once more, in a re-creation of the scene of "Zizi's" transvestism at the hands of Nana, who made him her

feminized sex toy during the country escapade. The *ombrelle* personifies the desired woman and so expresses the brothers' sexual rivalry,
but more crucially, it incarnates Nana's sexual power and points to the
instability of gendered categories as it passes from its normative function and possessor.

The social drama of Nana's infiltration of the elite echelons is rehearsed as well in the scene at Longchamp as she penetrates the forbid-
den hippodrome of the racetrack on the arm of Count de Vandeuvres.
The personal-professional rivalry between Nana and Rose Mignon,
from whom she had usurped the coveted role of respectable womanhood in the play *La Petite Duchesse*, also unfolds in this scene. Both the
broader social drama and the personal rivalry, which are, in a sense,
mirrors of each other, are played out in the symbolic combat of the
ladies' *ombrelles* at the races. While all of the other *ombrelles* at Longchamp in the panoramic scenes of the crowds remain open like shields
in the gesture appropriate to the imperative of protecting delicate white
skin in this elite outdoor setting ("Et tout flamba de nouveau, les ombrelles des femmes étaient comme des boucliers d'or, innombrables, au-
dessus de la foule" [381] [everything sparkled once more. The wom-
en's parasols looked like innumerable shields of gold above the crowd
(352)]), Nana's remains closed, functioning phallically, like a sword),
or at the very least, not performing its requisite function of shielding
white skin from the darkening effects of sunlight. To pick up Gilman's
argument again, in light of the distinction between cosmetics and *ombrelles* in the construction of whiteness, Nana's *ombrelle* is of no use in
protecting her essential whiteness, since she is not white but only concocted as such theatrically with heavy clouds of *poudre de riz*.

In protecting whiteness, the wall of *ombrelles* held by the society ladies in the stands of the racetrack also protects their status and the
value system they stand for against the infiltration of the courtesan-
actress, who has shown herself capable of destabilizing both class and
gender throughout the novel.[49] Upstaged yet again, and doubling the
elite crowds of women in the stands, Rose Mignon, a bourgeois married lady and Nana's theatrical rival, "dans un mouvement de rage"
even breaks her own *ombrelle* in her frustration over Nana's shatter-
ing success at the races (387). In the Longchamp scene, Nana's gender
transgression is marked in the details of her inappropriate uses of her
ombrelle, and her castrating power over men like the Comte Muffat ex-
tends also to women, apparently, as her absolute victory in the public's
eye over her longtime rival is solidified in the emblematic breaking of

Rose's *ombrelle*.[50] Nana's repeated misuse of the *ombrelle* in Zola's parodic rendering of these scenes of elite and bourgeois leisure shapes her affront to social and gender orders in the Second Empire France that Zola depicts. If, as I have shown, the *ombrelle* represented the most visibly feminized fashion accessory that could be both classed and raced to bolster a hegemonic domestic ideology, then Nana's masculinized deformation of her *ombrelle* both challenges that ideology and supports her marginalization as a prostitute. The horror of Nana's decomposing face, "d'un aspect grisâtre de boue" (with the grayish aspect of mud), as Gilman and Dolan have both observed, exposes her essential blackness, her incapacity to perform the duty of woman as mother, wife, and icon of the nation (476).

In this chapter, I have demonstrated the *ombrelle*'s particular function to naturalize standards of beauty, foremost among them being fair skin as it was linked to the value systems of leisure and domesticity. That the *ombrelle* was a staple of the feminine silhouette in the nineteenth century is apparent from the visual evidence provided by fashion plates and caricatures and by fashion discourse attesting to its importance. But the *ombrelle* was also a crucial tool in the production of a classed and raced ideal of the feminine. The drive to maintain visible signals of social class and gender categories surfaces even in a 1912 children's book, the genre perhaps best suited to the project of ordering class and gender given the role of children's literature in the transmission of cultural values. In *Monsieur Parapluie et Mademoiselle Ombrelle*, we discover, alongside a fanciful genealogy of the most bourgeois of accessories, the *parapluie*, an allegory of properly gendered behavior combined with clearly demarcated social roles, in which little Mademoiselle Ombrelle stars as the most tiny, most delicate, most aristocratic of accessories, "la fille de M. Parapluie."[51] As Papa narrateur explains to his dazzled brood of children stuck inside on a rainy day, there is a class of *ombrelle* for all types: "l'immense parapluie rouge du marchand forain, sous lequel il abrite son étalage; le parapluie de coton bleu à grosses baleines de la bonne, rapportée du fond de sa Bretagne, le parapluie à manche recourbé de grand-père" (13) and "le chef-d'œuvre de grâce et de bon goût . . . [la] toute petite, toute menue, toute frêle . . . Mademoiselle Ombrelle" (12) ("the fair merchant's immense red umbrella, under which he shields his goods; the maid's blue cotton umbrella with big ribs, brought back from the depths of Brittany, the grandfather's curved-handled umbrella . . . and the masterpiece of grace and good taste . . . the teensy, tiny, frail . . . Mademoiselle Ombrelle"). If the *om-*

brelle expressed idealized bourgeois femininity as constructed through whiteness, leisure, and social *savoir faire*, and through a personification of the *ombrelle* as woman herself, the next accessory I will consider, *l'éventail* (the fan), fetishized female sexuality just as it distilled into a single overdetemined object Old Regime nostalgia for clearly marked social boundaries imperiled by modern access to wealth and mobility.

CHAPTER FIVE

Fan Fetish

Gender, Nostalgia, and Commodification

Parmi tous ces bijoux de l'ornementation féminine, l'Éventail devait avoir la priorité, car, au pays de la grâce et de l'esprit, il brille encore au premier rang.

OCTAVE UZANNE

... il est bavard l'éventail!

LA BARONNE STAFFE

When Emma Bovary makes her début at the Vaubyessard ball at the end of the first part of Flaubert's *Madame Bovary* (1857), she gains valuable insight into the social class to which she yearns to belong by reading the material objects of fashion through which the aristocratic ball-goers communicate and construct their identities. She learns, for example, that although provincial ladies do not drink at dinner and signal their abstinence by placing their gloves in their wine glasses, ladies up to date on Parisian manners do indeed drink. Likewise, the number of flounces on a lady's ball gown is a measure of her fashionability, and gentlemanly elegance can be contained and expressed in an embroidered cigar case that tells its own love story.[1] Most important of all, however, Emma learns her first lesson in adultery by observing the studied carelessness and erotic trajectory of a lady's fan.

> Une dame, près d'elle, laissa tomber son éventail. Un danseur passait.
> —Que vous seriez bon, monsieur, dit la dame, de vouloir bien ramasser mon éventail, qui est derrière ce canapé!
> Le monsieur s'inclina, et, pendant qu'il faisait le mouvement d'étendre son bras, Emma vit la main de la jeune dame qui jetait dans son chapeau quelque chose de blanc, plié en triangle. Le monsieur, ramenant l'éventail, l'offrit à la dame, respectueusement; elle le remercia d'un signe de tête et se mit à respirer son bouquet. (85)

> [A lady, close by, dropped her fan. A man was passing.

—Would you be so kind, sir, said the lady, as to pick up my fan from
behind this sofa?
    The man made a bow, and, as he was reaching out his arm, Emma
saw the young lady's hand drop something white, folded in a triangle,
into his hat. The gentleman, retrieving the fan, presented it to the lady,
ceremoniously; she thanked him with a nod of her head and made a
show of inhaling the scent from her bouquet. (41)]

This *éventail*, or fan, it turns out, doubles and conceals a *billet doux*,
a love letter, both through its folded triangular shape, which the folded letter mimics, and through its expression of illicit, erotic communication, the implicit function of the letter. Emma's one-time entry at
the Vaubyessard ball into what she perceives as the closed and precious
world of Old Regime aristocracy offers a unique window into the fetishization of an imagined historical grandeur, inextricable from the
seductions of gallantry, that crystallizes around the provocative object
of the fan.
    Emma's experience at the ball paradoxically holds both the promise
of social mobility and the nostalgia for Old Regime stability. It is here
that she learns to perfect her social performance, and the brief flash of
the fan cues the reader to her *apprentissage*. Now, the much-studied
embroidered cigar case that Charles finds on the road home to Tostes
after the ball and that Emma hides in an armoire, retrieving from time
to time to rekindle her memories of the ball, is certainly the more explicit emblem of Emma's fetishistic attachment to material objects. But
the Vaubyessard fan actually works both more subtly and more generally to link fetishization with nostalgia, a romanticized longing for
an idealized past. Such a nostalgic yearning overinvests certain objects
with emotional powers, and the object is thus fetishized. This linkage
of fetishization and nostalgia recurs throughout the novel and defines
Emma's character in important ways.[2] The fan serves as the cigar case's
feminized double, for just as Rodolphe Boulanger will later incarnate
the waltzing vicomte who dropped his cigar case on the road home
from the ball, so will Emma appropriate the behavior of the clever *dame*
who let her fan drop at the Vaubyessard ball when she communicates
with her own lovers and idealizes adultery. And just as the cigar case,
with its phallic symbolism, becomes the material catalyst for Emma's
reveries of the fantasized world of the vicomte, the fan points fetishistically to that world's feminized counterpart.[3]
    Elaine Freedgood asserts that "fetishism in realism . . . finds a particu-
larly comfortable home because of the predominance of things, of details,

of qualities—in short, of metonymy—in its figural ground. . . . Readers of metonymy routinely and unconsciously recuperate all kinds of relationships between the thing in the text and those things outside the text with which it can be connected" (101). Emma Bovary is just such a reader, and her reading of the fan in this primordial scene at the Vaubyessard unfolds to project her own sentimental adventure modeled on the performative and sentimentalized gallantry of the past that was often the very painted subject matter of fans themselves (Figure 19).[4] In her later encounters with her lovers, set in motion in part by the Vaubyessard ball scene, she vainly tries to enlist them into the stylized performance of gallantry. She prepares for her "enlèvement" by Rodolphe, for example, by purchasing fashionable travel items and anxiously verifies that he has his "pistolets" in the event of a duel; she also demands "des vers" from Léon and tries with him to recreate the scene of Lamartine's elegiac love idyll, "Le Lac," while floating on a punt in the port of Rouen. Emma's insatiable desire for fashionable accoutrements corresponds to her need for the fetishistic props of her fantasies. She represents the nostalgic longing for something she never possessed in the first place, just as she and Léon recreate Lamartine's scene of death and loss in a disfiguring appropriation of his early romantic poem.[5] Nostalgic fetishism reaches back through loss by way of an object endowed with the symbolic power to reproduce a scene—for Emma, a scene conjured by the most famous poem of the period, by a reproduced keepsake image, or by a fashion accessory like a fan, complete with painted scenes.

If *Madame Bovary* is the nineteenth century's quintessential novel of adultery, then this brief quasi-voyeuristic scene of the dropped and retrieved fan contained within the "enchantement" of the Vaubyessard ball becomes monumental in terms of the novel's development: the fan plays a central role both in Emma's education but also in a broader cultural experience of nostalgic fetishism.[6] As Emma plots her own novelistic turn to adultery, which is deeply marked by her *apprentissage* at the pseudoaristocratic ball, this well-placed object—at the heart of Emma's fantasy of Old Regime aristocracy—with all that it obscures and communicates becomes a fetish object embodying a nineteenth-century nostalgia for an imagined aristocratic grace as well as a kind of sexual fetish, opening the sealed chamber of bourgeois marriage to adultery and signifying female sexuality.

In many ways, the fan also reflected the paradoxical status of women in the nineteenth-century imagination. Like other fashion accessories associated with the feminine, the fan was linked both metonymically

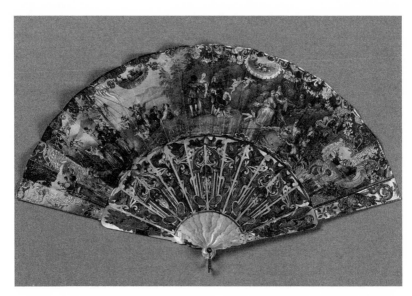

Figure 19. Nineteenth-century fan after Antoine Watteau; paper leaf, litho-
graphed, embossed, gilded and painted with watercolor; mother-of-pearl sticks
pierced and incised with gilt; brass. Guard: 28 cm (11 in.); maximum open: 52 cm
(20.5 in.); arc: 160°. Museum of Fine Arts, Boston; gift of Miss Mary Lee, in memory of Miss Alice Lee, 56.131.

to the female body and metaphorically to cultural fantasies of womanhood.[7] The fan was anthropomorphized linguistically, possessing a
pied (foot), a *tête* (head), and a *gorge* (bosom). The *gorge* was the term
used to designate the part of the *monture* (frame) that was not covered
with the painted *feuille* (leaf), thus consolidating the erotic anthropo-
morphism suggested by the fan's terminology. Indeed, as Valerie Steele
has documented, in eighteenth-century English, the word *fan* was slang
for the female genitals, further multiplying the erotic potential of this
"female toy."[8] The fan's delicate folding structure, its triangular shape,
its capacity to open and close flowerlike, and its deep associations with
icons of feminine sensuality such as mistresses to the king and Venus
herself work together to construct the erotic symbolism of this accessory. Poet Henry Vesseron refers to the tradition linking fans to Venus
in his poem "Sur un éventail":

> Les Grâces, certain jour, réclamaient de Vulcain
> Un bouclier léger, fait pour leur faible main,
> Et qui pût protéger leur jeunesse et leurs charmes,

À la fois contre Amour, son audace et ses armes.
De ses noirs arsenaux visitant l'attirail,
Le dieu ne découvrait rien à leur convenance,
Quand Vénus, en riant, aux trois sœurs sans défense,
Au lieu d'un bouclier donna son éventail.

[One day, the Graces demanded from Vulcan
A lightweight shield, made for their weak hand
And that could protect their youth and charms
At once against Love, his daring and his weapons.
From his black arsenals visiting the gear
The god discovered nothing that would do
When Venus, laughing, to the three defenseless sisters
Instead of a shield gave her fan.][9]

The fan thus became "an ornament, a bibelot, a kind of fetish object" both in the anthropological sense, that is, a talismanic object with seemingly magical properties, and in the psychological sense, that is, an object that stands in for something that is absent or must remain hidden from view.[10] In the cultural sense, as I am understanding it, the fan as fetish combines these two notions and overlays the key element of nostalgia, implicit in any figuration of the fetish.

This chapter analyzes the fan in these multiple contexts through a preliminary reading of Flaubert's ball scene in conjunction with a sociohistorical analysis of the fan, followed by a primary reading of Balzac's 1847 novel *Le Cousin Pons*. I conclude my discussion of the fan with a brief juxtaposition of scenes from Zola's *Au Bonheur des Dames* (1883) and Proust's *À la recherche du temps perdu* (1913–27) in order to mark the move toward the fan's commodification, on the one hand, and its aestheticization, on the other.

The fan exerted considerable cultural leverage in nineteenth-century bourgeois phantasms of the *Ancien Régime*; it was an object deeply associated with visual representations of eighteenth-century gallantry (see Figure 19) just as it was an indispensable accessory for the most aristocratic of leisure activities, ball-going. A *mise-en-abîme* of aristocratic leisure and libertine activity and a required accoutrement in the ballroom, the fan in the nineteenth century would also become emblematic of the work of art in the age of mechanical reproduction—a reproducible commodity. Elizabeth Outka has coined the term *commodified authentic* to refer to a modern paradox that unites "desires for permanence, or commercial purity, or for the absolute original, with the promise that despite appearances such things might be endlessly remade, constructed, reproduced, and exchanged" (5).[11] The fan was an object poised between these two trends, at once a nostalgic referent to the aristocratic world of the Old Regime and a rapidly developing commodity, whose mastery could grease the wheels of social mobility. A crucial component of feminine fashion, it was, in short, an evocative object metonymically linked to the woman who carried it, functioning primarily in the eroticized space of the ballroom and referring nostalgically to Old Regime aristocracy.

THE CHATTY FAN

Flaubert was not alone in writing a range of meanings into this symbolically charged accessory. "A quoi l'éventail ne sert-il pas?" (what function does the fan not perform?), muses the author of the chapter "Accessoires féminins" of *Les Coulisses de la mode*, a volume in the series *Paris-vivant* treating different segments of Paris society.[12] "A la rigueur les femmes s'en servent pour s'éventer, mais aussi pour chuchoter, pour médire et pour rire à leur aise. C'est un objet de maintien et c'est un appareil télégraphique" (236) (At the very least women use it to fan themselves, but also to whisper, to calumny and to laugh at their leisure. It is an object of etiquette and a telegraphic tool). The skillfully timed dropping of one's fan guaranteed that the nearest gentleman would retrieve it, as etiquette required; and thus at the Vaubyessard ball, Flaubert doubly inscribes the fan's sentimental communicative function: it both effects the exchange between the lovers and instructs Emma in the still-flourishing art of gallantry so celebrated in the eighteenth century.[13] "Le langage de l'éventail" was widely known, even if its mystique is understood today only as an invention of market-savvy nineteenth-century fan makers such as Duvelleroy.[14] Circular gestures or tapping with the fan could indicate the assignation of a rendezvous, just as the fan's disposition, open or closed, could indicate its owner's desires: "Trois compartiments ouverts veulent dire: 'Je vous aime'. C'est un aveu—Deux compartiments indiquent une excessive sympathie—Un seul la chaste amitié. Même dans les pays intertropicaux, on n'ouvre jamais plus de trois compartiments pour cette télégraphie; si le fait se produisait, ce serait inadvertance ou indice d'une passion non pas brûlante,—dévorante" (Three open compartments mean: "I love you." It's an avowal—Two compartments indicate an excessive attachment—One, chaste friendship. Even in semi-tropical countries, one never opens more than three compartments for this telegraphy; if this happened it would be by error or a sign not of a burning passion, but an all-devouring one).[15] The requisite silence of nineteenth-century female voices was thus quietly inverted by the fan's gestural chattiness.

Just as the fan could be used to communicate by signaling to a lover, it could also conceal less than ladylike conversation. Gustave Droz in his 1883 fictional piece *Entre nous* recounts an anecdote he calls "Sous l'éventail" in which the male narrator satisfies a voyeuristic desire to get inside young girls' minds (and ultimately, into their beds) by eavesdropping on a group of young ladies gossiping behind their *éventail* at a ball.[16] Spying from across the room "un petit groupe de trois jeunes filles, perdues dans des flots de mousseline blanche et causant avec tant d'animation, derrière leur éventail" (189) (a small group of three young ladies, lost in a white muslin froth and chatting with such animation behind their fan), he cannot resist listening in on what is being communicated behind the *éventail*. As we might expect, the young girls are dissecting the gentlemen of the ball in minute detail, gossiping about the potential marriages of their friends, and revealing their secret desires— "Sais-tu qu'on a un grand avantage quand on est mariée, ma chère? On peut se décolleter franchement, et on doit avoir bien moins chaud" (201) (Do you know, my dear, that being married has its advantages? One can lower one's neckline openly, and one must be much less hot). The narrator's winking voyeurism yields a projected pleasure, as he imagines the girls later that night in bed: "Ces trois petits anges, encore tout frémissants, joindront pieusement les mains sous la couverture,— pour être plus chaudement [*sic*],—et remercieront Dieu de tout ce qu'il vient de faire pour elles" (202) (these three little angels, still trembling, will join their hands under the covers—for warmth—and will thank God for everything he has just done for them). The preposition shift (from *derrière* [behind] to *sous* [under]) indicates the phantasmic shift from the verticality of standing at the ball to the horizonality of lying under the covers in bed. Whether the narrator imagines the young girls praying or masturbating, or that he joins them in their undercover adventures, "*Sous* l'éventail" ends on the image of "*sous* la couverture," thus reinforcing the erotic symbolism of the fan as the voyeur-narrator penetrates the virginal space of the eager *demoiselles*.

The fan was a ubiquitous lady's fashion accessory, but it was also a painting, even a jewel. Like other luxury articles, such as the cashmere shawl, the folding fan arrived in France circuitously from Japan via Portuguese trade routes in the sixteenth century and began as a royal trend. Catherine de Medicis introduced the fashion of fans to France when she came from Italy in 1533 as Henri II's wife, and they were obligatory accessories regardless of season at the court of Louis XIV in the seventeenth century.[17] It was Louis XIV who created the French fan maker's guild, thereby solidifying France's preeminence in this luxury production.[18]

The fan was put to work linguistically, aesthetically, and erotically as it entered the realm of female fashion in its first golden age in the eighteenth century, particularly during the so-called Pompadour period (1745–64), a period that gained enormous prestige in the nineteenth century through publications by authors like the Goncourt brothers.[19] It was nineteenth-century commentators who established the importance of the preceding century to discussions of the fan. As one of the jurists of the Exposition universelle of 1851 explains, the Parisian fan achieved its greatest beauty and craftsmanship during the eighteenth century. His judgment illuminates the valuation of the eighteenth-century fan for a nineteenth-century public: "Nous arrivons au XVIIIe siè-cle. L'éventail est partout à la mode, en France, en Angleterre, en It-alie, en Espagne, et la vogue est de plus en plus assurée aux éventails de Paris. C'est à Paris que la fabrication fait le plus de progrès, et, dès les premières années du règne de Louis XV, nulle part on n'imagine des modèles aussi élégants et l'on ne sait réunir autant de goût dans l'enjolivement à autant de délicatesse dans le travail" (Now we come to the eighteenth century. The fan is fashionable everywhere, in France, in England, in Italy, in Spain, and the fashion is more and more sustained through Paris fan making. It is in Paris where fan manufacture makes the most progress, and from the first years of Louis XV's reign, nowhere else were more elegant models imagined nor could anyone elsewhere possibly unite so much taste in the beautification with so much delicacy of craftsmanship).[20]

Whether small or large, fans were indispensable at balls throughout the nineteenth century, as nearly every illustration of fashionable ball attire attests (Figure 20). Flaubert gives this "accompagnant obligé des toilettes de bal" (compulsory accessory to a ball gown) a prominent position in Emma's first glimpse of the ballroom: "Sur la ligne des femmes assises, les éventails peints s'agitaient, les bouquets cachaient à demi le sourire des visages, et les flacons à bouchon d'or tournaient dans des mains entr'ouvertes dont les gants blancs mar-quaient la forme des ongles et serraient la chair au poignet. Les garni-tures de dentelles, les bracelets à médaillon frissonnaient aux corsag-es, scintillaient aux poitrines, bruissaient sur les bras nus" (82) (Along

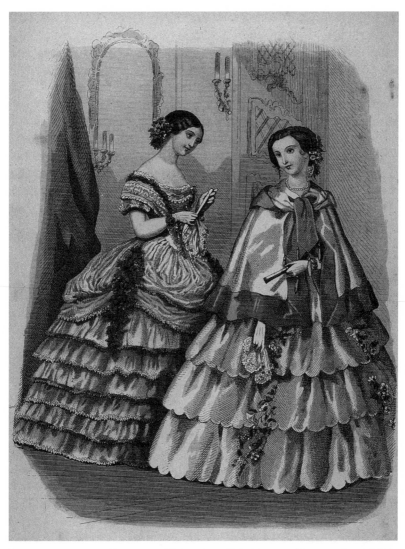

Figure 20. *Evening Dress, 1856*, University of Washington Libraries, Special Collections, UW 28236z.

the rows of seated women, painted fans were rippling, bouquets of flowers were screening smiling faces, and gold-capped scent-bottles were tilting in unclasped hands with white gloves that revealed the shape of the fingernails and marked the skin at the wrist. The lace frills, the diamond brooches, the medallion bracelets were quivering on every corsage, gleaming on every breast, chiming out from each bare arm [39]). Here the fan takes first position in the long list of feminine accessories, which seem to become animated, obscuring and fragmenting the ladies who possess them.

The fan's use value was critically tied to the space of the ballroom, where, overheated from dancing, ladies needed to cool off after their exertion. This link to the social space of the ball is particularly significant in the Vaubyessard ballroom, which is so stifling that servants must break windows to let in the breeze. Here, the theme of Emma's potential social mobility joined with the aristocratic nostalgia of the ball is nearly derailed by the apparition of her peasant doubles at the broken window. Doctor J.-B. Fonssagriues, discussing the dangers of fans for young ladies because of their supposed role in the production of both cavities and pulmonary ailments, nonetheless acknowledges that "l'éventail est devenu un moyen de soulagement contre les chaleurs étouffantes de l'été et la température des salons, en même temps qu'une grâce expressive et presqu'une langue" (the fan has become a relief from the stifling summer heat and the temperature of salons, as well as an expressive grace and almost a language).[21] The demure and diaphanous lady pictured in Figure 21 in "L'Éventail" is suggestive of the multiple uses of the fan. Dressed in evening clothes, she cools herself even as she gazes longingly at some distant object of desire. The fan's open fluttering increases the expressivity of her pose.

Nineteenth-century commentators, collectors, and fashion writers alike were well aware of the fan's preeminent place both in the *toilette d'une femme* and in the broader cultural signifying processes of their day. Its eighteenth-century values were still in circulation even as new values would be added. In the eighteenth century, the fan had become intimately linked to both female sexuality and propriety in France. For example, fans were codified according to a woman's "condition"—married or marriageable. Elaborate wedding fans were produced to commemorate betrothal and marriage ceremonies—even wedding contracts and banquets were often represented on fans.[22] Simple white fans were often carried by unmarried ladies, and more detailed fans were designed for married women. Commemorative fans were also standard gifts for female attendants at weddings. It was a paradoxical object, both concealing and revealing, both modest and sexy; its properly subtle deployment resulted in "le langage de l'éventail," discussed above; and the fan itself, in a less prim symbolic turn, came to represent female sexuality as well as the more demure art of seduction.[23]

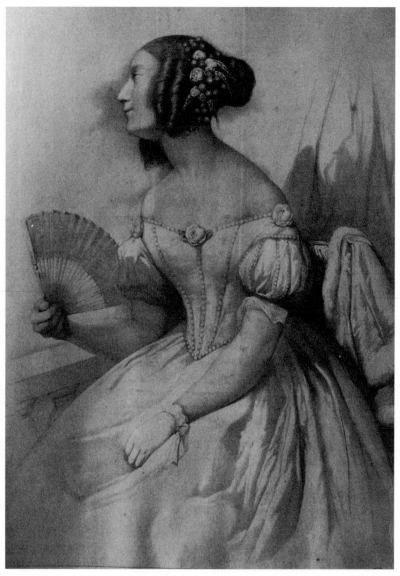

Figure 21. "L'Éventail," Maciet Collection, Bibliothèque des arts décoratifs.

The fan thus embodied the duplicitous ideology of the feminine flourishing in the nineteenth century. On the one hand, according to Madame de Genlis, former governess of the Orléans branch of the monarchy and ever praising the superior morals of the lost eighteenth century, the fan signified modesty: "Dans le temps où l'on rougissait souvent, où l'on voulait dissimuler son embarras et sa timidité, on portait de grands éventails; ils servaient de voile et de contenance. Une femme se cachait en agitant son éventail. Aujourd'hui l'on ne rougit pas et l'on n'a plus de timidité; on n'a aucun désir de se cacher, et l'on ne porte que des éventails imperceptibles" (At the time when one blushed regularly, when one wished to hide one's embarrassment and shyness, one carried large fans; they served as veils and as attitudes. A woman hid herself by moving her fan. Today, no one blushes and there is no more shyness; one has no desire to hide oneself, and one wears only tiny fans) (Figure 22).[24] The 1820 fashion plate pictures the kind of dainty, almost imperceptible fan to which Madame de Genlis objects, zooming in on the fan as barometer of moral rectitude.[25]

But fans were also quite clearly perceived as instruments of seduction, even female weapons, a function amply demonstrated by the fan's recurrence in many occasional poems, such as Gabriel Marc's 1875 "L'Éventail":

J'ai retrouvé ton éventail;
Tu pourras t'éventer encore.
Dans tes mains, enfant que j'adore.
Il brillera comme un émail.
Du Japon c'est du pur travail,
Couleur d'améthyste et d'aurore.
J'ai retrouvé ton éventail;
Tu pourras l'égarer encore.
Ma chambre se change en sérail.
Ton éventail multicolore,
Ouvert à demi la décore,
Etincenant comme un vitrail.
J'ai retrouvé ton éventail;
Tu pourras m'en frapper encore.

[I found your fan;
You can fan yourself once more.
In your hands, beloved child,
It will gleam like a Japanese enamel.
It is pure workmanship

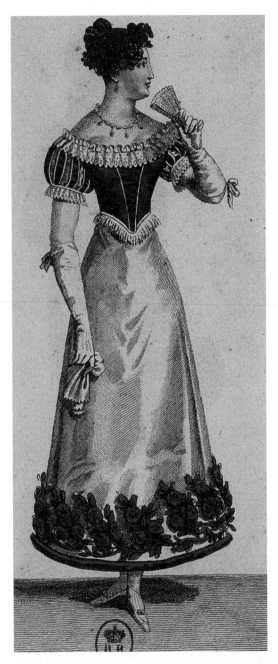

Figure 22.   *Costume parisien*, 1820, Bibliothèque nationale de France.

In the colors of amethyst and dawn.
I found your fan;
You can mislay it again.
My room is transformed as seraglio.
Your multicolored fan,
Slightly open decorates it
Shining like a stained-glass window.
I found your fan;
You can strike me with it again.][26]

In this poem, as in many others of the same genre, the fan literally works fetishistically to conjure the poet's absent mistress: the poet develops the fan's power in a movement from its original functional value (*éventer*) toward its aesthetic value (*émail, améthyste*) to end with its erotic fantasy value (*sérail, ouvert à demi, me frapper*).[27]

As demonstrated above, nineteenth-century French fashion plates, descriptions of ladies' *toilettes* in fashion journals, and manuals of *savoir-vivre* are filled with fans.[28] These indispensable accessories may seem to flutter only at the margins of male-dominated literary discourse, appearing as peripheral to the realist novel's central claims, the props of realist décor. Yet, as we saw in our first look at the Vaubyessard ball in *Madame Bovary*, the fan both contained and helped readers to visualize a fantasized past; it coded a system of behavior and communication; and it projected externally the most hidden of female body parts. Most important, however, in *Madame Bovary*, the fan is directly linked to Emma's erotic fantasy of the vicomte, since it is with him that she waltzes into a spinning frenzy, panting from both pleasure and exertion, and it thus becomes the feminized double of the vicomte's signifying cigar case.[29]

Emma and the vicomte break all the rules of ballroom propriety as they waltz, a fact that the reader understands, even without having encountered the innumerable manuals of *savoir-vivre* produced during the nineteenth century explaining what was and was not permitted on the dance floor. Decorum dictated that a lady's dance partner ought not to whirl her to the far end of the room (as the vicomte does), away from her chaperone's view, nor hold her quite so close, looking directly into her eyes; and likewise, Emma most assuredly ought not to rest her head against her dancer's chest, no matter how dizzy she may be: "Un homme bien élévé ne serre jamais sa danseuse contre lui. . . . [I]l ne s'offre à tenir ni son bouquet, ni son éventail, quelque embarrassée qu'elle en puisse être. . . . Toute femme bien élévée doit s'en abstenir, tout aussi

bien que de prendre une attitude trop abandonnée sur l'épaule du dan-
seur" (A well-bred man never holds his partner against his body. . . .
[H]e does not offer to hold her bouquet, nor her fan, no matter how in-
convenienced she may be. . . . Every well-bred lady must abstain from
this, as well as from appearing too enraptured on the shoulder of her
partner).[30] Although Emma's own fan goes without mention in this
scene, the gallant exchange centered around the telegraphic fan she
carefully observes before the dancing begins sets the stage for the erotic
initiation of her "orgasmic waltz" with the vicomte.[31] The fan, "au bal un
objet de nécessité" (a necessary object at a ball), according to Baronne
Staffe, thus references and acknowledges the sexual charge of ballroom
activity, the memory of which, for Emma, becomes the touchstone of
many of her most powerful desires and fantasies, and the vicomte's cigar case the fan's tangible corollary and gentlemanly double. And yet
Emma's fan is curiously absent from this scene. How are we to interpret
this representational absence, given the fan's integral function to the
ritual of the ball and Emma's careful performance of aristocracy if not
as the inscription of an absence? Emma can certainly read the language
of the fan, but her behavior suggests that she cannot wield it properly, authentically. Indeed, Emma's absent fan expresses the fallacy of
her nostalgic fetishism; and her nostalgia for something she never had
(like the later botched appropriation of the Lamartine poem) suggests
a more generalized bourgeois nostalgia for a status never possessed but
much desired.

The sexual fetish incarnated by the fan is inseparable from its nostalgic power—its function as a historical fetish. Flaubert's treatment of the
marquis and marquise d'Andervilliers, who invite the Bovarys to their
ball to curry favor with the provincial voting public, and of the old duc
de Laverdière, half-deaf and drooling, serves up an aristocracy poised
between bourgeois self-interest and faded authenticity, between modern "progress" and nostalgic pining.[32] Emma is in rapture, however, and
easily succumbs to the fantasy of aristocratic superiority as she contem-
plates the old duke at the head of the table, who "courbé sur son assiette
remplie, et la serviette nouée dans le dos comme un enfant . . . mange-
ait, laissant tomber de sa bouche des gouttes de sauce" (80) (hunched
over his filled plate, wearing his napkin around his neck like a child and
letting drops of gravy fall from his mouth as he ate [38]). In spite of the
old man's decrepit appearance, Emma is transfixed by his aristocratic
pedigree, which is in turn linked to a romanticized, erotic past: "C'était
le beau-père du marquis, le vieux duc de Laverdière, l'ancien favori du

comte d'Artois, dans le temps des parties de chasse au Vaudreuil, chez
le marquis de Conflans, et qui avait été, disait-on, l'amant de la reine
Marie-Antoinette entre MM. de Coigny et de Lauzun. . . . Il avait vécu
à la Cour et couché dans le lit des reines!" (80) (This was the Marquis's
father-in-law, the old Duc de Laverdière, once the favourite of the Comte d'Artois, in the days of the Marquis de Conflans' hunting-parties at
Vaudreuil, and he, so they said, had been the lover of Marie-Antoinette,
in between Monsieurs de Coigny and de Lauzun. . . . He had lived at
court and slept in the bed of a queen! [38]).

The text's limber slippage in the last sentence of the passage into free
indirect discourse confirms Emma's unbridled enthusiasm for an earlier era—an era ironically condensed by Flaubert into a shorthand of "du-
els, wagers and abducted women" but remystified by Emma into tran-
scendent amorous adventures with royalty. As Larry Riggs has argued,
here Flaubert is engaged in exposing "the great irony of social mobility: having destroyed the aristocracy as social substance, the bourgeoisie restores it as *style*, as *phantasm*" (44). The duc de Laverdière is the
last remnant of the eighteenth century, a relic of Old Regime splendor,
linked to none other than the "queen of fashion" herself, Marie-Antoinette.[33] It is amid this nineteenth-century referencing of Old Regime
glory that the fan, the fashion accessory most linked to the eighteenth
century, acquires its importance in *Madame Bovary*. Emma's surrepti-
tious education via the fan scene opens up the world of adultery cou-
pled with gallantry and *savoir-vivre*. The scene at the Vaubyessard ball
offers, by way of Emma's fetishizing process, a view of a broader cultural fetishizing of the more splendid eighteenth century, both celebrated
and lamented by authors such as Balzac, the Goncourt brothers, Dumas, and Octave Uzanne.[34]

The analysis that follows builds on my discussion of nostalgia and
fetishism in *Madame Bovary* and focuses on novels that illustrate how
in nineteenth-century France the fan functioned as a tool with which
people could assess the value of both things and each other, thus initiating a discourse of commodification in spheres not normally associated with consumerism. The primary focus of the following discussion
is a detailed reading of Balzac's last completed novel, *Le Cousin Pons*
(1847), a novel in which a fan figures as a key organizational and symbolic object that signifies both the increased pace of commodification
and the erasure of visible markers of social hierarchy and even of gendered spheres. The Pons fan is also profoundly linked to the fetishizing
of the past discussed above in connection with *Madame Bovary*, as we

shall see, and this nostalgic impulse for the fixed structures of the past is paradoxically inseparable from the object's commodification, its link to social mobility. I then offer brief readings of the material and symbolic presence of fans in two later novels (Zola's *Au Bonheur des Dames* and Proust's *À la recherche du temps perdu*) and consider how the modern impasse of nostalgia and change, of aestheticism and commodification Balzac's novel portrays through the fan evolves, even as the fan continues to serve as a cultural fetish, a metonymy of the female, and ultimately, an emblem of fashion's own dialectical character.

THE "COMMODIFIED AUTHENTIC" IN *LE COUSIN PONS*

In modern France, collecting, or the "appropriate consumption for bourgeois men," as Leora Auslander has argued, was a sanctioned male activity and "was deemed to be highly individual and often authenticity-based, a creative, self-producing, order-making activity," while the principal form of female consumption was shopping for fashions both for herself and for her home.[35] After the Revolution disseminated into the open market masses of objects once belonging to aristocrats, bourgeois buyers, insecure about their place within the regrouping hierarchy, began to collect items associated with an Old Regime past. The true collector, linked with the artist, masculinity, and elite classes through his recognition of the authentic value of the art object, is distinct from the consumer, or decorator, who is associated with women and the bourgeoisie and as such is concerned with an object's referential value and may not be capable of distinguishing a reproduction from an original.[36] The prestige of the authentic is played out in the gendered field of consumption.[37] In the masculinized activity of a burgeoning culture of collection, authentication confers value; and in the feminized culture of fashion, originality competes with imitation to produce style.[38] Although clearly related to one another, the activities of collection and consumption, like their objects, art and fashion, remained worlds apart. Fashion was explicitly coded as feminine and was not to be confused with art.[39]

An object both collectible and consumable, the fan, then, is hard to place within the dichotomy of art and fashion, elite and mass cultures, male and female, and it thus presents a challenge to this nineteenth-century gendered hierarchy. Already overdetermined by the nineteenth century, the fan gradually assumed a commercial role, for its erotic symbolism was deeply bound up in the relationship between women and fashion in nineteenth-century France. Like so many other feminine fashion accessories, the fan could silently speak of the social virtuosity of its possessor. A woman's skilled manipulation of her fan was "sufficient by itself to distinguish between a princess and a countess, a marchioness and a plebeian."[40] Fans could also publicly communicate what virtuous ladies were prohibited from uttering aloud. Thus fans could remonstrate, flirt, invite, or even conceal a love letter, as we have seen. Their coupling of virtuosity and virtue enacted precisely the paradoxical status of nineteenth-century femininity. This constantly resurfacing object, in the hands of the bourgeois subject, came to mediate the developing tensions of modernity itself as both fans and women emerged as commodified objects of circulation.[41]

Published in the last years of the July Monarchy (1830–48), *Le Cousin Pons* has traditionally been read as an important example of Balzacian nostalgia for older (legitimist) values that had been swept away by the modern tides of a new economy and social order.[42] And while Balzac is well known for his contributions in the realm of fashion—as we have seen in earlier chapters, he published in the magazine *La Mode*, was the author of one of the first fashion manuals, *Le Traité de la vie élégante*, and included detailed accounts of contemporary fashions in many of his novels—*Le Cousin Pons* is not a novel normally associated with the theme of fashion. Yet the very discussions of collecting and art traditionally linked with this novel and focused around the key symbolic object of the fan cannot be divorced from the context of women, commodities, and fashion.

The novel tells the tale of Pons, an unattractive art collector and musician who won the Prix de Rome in his youth but who is now impoverished, working in a boulevard theater and living with Schmucke, his best friend and a pianist with whom he also works. Pons is the cousin of the *président* Camusot de Marville, a judge, head of a status-conscious bourgeois family who is trying to find a suitable husband for their daughter Camille. Marrying her off is no small task because of their financial straits, brought on by overextensions in land purchases. Pons, a gourmand, wishes to frequent the Camusot dining table and so ingratiates himself, first with the gift of an antique fan, then with the introduction to their daughter of a wealthy bachelor, Brunner. The hoped-for engagement never follows, and Mme Camusot blames Pons and snubs him. Stunned by his exclusion, Pons falls ill and is "cared for" by his housekeeper, la Cibot, who has designs on his art collection, which, she has learned, is valuable. Other contenders for the valuable collection, including the Camusot family, surface and begin to work to swindle Pons, and an elaborate plot evolves around the competing swindlers and the moribund Pons. Finally, on Pons's death, because his will has been lost (or rather, stolen), the collection goes to the Camusots as the closest kin, who promptly sell it to Popinot, a wealthy bourgeois who, while able to appreciate the aesthetic value of the collection, nonetheless participates in the *embourgeoisement* of art through his purchase.[43]

The novel mourns the lost ideal of a separation between the aesthetic and commercial spheres. Instead of this longed-for separation, the novel finds only the commodification of the aesthetic and the consequent blurring of lines between the world of art and the world of commerce.[44] The vehicle for Balzac's commentary on this blurring is the fan. Functioning both aesthetically and commercially, it frames the tale and surfaces at key moments in the text—at the court of Louis-Philippe and in the failed marriage transaction. While it is true that the fan is an artifact—aestheticized, priceless, and noncirculating—and a metonymy for Pons's art collection as well as for an idealized Old Regime past, it is an especially loaded one. Scholars have been sensitive to *part* of Balzac's message regarding the fate of the objet d'art, but without taking the gendered nature of the object into account, they have failed to grasp its more unsettling implications. Typically, analyses of the text have treated this fan, purportedly painted by Watteau, as a decorative art object tangled up in the destructive chaos of emerging modern culture. In his *Mythes balzaciens,* for example, Pierre Barbéris reads the novel as driven by an opposition between the commercial and the aesthetic that lines up with the development of a moneyed bourgeois society and the extinction of the aristocracy. Barbéris's discussion of the fan focuses primarily on its auratic value as "pure" art, painted by the eighteenth-century master Watteau.[45] But its function as antique collectible is unbreakably linked to its role as feminine fashion accessory, a role overlooked in the terms that discussions of the novel tend to use. To get at Balzac's implicit if perhaps unconscious critique, we need to recognize that by having Pons choose a fan as his gift, Balzac has his hero participate in a particularly feminine economy of material signification. This gesture also launches a conversion of art to fashion and of gift to commodity.

The fan embodies the fissure between the commodified and the aesthetic that animates this novel and, likewise, the split between fashion and art that will become more heatedly contested later in the century.[46] Its paradoxical status is signaled from the novel's opening pages, which painstakingly detail the outdated fashions of the "homme-Empire."[47] Pons crosses town in 1844 with the charge of delivering the fan, characterized mysteriously only as "l'objet précieux" (48) (that precious object [25]).[48] It is *précieux* not only because of its cost but also because of its delicacy and craftsmanship. Thus, even before Balzac tells us what kind of object Pons carries, it is classed as already belonging simultaneously to the economic and the aesthetic worlds.

The tension implicit in the "preciousness" of the object that sets the plot in motion prefigures the narrative conflicts between the rising bourgeois family (Camusot) and the poor declining art collector (Pons). Among others in the family, Madame Camusot (the *présidente*, as she is known) and her dowry-poor daughter Cécile underappreciate the fan's aesthetic and historic lineage (neither woman recognizes the name Watteau, nor does either seem to recognize the name Pompadour—for Cécile, in fact, "le bijou paraissait trop vieux" (57) (the trinket was an old-fashioned thing [33]).[49] Ignorant of both history and art, both women utterly miss the point of the fan's antique value and crystallize a continuing theme throughout the novel: the exclusion of women from the aesthetic realm and their consequent connection to the aesthetic's apparent opposite—the commodity. Cécile and her mother commonly refer to the fan and, by extension, Pons's collection as "cette petite bêtise" ("this little trifle" [29]), looking ahead to the *portière* Madame Cibot's designation of all of Pons's treasures as "biblots" [*sic*] (52).

For Pons, however, the fan possesses the divine status of all authentic and "ravissants chefs-d'œuvre" (56) ("exquisite masterpieces"). As he recounts the story of his acquisition of the fan, he personifies the art object, romanticizing the shopping experience (which he calls *collecting*) as he lovingly asserts: "Moi je crois à l'intelligence des objets d'art, ils connaissent les amateurs, il les appellent, ils leur font 'Chit! Chit!'" (57) ("Well, I myself believe that there is an intelligence in works of art; they know art-lovers, they call to them 'Cht-tt!'" [33]). Not only does Pons personify the fan, he genders and sexualizes it as well, imbuing it with the qualities of an adored mistress, a soul mate, or, should we presume, a streetwalker, for who else would have been sanctioned, after all, to call out to a man on the street?[50] Pons repeatedly refers to the signs of the fan's authenticity—*la signature* and the trademark *bergeries* of Watteau, along with the reputation of Madame de Pompadour, for whom "on faisait tout *unique*" (58) ("a unique specimen, made solely for Mme de Pompadour" [34]). Women, and this includes even Madame de Pompadour as consumer, are thus associated with a bourgeois commodity culture for whom the fan could only exist as a pretty accessory, not as an objet d'art, while men are linked to the aesthetic world through Pons, the knowledgeable collector, and Watteau, the producer of art.

Although strictly speaking it never belongs in the Pons collection of some 1,900 objects because he gives it away, the Watteau-Pompadour fan serves as the metonymic figure for this collection.[51] The fan is a composite object, a *plissé* (or folded) fan, composed of *branches* (branches) and *feuilles* (leaves). It is at once a painting, an ornament, an artifact, a *bijou*. Pons's initial description to his philistine cousin articulates its multiple values, just as it betrays a provocative zeal for authentification:

> —Watteau! ma cousine, un des plus grands peintres du dix-huitième
> siècle! Tenez—ne voyez-vous pas la signature? dit-il en montrant une
> des bergeries qui représentait une ronde dansée par de fausses pay-
> sannes et par des bergers grands seigneurs. C'est d'un entrain! Quelle
> verve! quel coloris! Et c'est fait! tout d'un trait! comme un paraphe de
> maître d'écriture; on ne sent plus le travail! Et de l'autre côté, tenez! un
> bal dans un salon! c'est l'hiver et l'été! Quels ornements! et comme c'est
> conservé! Vous voyez, la virole est en or, et elle est terminée de chaque
> côté par un tout petit rubis que j'ai décrassé! (59)

> ["Watteau, cousin. One of the greatest eighteenth century painters in
> France. Look! Do you not see that it is his work?" (pointing to a pasto-
> ral scene, court shepherd swains and shepherdesses dancing in a ring).
> "The movement! The life in it! The coloring! There it is—see!—painted
> with a stroke of the brush, as a writing-master makes a flourish with
> a pen. Not a trace of effort here! And, turn it over, look!—a ball in a
> drawing-room. Summer and Winter! And what ornaments! And how
> well preserved it is! The hingepin is gold, you see, and on cleaning it, I
> found a tiny ruby at either end." (35)]

The fan thus combines the various elements of the Pons collection, which comprises paintings, sculpted objects, and *curiosités*.[52]

Just as the fan points metonymically to the elements of Pons's collection by standing for the aesthetic, it is also symbolically attached to the commercial world of the competitors for inheritance of the collection through the very components of its construction. Fans were constructed with a *monture*, the structural apparatus, made of metal, wood, ivory (as is the case here), or, often, *écaille* (tortoiseshell or mother-of-pearl), upon which was attached the leaf, which would have been made of various materials, such as vellum, silk, lace, or feathers. Each of Pons's antagonists, who are all trying to acquire a piece of his fortune, that is, trying to gain inheritance of the collection so that they can sell it at market value, is attached (either linguistically or materially) to one of the composite elements associated with the industry of fan making. La Cibot, the greedy *portière*, was an "ancienne belle écaillère" [former oyster girl] at the Cadran-Bleu (a popular restaurant) before marrying the tailor Cibot; Rémonencq, the *bric-à-brac* salesman, is also a *férrailleur* (ironworker), and the Camusot family had made its fortune as silk merchants. As a narrative symbol, the fan thus recuperates and unifies many of the disparate threads and characters of the novel. This subtle symbolic division of labor or parceling out of the raw materials of fan production among the interested parties in the novel underscores their opposition to Pons, who is devoted to the object in its integrity—the whole object as work of art. Their interest in the production, circulation, and growth of capital opposes Pons's devotion to the aesthetic value of the fan and the collection it represents.

Balzac situates Pons on the side of the aesthetic (against the commercial), and the novel reinforces that opposition in its pitting of Pons and Schmucke, musicians and friends, against nearly all of the other enterprising and conniving petit-bourgeois and bourgeois characters of the novel (la Cibot the *portière*, Rémonencq the scrap-metal shop owner, Fraisier the lawyer, and the Camusot clan). Pons wants to keep this collection intact, either as a dowry gift to Cécile, or later, after being disinherited from his family, as a legacy to the state or finally to his friend Schmucke,[53] whom he trusts to maintain the collection's integrity. But the collection will most probably not remain intact, as it passes to the Camusots, who view it only in terms of its market value. Closeted away in a secret room of his apartment, the collection preserves the objects from any form of circulation, even visual. Although the fan is clearly made to stand for this collection as a whole, and although Pons has been coded from the novel's outset as a champion of the aesthetic, it is nonetheless the old collector himself who first brings the fan into the economic world of circulation by attempting to exchange it against a standing dinner invitation to the Camusot house, where he hopes to satisfy his chronic *gastrolâtrie*, itself a form of art consumption.[54]

From the novel's first sentence, Balzac, too, problematizes Pons's aesthetic distance from commerce with the double simile he uses to describe Pons's self-satisfied look on having acquired the fan: he walked along "comme un négociant qui vient de conclure une excellente affaire, ou comme un garçon content de lui-même au sortir d'un boudoir" (21) (like a merchant who has just done a good stroke of business, or a bachelor emerging from a boudoir in the best of humors with himself [1]). This double simile unites pleasure and commerce, conjuring prostitution at the novel's outset. Pons may not know the "valeur vénale de sa collection" (its monetary value), but not because he is not preoccupied with the cost of things: on the contrary, Pons follows strict rules about the cost of items he purchases and brags to his cousin that he did not pay "la centième partie du prix d'art" (53) ("the hundredth part of its value as a work of art" [29]). For Pons, the fan is an indebting gift, and its extravagance, Pons hopes, will produce an equally extravagant gastronomic return. The gift of the fan is thus pure transaction, its market value literalized as meal ticket.[55]

Balzac uses the fan to illustrate the recurring modern theme of social mobility in a society in transition, a theme inevitably tied to women's virtue in nineteenth-century France. Pons's bon mot as he offers his gift—"Il est temps que ce qui a servi au Vice soit aux mains de la Vertu!" (60) ("It is time that it should pass from the service of Vice into the hands of Virtue" [35])—capitalizes on the ambivalent social function of the fan, which serves both demure and flirtatious behavior. This dual symbolism, tying the fan to both feminine modesty and seduction, emblematizes the impossible paradoxes of nineteenth-century ideologies of bourgeois womanhood, with their idealization of the "virginal" mother and its stigmatization of female sexuality even as the *maisons de tolérance* legitimized and capitalized on widespread prostitution. Pons's witticism also pretends to replace the aristocratic seductions of the Old Regime courtesan with the bourgeois decorum of domestic virtue. But his expression is loaded with irony, since Madame Camusot is actually quite vicious, a fact already made clear from her unkind exchange with her servant at Pons's expense, which Pons overhears. It also looks forward to the catty thoughts of a Russian lady visiting the court, who offers to buy this fan "de duchesse" to save it from the ignominy of bourgeois hands, thus effectively reversing the moral categories of Pons's witticism.

The fan literally and figuratively has *cachet*, as the *présidente* eventually learns when at last it achieves value for her as it circulates "de main en main" (from hand to hand) at the court of Louis-Philippe, winning her both compliments "qui flattèrent excessivement son amour-propre" (her vanity was not a little gratified by the compliments it received) and unnoticed slights such as Balzac insinuates (what was such a royal fan doing "en de telles mains?" (in such hands) thought the Russian lady) (91/63). Indeed, what was it doing if not performing fashionability and thus purchasing social status for its bearer? The fan undergoes a commercial conversion with its re-presentation at court, itself a kind of market, slipping into fashionable circulation, and nearly brokers a marriage deal, after Pons rescues it by buying it from the *brocanteur*. In the economy of status, however, Madame la Marquise de Pompadour, Louis XV's extremely fashionable mistress, the putative representative of vice, still trumps even an apparently wealthy, and putatively virtuous, *présidente* Camusot.[56] Old Regime cultural capital is as yet worth more than the rising fortunes of a politically savvy, but culturally deficient, bourgeoisie.

In the gendered economy of production and consumption that governs this novel, Pons and the aristocratic world represented by Watteau are linked to aesthetic value, while the *présidente* Camusot and the bourgeois world of consumption she stands for are linked to commodity value. But what of the fan itself, the art object brought into circulation? The gendering of the Pons fan can be traced to its highly symbolic origins as well as to these gendered cultural valences. Hidden in a "boîte divinement sculptée en bois de Sainte-Lucie" (52) ("this little carved cherry-wood box" [34]) and further concealed within a locked *bonheur-du-jour*, it was discovered at one of Madame de Pompadour's châteaux, recently *dépecé* [dismembered]. From the embodied Old Regime edifice of an aristocratic chateau plundered by postrevolutionary pirates, to the quintessentially feminized and secretive furnishing of the *bonheur-du-jour*, to the delicately adorned inner sanctum of the box, the excessive layering of secrecy surrounding this fan is erotically charged. If, as John Patrick Greene has argued, Pons's art and antiques collection is personified as his mistress, then the Watteau-Pompadour fan with its metonymic potential represents that mistress's sexuality. As an exchangeable object deeply linked to female sexuality, this association suggests the commodification and thus the corruption of women, as both objects and agents of consumption, along with the objects that constitute their adornment.

Already generically connected to marriage and marriageability but also clearly to sex and seduction, the fan is explicitly linked to another commercial transaction in Balzac's chapter heading "Où Pons apporte à la présidente un objet d'art un peu plus précieux qu'un éventail" (In which Pons brings the *présidente* a work of art a bit more precious than a fan), that is to say, that involving the German financier Brunner, the "phénix des gendres" (112) (phoenix of a son-in-law [83]). Pons announces in earshot of Brunner that Cécile will inherit his collection;

thus in effect offering Brunner the collection as Cécile's dowry. Pons even allows the faux lovers' first meeting to occur within the sacrosanct salon that houses his private collection; and when the deal is almost certain to be concluded, only then to falter inexplicably, it is to the Watteau-Pompadour fan, languishing in the *présidente*'s bedroom awaiting the next fashionable occasion, that Camusot *père* directs Brunner's waning attention, as if to remind him of what marriage to Cécile might materially bring him. Unfortunately for Cécile and, as it turns out, for Pons as well, Camusot's strategy backfires. Brunner recoils from bourgeois marriage, citing fears of the extravagant needs of spoiled only daughters.[57] As he retreats from the marriage contract, however, he continues to covet Pons's collection: the fan, he judges, is worth five thousand francs, but even this aesthetic treasure cannot convince him to take the hand of "une fille unique, si précieuse pour tout le monde" (116) (an only daughter, idolized by her parents [87], but not precious for him. Again, *précieuse*—but here, not of equal value to that of the collection: for Brunner, Cécile is *too* dear. Like her double Noémi, the chaste and sequestered daughter of Pons's rival collector Magus, Cécile is assimilated to the fan through the notion of *preciousness*. The link between luxury objects and women, and thus between marriage and commodification, is produced by the linguistic repetition of the word *précieux*. In *Pons*, the fan is personified as feminine and linked to the family "trésors" of Cécile and Noémi Magus—the unwed daughters of the novel. But here the fan's cultural and historical link to betrothal and marriage is ironized in this turn of events that sees the fan as a reminder of the excessive fashion expenses of spoiled young wives.[58] Fans are thus irrevocably linked to women's fashion and their role in consumption.

The Watteau-Pompadour fan Pons offers to his ungrateful social-climbing relative is clearly an overdetermined object. Its most sweeping value, however, may well be its inscription in one of the most obsessive debates of modernity, and one that informs fashion discourse as well: authenticity versus the copy. Fans began to be mass-produced at the end of the eighteenth century, when Martin Petit invented a molding system that permitted a rapid and uniform folding process, allowing the use of fragile silk in fan manufacture. Later, designs would be printed on the leaf and colored afterward; and during the Restoration (1815–30), lithographs would begin to be represented on fans.[59] Pons refers to such reproductions in the scene of the purchase of the fan from a Paris *brocanteur*. Using reverse psychology to convince the sales-

man that newer models are better in order to make off with the antique jewel at a good price, Pons insists: "On en fait des neufs, bien jolis.
On peint aujourd'hui ces vélins-là d'une manière miraculeuse et assez
bon marché" (58) ("you can buy miracles of painting on vellum cheaply enough" [34]). Pons's Watteau-Pompadour fan is clearly not one of
these "industrial" fans so popular during the Restoration, and Pons obviously values it for its uniqueness, even if he verbally cheapens it to get
a bargain.

Yet, although Pons presumes his fan to be authentic, the question
of authenticity that surfaces with the attribution of the fan to Watteau,
who presumably produced it for Madame de Pompadour, is significant.
Critics have shown the impossibility of the historical veracity of the
Watteau-Pompadour connection as Watteau died in 1721, the year of
Madame de Pompadour's birth.[60] Beyond this obvious historical inac-
curacy in Pons's account of the fan's origins, however, there is also evidence in the history of fan production and the guild laws governing it
that would preclude a painter such as Watteau from painting a fan.[61]
The style and themes of paintings by Watteau, Boucher, and Fragonard
were copied on many eighteenth- and nineteenth-century fans, suggesting that what Pons may have taken as original was in fact a high-
quality copy.[62] But even Watteau himself, seen in the latter half of the
nineteenth century as the consummate artist of an idealized eighteenth
century, was not above commercial gain, and his trademark *bergeries*
were, of course, stylized aristocratic performances of the pastoral.[63]
Balzac thus builds the problem of legitimacy right into the key object
around which the plot develops.

Social authenticity and political legitimacy are recurring twin anxieties throughout Balzac's work, which repeatedly illustrates a society
in shift from heredity to meritocracy. In this disturbingly changeable
Balzacian universe, women become the flash point around which this
anxiety circles. Through its ambiguous use of the fan as simultaneously
fashion accessory and art object, and through the fan's association with
an ideology of the feminine, *Cousin Pons* participates in the structuring
of the female as both agent of commodity culture, the consumer, and
as commodity herself, a rarefied, idealized object. In this novel, women
like La Cibot and the *présidente* Camusot ignore aesthetic value and
are interested only in market value, whether monetary or social. The
hapless Cécile, on the other hand, like the fan, is reduced to exchangeable commodity on the marriage market, which is itself another incarnation of the financial and status markets the novel portrays.[64] The

sale of Pons's collection at the end of the novel and the enriching of his bourgeois relatives that Pons's death brings about mark a transition to a modern commodity society, which was in fact already nascent in Pons's paradoxical relationship to the fan.

The brief readings that follow outline a dual development of the status of the fan as Balzac constructs it. While Balzac in *Cousin Pons* begins to propose an organic connection between women and commodity culture through his focus on the essential feminine accoutrement of the fan, Zola links the two quite explicitly in his 1883 novel *Au Bonheur des Dames* surrounding the emergence of the modern department store in 1860s Paris.[65] Zola's novel, and within it, his treatment of the fan, stand for the move to increased commodification, thus pointing toward the appearance of *prêt-à-porter*. Proust's novel, *À la recherche du temps perdu*, on the other hand, uses fans to illustrate a countermove toward greater aestheticization, echoing fashion's elite expression as *haute couture*. Zola and Proust, both deeply engaged with fashion as a manifestation of modernity, thus confront the conflict between aesthetics and commodification, which Balzac's novel raises, in different ways.

GENDER IN THE MARKET: ZOLA AND PROUST

The duality of aesthetic and commodified, already revealed in Balzac's novel to be interconnected, is fully dramatized and accomplished in Zola's novel of the triumph of consumerism, *Au Bonheur des Dames*. In an early scene, a fan subtext becomes an allegory of mass production and marketing; and the fan itself, far from being a rare, priceless art object, is characterized almost exclusively in terms of its cost. This pivotal scene, which occupies chapter 3 of the novel and contains Mouret's famous explanation of the *démocratisation du luxe* (democratization of luxury) on which the success of the department store and indeed modern shopping hinges, stages a feminine postshopping spoils fest and a masculine preshopping sales pitch.

Octave Mouret, proprietor of the Bonheur des Dames, a fictional department store modeled on Paris's Au Bon Marché, arranges to meet Baron Hartmann at the afternoon tea of Mouret's mistress, Henriette Desforges, who has brought her new fan into her drawing room for inspection by her lady friends. This scene echoes the court scene in *Le Cousin Pons*, where the Pompadour fan passed "de main en main" and earned for Madame Camusot the compliments of high society and with it a status raise thanks to the "beauté des dix branches d'ivoire dont

chacune offrait des sculptures d'une finesse inouïe" (91) (the beauties
of the ten ivory sticks, each one covered with delicate carving [63]). In
Zola, Madame Desforges's black Chantilly lace fan with its simple ivory
monture also earns compliments—not for its unique artistry, though,
but rather for its having constituted such a good buy. Madame Desforges had purchased the lace directly from the laceworker in Normandy,
famous for its production of black Chantilly lace, for only twenty-five
francs and had it mounted herself. Lace (and later, feathers) was extremely popular for fans in the latter half of the nineteenth century.
Lace is also the weakness of Madame Deforges's good friend, Madame
de Boves (a shabby aristocrat trying to secure a match for her daughter),
a detail that becomes significant in the novel's *dénouement*, when she is
caught shoplifting. The fan's ivory *monture*, we learn, however, cost two
hundred francs, which undoes any bargain benefit Madame Desforges
might have gained through her "smart" shopping.

Zola uses Madame Desforges and her piecemeal fan manufacture
to illustrate the evolution of fashion in the postindustrialist era. Her
activity reproduces the old style of shopping, which involved multiple
boutiques and artisanal crafting of individual pieces of what might be
a composite final product. A new form of production and consumption is emerging, and Mouret is its great exploiter and promoter. One
could find "à cent vingt francs les mêmes éventails tout montés" ("Similar fans could be found already mounted for 120 francs"), suggests a
friend.[66] In effect ironically mimicking the scene at court in *Pons*, as
the fan passes from hand to hand, it is *devalued* precisely because it
cost too much.

This critical early scene illustrates the conversion of a seductive instrument of feminine fashion into masculine commercial instrumen-
tality, a process that exposes the feminine fashion accessory as metonymy for the woman herself. In light of the fan as a metaphor for female
genitalia, as it was construed in the eighteenth century, this scene becomes increasingly readable in terms of fashion, consumerism, and female sexuality. Mouret's liaison with Henriette Desforges is motivated
by his desire to procure social and business connections, notably with
Hartmann, a former lover of Madame Desforges. As Mouret the shopping oracle prepares to announce his own evaluation of his mistress's
fan, a series of guests, including Baron Hartmann, enter, and Mouret
must instead make his pitch for the banker's support in his attempt to
acquire the properties surrounding his *magasin* so that he can realize
his massive expansionist dreams: "Nous bâtissons sur les terrains une

galerie de vente, nous démolissons ou nous aménageons les immeubles, et nous ouvrons les magasins les plus vastes de Paris, un bazar qui fera des millions" (78–79) ("We'll building a shopping arcade on the sites, we'll demolish or convert the houses and we'll open the most enormous shops in Paris, a bazaar which will make millions" [72]). The feminized fan text is thus interrupted by a masculine property drama.

But the fan text is eventually what concludes the property drama; in fact, they are inextricably linked. To illustrate his point to a cautious and skeptical Hartmann that women are the new exploitable consumers and that high volume at low cost is the new value, Mouret seizes the fan and explains, "Eh bien, le chantilly n'est pas cher. Pourtant, nous avons le même à dix-huit francs. . . . Quant à la monture, chère madame, c'est un vol abominable. Je n'oserais vendre la pareille plus de quatre-vingt-dix francs" (87) ("Well, the Chantilly isn't expensive. But we have the same one for eighteen francs. . . . And as for the mount, my dear lady, it's pure theft. I wouldn't dare to sell one like that for more than ninety francs" [81]). The fan begins to circulate again: "Quatre-vingt-dix francs! murmura Madame de Boves, il faut vraiment ne pas avoir un sou pour s'en passer" (87) ("Ninety francs!" murmured Madame de Boves. "One would have to be very poor not to buy one at that price" [81]). Ironically, it is Mouret's discount price that revives the fan as *objet précieux* in the eyes of the luxury consumer and that simultaneously clinches the deal with Hartmann. Madame de Boves, who covets Madame Desforges's fan here, incarnates the female consumer drive at the end of the novel when she finally satisfies her lust for *luxe* by shoplifting, among many other *nouveautés*, a fan, which are discovered "dans la gorge, aplatis et chauds" (435) (squashed and warm in her bosom [422]).

While Zola places his discussion of the fan as pure fashion accessory squarely within modern commodity culture's race for profit through the creation and cultivation of the female consumer, in *À la recherche du temps perdu*, a veritable fashion show of the Belle Époque, Proust resurrects the art fan as fashionable and converts fashion into art. Proust's novel, whose action takes place between 1877 and 1925, is rich with details of contemporary fashion as it portrays the elegant social labyrinth of the finale of nineteenth-century France, and fans appear with great frequency in discussions of ladies' *toilettes*.[67] "Social miscegenation," authenticity, snobbery, and female virtue are all principal and interwoven themes in Proust's novel, and as did Balzac before him, Proust consistently articulates these themes through references to fashion.[68]

Fans appear throughout the *Recherche*, as we would expect, given
Proust's interest in fashion and given the great revival of the fan, the
so-called *miroir de la Belle Époque* (mirror of the Belle Époque) during the period portrayed in the novel.[69] For example, in *Un Amour de
Swann* (1913) Oriane de Guermantes taps her folded fan rather loudly
and offbeat during a musical performance to signal her fabulously aristocratic and disingenuously wallflowery presence. In *Du Côté de Guermantes* (1920), we learn that Baron Charlus, dandy extraordinaire, had
dabbled briefly as an *éventailliste* to paint a magnificent fan with yellow
and black irises for Oriane.[70] Pons's implicit homoerotics becomes explicit in the figure of Charlus. Curiously, Charlus is the only fan painter
in this novel; and yet, perhaps the central figure in Proust's representation of the irrevocable social change of his era, the *bourgeoise* Madame
Verdurin, who morphs into the princesse de Guermantes by novel's
end and who is portrayed as devoid of any authentic artistic talent, was
modeled on Madeleine Lemaire, a prominent artist, social hostess, and
fan painter.[71]

Along with folding fans, autograph fans, feathered fans, fans used
in lieu of bodies to reserve seats, and metaphorical fans that describe
the unfolding countryside, we also find display fans in the *Recherche*.[72]
Odette de Crécy, the accomplished courtesan and future wife of both
the Jewish aesthete Charles Swann and the comte de Forcheville, uses
fans to adorn the alcove of seduction in her trendy drawing room. In
Un Amour de Swann, Odette has placed photographs, ribbons, and fans
on a decorative screen to create an intimate corner in her "oriental"
salon, the space where she first seduces Swann. Odette's use of fans as
both displayable and personal, in conjunction with photographs, another suspect art form that straddles the intimate and the public, the
aesthetic and the quotidian, calls attention to the fan's hybrid status.
Situated between art and fashion, Odette's display fans double her own
hybridity. She is located on the fringes of polite society, somewhere
between respectable and loose, and even on the margins of normative gender coding, as she is both man-eater and lesbian. Paired with
the elitist art connoisseur Charles Swann, Odette the courtesan with a
checkered past emerges as Proust's incarnation of fashion as art. From
Charlus's aesthetic creation to Odette's fashion accessories displayed as
décor, Proust integrates fan fashion and art, suggesting a creative commerce between the two.

Descended from the Pons fan discussed above, the Proustian fan
belonging to the reine de Naples in *La Prisonnière* (1923) suggests the

staying power of aristocratic nostalgia in the face of certain disintegration. As Michael Angelo Tata has convincingly set forth in his essay entitled "Post-Proustian Glamour," this fan serves to crystallize both the closing of ranks around an aristocracy in peril, represented here by his rival Madame Verdurin's denouncing Charlus to his lover, and the inevitable vaporization of that aristocracy into oblivion. Left behind at Madame Verdurin's musical gathering and high society début, possible only through a collaboration with Charlus, the lover of the musician Morel, whose talents are being showcased at the gathering, the queen of Naples's fan signals at once the obsolescence of the old aristocracy and its revered status.

The queen of Naples is Madame Verdurin's closest brush thus far in the novel with aristocracy. The fictionalized *reine* attends Madame Verdurin's salon at Charlus's invitation to hear Morel play, and she subsequently leaves behind her fan. With it she leaves behind the metonymy of herself, a trace of the aristocratic splendor so tantalizingly unattainable for Madame Verdurin. Charlus, however, recognizes the shabbiness of that splendor as he comments on the fan's hideousness: "Il est d'autant plus touchant qu'il est affreux; la petite violette est incroyable!" (It's all the more touching that it's hideous; the little violet is incredible!).[73] That "little violet" dates the fan for us. Extremely popular during the first half of the nineteenth century, violets symbolized modesty. This dainty romantic flower is no match for the giant flaming irises Charlus had painted on Oriane de Guermantes's fan.

Charlus continues to tease, referring to the "relic" as destined for the auction block, poor as the reine de Naples is; and finally, playing Pons to the reine de Naples's Madame de Pompadour, he proposes that he himself purchase or steal it, so as to bequeath it to a museum. Pons's dream of preservation is realized in Charlus's ironic fantasies about a fan transformed from dated fashion accessory into objet d'art and historical remnant. In a gesture just verging on parody, Charlus the fan painter doubles both Watteau and Madeleine Lemaire; Charlus the fan amateur doubles Pons the collector; and Charlus the homosexual aristocrat doubles his own nemesis, the bourgeois social-climbing Madame Verdurin, in his commodification of the aesthetic in the service of social supremacy. For at the music party both stage a social coup, the centrality of which reduces the music to mere background noise. Through Charlus's mocking reference to Pauline de Metternich's patronage of Wagner, Proust links the reine de Naples's fan to music and the promotion of art by socially powerful women: as Tata has argued, "the fan is used to rearticulate a latent social structure."[74] With this fan Proust effects, albeit ironically, the movement of fashion into art captured in the final metaphor of the novel's production, that of the *couturier* sewing a dress.[75] And with this metaphor Proust inscribes women and fashion indelibly into the story of modernity.

CONCLUSION

The fan's trajectory over the course of the nineteenth century typifies the development of modernity in France as it leads inexorably either to its place in mass commodity culture or to a position as exclusive art object, the reproduced or the authentic, reflecting both the cultural hierarchy of fashion and art and ultimately fashion's own progressive split into *prêt-à-porter* and *haute couture*. From Balzac and Flaubert to Zola and Proust, the fan's narrative and social value shifts, but its fate in the nineteenth century marches toward modernity and is undeniably and simultaneously linked to the fetishization of the past, the marketing boom of the future, and the inscription of woman as principal signpost in the consumption and maintenance of cultural value.[76] As my analysis of these canonical nineteenth-century novels dealing with the rise of consumerism and modernity in nineteenth-century France shows, the fan functions not only as social marker and cultural capital but also as economic asset and narrative currency. These novels make use of fans as organizing plot devices, aestheticized but circulating commodities, sexual fetishes, and nostalgic referents to the Old Regime. Each novel capitalizes on the status of this luxury object, alternatively commodifying the aesthetic or aestheticizing the commodity.

In spite of a second golden age of the fan during the Second Empire (1852–70), whose penchant for opulence, led by the Spanish-born empress Eugénie, tried to equal that of the eighteenth century, fan fashion ultimately moves toward the fate Zola's novel logically forecasts. After the Belle Époque, the fan becomes pure marketing tool, as the proliferation of fans advertising anything from department stores to laxatives attests.

Even by the 1880s, when Zola's and Uzanne's works were published, paper fans were already mass-produced, imprinted with images of *brasseries* or *grands magasins*, and sold cheaply as advertisements for the very mass culture they represented, thus reproducing another form of nostalgia—commemoration and tourism.[77] The fan had become an empty signifier, an advertising phenomenon, a souvenir rather than a memory. Octave Uzanne's fin-de-siècle panegyric to the fan that serves as an epigraph to this chapter thus reads as an appeal to the fan's mythology, to the legacy of the *Ancien Régime* it recalls, an attempt to reclaim the glory of a fashion and of an era in the face of its degradation as marketing vehicle.

The fan intervened critically in the dialectical exchange between nostalgia and the *nouveauté*[78] that produced fashion and participated in the evolving relationship of fashion to the feminine in nineteenth-century France. At once collectible antique and fashionable accessory, the fan operated on the border of gendered forms of consumption, of the aesthetic and the commercial worlds, of art and fashion. It thus became a cipher for modernity, a repository for anxieties about gender, social mobility, and the transformation to a modern economy in nineteenth-century France. "Eussiez-vous pensé que l'éventail dans la main d'une femme put signifier tant de choses? Vous n'imagineriez pas de même tout ce que peut renfermer d'objets étranges le petit sac en cuir que la mode leur a remis, pendant un certain temps, dans la main. Déjà sous le premier empire, cette mode avait fait son apparition" (Coffignon, 238) (Would you ever have thought that the fan in the hand of a woman could mean so many things? You would also not imagine all the many strange objects that can contain a little leather handbag, which fashion has brought back into the hand, for a little while now. This fashion had already appeared during the first empire). The commodity fetish represented by the fan leads to the final accessory analyzed in this study, the quintessential tool of female consumption, the *sac à main*.

CHAPTER SIX

Between Good Intentions and Ulterior Motives

The Culture of Handbags

Why should I not wear a reticule like this, as it is now the fashion to do so?

DORA, qtd. in Sigmund Freud, *An Analysis of a Case of Hysteria*

Jean-Luc Godard's scathing indictment of acquisitive bourgeois culture and "serial consumption," the 1967 film *Le Week-end*, channels Balzac through intertitles like "Scène de la vie parisienne" and through its commentary on the sham of bourgeois propriety, embodied in the self-centered couple Roland and Corinne. As they travel to the country one weekend to wrest an inheritance from Corinne's parents, they are blithely oblivious to the many horrific scenes of human suffering they either pass or create along the way.[1] Eventually, they themselves crash on the highway; and as husband and wife drag themselves from the wreckage, bloodied and distraught, the car in flames, Corinne, with a classic gesture of horror, screams in anguish for what is trapped inside. In one of her few expressions of affect in the film, Corinne doesn't cry out what we might expect—"Roland!" or "My baby! My baby!"—but, rather, screams to lament an entirely different kind of loss: "Mon sac de chez Hermès!" ("My Hermès bag!"). Godard captures in this critique the essence of luxury consumption and its subsuming of other value systems.[2] This scene, however, also illustrates a shift in defining the feminine that had been developing over the course of the nineteenth century and into the twentieth: Godard's Corinne demonstrates that woman's societal function as wife and mother is now usurped by her new role as consumer of luxury fashion products.[3]

In this chapter, I focus on the *sac à main* (handbag) to demonstrate this shift. Nineteenth-century fashion journals do not describe or illustrate the *sac* and its variants with the same frequency as the other fashion accessories I consider in this study, but they do follow trends in bags—such as the leather shell bag of the 1820s, the *châtelaine* bags of the 1880s, and the reemergence of the reticule at the fin de siècle. The *sac à main*, however, has emerged as today's iconic feminine fashion accessory, and it is indicative of consumption on two levels.[4] Itself a luxury object and fashion accessory, thus signaling consumption in its very object status, it also signals consumption because it is shopping's instrument, containing both the means for purchase (money and its forms) and many of the purchases themselves (the portable accessories of femininity).[5] It is both a metaphor for consumption, the *grand magasin* in miniature, as we shall shortly see, and a prized object of desire—the metonymy of luxury fashion and emblem of female pleasure. The story of the *sac à main* incarnates the paradoxical doubleness of women's role in consumption: like the ornamental idealized woman of the nineteenth century, the *sac* and its ancestors are decorative objects of desire. And yet, like the *nouvelle femme* of the fin de siècle, the *sac à main* becomes the vehicle and emblem of a new female autonomy that looks ahead to economic independence from patriarchal structures.[6]

The *sac à main*, a term that gained currency only in the early years of the twentieth century, serves as a pendant to the *corbeille de mariage*, the other container object in the female fashion repository, with which I began this book. Each object contains the props and seductive accoutrements of femininity, and the *bourse de la mariée* (bridal purse) as well as the *aumônière* (alms bag), both versions of *sacs*, were often included in the *corbeille*, as we shall see. Yet in spite of the close relationship, at once functional and symbolic, of these two objects, the *sac* represents a departure from the associations of the *corbeille* in radical ways. While the *corbeille*, containing the little luxuries of the married lady, was a static object destined for the domestic interior, like the wife who received it, the *sac à main* and its cousins were mobile and ventured out in public, like the new woman of the fin de siècle. Additionally, the *corbeille* contained wedding gifts offered by the groom and was inseparable from the institution of marriage; but the *sac à main* often contained items of women's own selection and became emblematic of their new autonomy, mobility, and public presence. Finally, unlike the *corbeille*, which was intended to be opened, its contents viewed, inspected, and evaluated, the *sac à main* was a seductive accessory, the sacrosanct "boîte à féminité" stashing away "les instruments personnels, les objets privés des femmes, leur monde intime" (a box of femininity . . . the personal tools, private objects of women, their intimate world).[7] The ambiguity of the handbag—both publicly displaying the existence of the props of femininity and keeping those items guarded and hidden—makes this accessory particularly poised as the liminal object signaling the transition from traditional to modern femininities.

Perhaps more than any of the other accessories I have discussed, the *sac à main* engages in the seductive game of hiding and revealing a woman's secrets. Certainly, of all the fashion accessories I analyze here, the handbag is the only one with real staying power, and so I conclude my analysis of women's fashion accessories with this one object that still survives, and indeed thrives, in today's fashion world. One of fashion's most mocked accessories, the handbag went in and out of fashion over the course of the nineteenth century depending on the vagaries of the silhouette. I consider here several types of interrelated bags, each of which is tied to the idea of bourgeois femininity in the nineteenth century and each of which illuminates the definition of women's roles through their relationships with objects. The *aumônière* and its close relation, the *bourse de la mariée*; the *sac à ouvrage* (sewing bag); and the *réticule* (reticule) are all ancestors of today's *sac à main*.[8] It became universal toward the end of the nineteenth century, when women entered the world of consumption, attesting to their new mobility and most conspicuous new leisure activity: shopping.[9] It is now the single most important retail object of the couture houses, keeping afloat through its accessible aura of status the erstwhile glory of the great fashion houses founded in nineteenth-century France.[10]

In this final chapter, I argue that by examining the genealogy of the handbag, we can uncover the paradoxical struggles of an emergent modern femininity. Unlike the *corbeille de mariage*, which needed critical resuscitation precisely because of its extinction, the handbag needs to be recovered because of an excess of familiarity. To retrieve the rich significance of this now too-familiar object, the first part of this chapter is devoted to a discussion of the object itself, making visible the links to some of the defining themes and roles of the feminine in nineteenth-century France. The handbag has a history that corresponds to real material conditions of women and reveals the performance of the social functions of femininity—whether virtue, seduction, beauty, or consumption. This genealogy summons remarkable links among these apparently dissimilar functions—pointing ultimately to one of the key threads of my argument throughout this study—namely, the fashion accessory's complicity in the performance of the feminine.

Through brief analyses of two novels by Balzac, the second part of the chapter develops the role of the *bourse*, or purse, in the central drama of the nineteenth-century woman—her marriage. As the examples from Balzac reveal, the *bourse* is still closely linked to marriage, even though it serves to "purchase," in a sense, a husband. The third section shows the object's shift into the public sphere, into shopping, as it follows the emergence of the woman consumer incarnated by Zola's Madame Marty. The prototypical shopaholic of his 1883 *Au Bonheur des Dames*, Madame Marty wields a handbag that is the very instrument of the consumer revolution, even if it is not yet a commodified good itself. Madame Marty offers a variation on Freud's Dora *avant la lettre*, chasing feminine pleasure, bag in hand. Finally, I conclude with a brief discussion of the revival of the handbag in Belle Époque France (after which it never retreated), considering the detailed descriptions of handbags in the women's magazine *Fémina* (1901–56).

This chapter reveals the emergence of the *sac à main* as portable foyer, as scandalous instrument of female pleasure, and as ultimate luxury accessory. Tracing the *sac à main* in this way from the early nineteenth century through the fin de siècle allows us to see how the object's use value, originally linked to women's independence and practicality, is ultimately co-opted by consumerist fashion. The handbag potentially turns the hidden pockets of previous generations inside out, displaying publicly what once had been carefully guarded under the skirts of women. But it also traces its own genealogy through the painstaking needlework and virginal wedding purses of generations of young girls. From alms purses to pockets to sewing bags to handbags, the last of which we recognize today as the key entry point into *haute couture*, the handbag's genealogy both refers to the virtue of woman's work and contains the accoutrements of her fashionability, just as it also signals her commerce with the public world of consumption.

A GENEALOGY OF THE HANDBAG

While the handbag is highly feminized today, it was viewed as scandalous in its earlier incarnations for its unfeminine attributes and for its associations with female independence. When in 1901 Freud famously unmasked Dora's secret sexual activity by observing and interpreting her manipulation of her newly (again) fashionable reticule, he articulated the symbolic content behind many nineteenth-century reactions to the reticule. "Dora's reticule," Freud tells us with smug authority, "which came apart at the top in the usual way, was nothing but a representation of the genitals, and her playing with it, her opening it and putting her finger in it, was an entirely unembarrassed yet unmistakable pantomimic announcement of what she would like to do with them—namely, to masturbate" (69).[11] Building on his analysis of the reticule, Freud goes on to identify a nexus of visible feminized objects of everyday life as referring symbolically to the sexuality of women: "The box—*Dose, Pyxis*—like the reticule and the jewel-case, was once again only a substitute for the shell of Venus, for the female genitals" (69). Freud's analysis of Dora's reticule, along with the other boxes of her dreams, offers a lesson in one kind of reading of the social symbolism of objects that both convenes and exposes at the fin de siècle an ideology of the feminine that depended on the repression of sexuality for the potency and longevity of its influence.[12]

Poches, or pockets, as one might expect, were just that—pockets made of simple unadorned white, black, or printed cotton or canvas (Figure 23). They were affixed to a sash and attached to a lady's waist under her dress, which had small slits along the sides for access to the pockets. A *réticule*, by contrast, was an early form of the handbag, held by a cord from the hand or arm (Figure 24). It took its name from the latin *reticulum* (little net) and was coined during the First Republic, a time when references to Roman republicanism, including slim gauzy dresses, were very fashionable.[13] Like many new fashion trends, the *réticule* was mocked in the press and renamed *ridicule* (Figure 25). Already, as the caricatural image reveals, the *réticule* was a commodity coveted by old and young women alike and was available in a wide inventory for consumption. The conflation of object and female bearer (*ridicule*) is made evident in the unflattering depiction of women in the shop being potentially ogled by the *incroyable* (fashionable man) with his *lorgnon* (eyeglass) who shares the space with them.[14] Ankles and bosoms exposed, along with every contour of their bodies, these female shoppers with their grasping, clawlike hands look intently around at the vast inventory of boxed and unboxed reticules that reaches up to the ceiling in this space of abundance. The other object of desire, the young man in the foreground, hand suggestively deep in his pocket, seems to float in a sea of reticules, conflating the sexual and consumer desire, a joining that would prove potent in the latter half of the century and would become the motor of Zola's *Au Bonheur des Dames*, which I will consider at greater length below. The image both genders and eroticizes the reticule, whose vogue in the early part of the nineteenth century waned and which would not make a comeback as a desirable commodity until about a century later. It was, however, all the rage in the early years of the nineteenth century.

In his popular *Almanach des modes* of 1815, fashion publisher Pierre de la Mésangère printed an imaginary dialogue between a pair of ladies' pockets and a reticule (ridicule), also known as an *indispensable*.[15] In the fashion journal's account of this "Dialogue en prose entre une paire de poches et un ridicule," the conversation is supposedly overheard by one M. Desarps, who has quite indiscreetly penetrated the bedchamber of an elderly dowager to eavesdrop. And here these personified accessories of ladies' fashion come to life and bicker over questions of propriety, fashionability, and femininity. The pockets, which are staid, plain, and hanging from a *prie-dieu* (kneeling bench), belong to the elderly lady, who is out hearing mass. The flashy reticule, on the other hand, which is carelessly lounging on an armchair, belongs to her stylish granddaughter. Outraged by the reticule's slight that they are "gothic" and ugly, the demure pockets strike back with an insult that compares the reticule to a huntsman's game bag (*carnassière du garde-chasse*) or a porter's powder pouch (*sac à poudre du vieux portier de l'hôtel*). In both cases, the reticule is distinctly classed down and, even more scandalously, masculinized. What had been as invisible as undergarments in the form of pockets, "happily" if obscurely placed under paniers and yards of silk, has now been externalized in the reticule; it is carried in plain sight and passed promiscuously "from hand to hand."

Safely concealed beneath the voluminous skirts of the older generation and tucking away a lady's secrets in the folds of her dress, the modest pockets signify respectable femininity. The invisible repositories of fans, hankies, money pouches, even love letters, the pockets have seen it all but have been seen only by a few: "a reckless hand would never have dared to dig around in the folds where we hide her secrets," the pockets claim. In contrast, the wanton reticule exposes all the mysteries of its "imprudent" proprietress, opening up willy-nilly, sharing her secrets indiscriminately, letting it all hang out. It reveals the existence of the accoutrements of femininity and contains the arsenal of feminine seduction, which surely ought not to be made public, exposing the feminine as performance. As the dialogue makes clear, the reticule is also objectionable in large part because it blurs gender lines. Unlike most luxury accessories associated with upper-class women in nineteenth-century France, the handbag has humble and practical origins, but it also makes visible a relationship with money that propriety dictated was the sphere of men, not women.[16] This dialogue develops as a classic female generational conflict—the modesty of a discreet, traditional

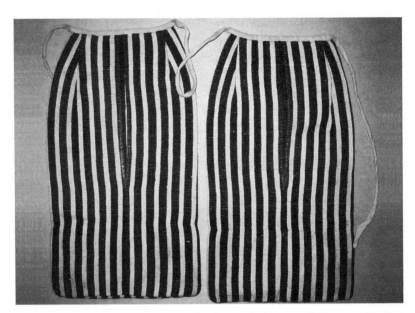

Figure 23.   W2997, "Pair of Pockets of Indigo and Blue-striped Cotton on Twilled Off-white Cotton Tape," French, nineteenth century, Cora Ginsberg Gallery, LLC, New York.

femininity is scandalized by the youthful affront of the ostentatiously new. But with its thinly disguised sexual innuendo and its explicit engagement in debates about female respectability, the dialogue also nuances the history of evolving femininities in nineteenth-century France by giving voice to an otherwise silent repository of female roles and agencies.

Yet before the pockets ultimately evolved through the reticule into the handbags of today, there were several other feminine *sacs* that were not so disreputable. In every *corbeille de mariage*, we recall, a fiancé was required to include (along with jewels, fans, gloves and glove boxes, silks, laces, and cashmere shawls, etc.) a purse of gold coins that had to be newly minted, indeed, virginal, and that were intended for giving alms on the bride's wedding day (Figure 26). The fashion plate of 1873 depicts the bride as she leaves church on her wedding day, dispensing coins to a beggar from her white satin *bourse de la mariée*. Because mothers or other female relatives and friends of the groom were frequently charged with selecting the contents of a *corbeille de mariage*, it is no surprise to find descriptions of bridal purses in fashion

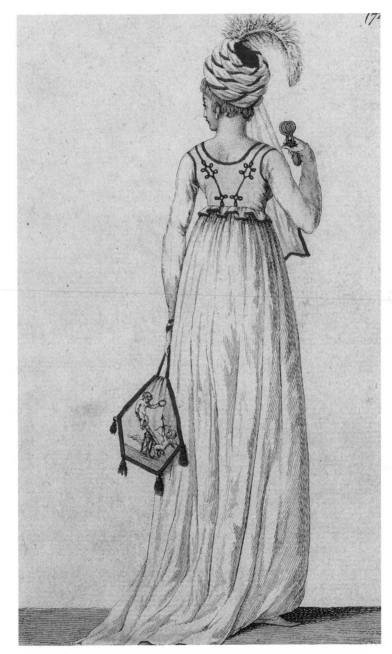

Figure 24. *Costume parisien*, 1798, Bibliothèque nationale de France.

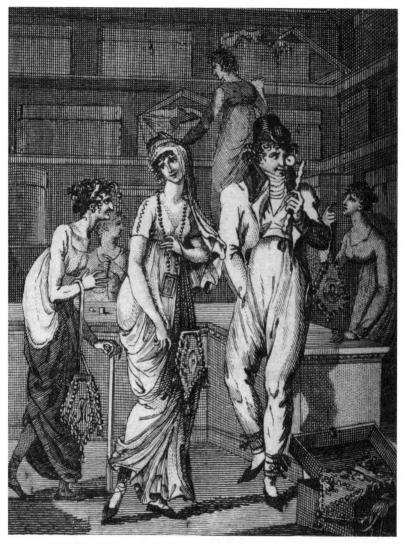

Figure 25. "Magazin de Ridicules et d'Indispensables," Washington University Libraries, Department of Special Collections.

journals. An August 1862 "Bulletin de la mode" segment of the widely subscribed *La Mode illustrée* describes "la plus élégante de toutes les bourses ... faite en soie blanche, en partie à jours, en partie à mailles serrées; sur celles-ci se trouvent un semé de boutons de roses encadrés par une bordure d'or. . . . Il vaudrait mieux, cependant, adopter celle-ci, si l'on destinait cette bourse, par exemple, à être donnée en présent à une mariée" (273) (the most elegant of all purses . . . made of white silk, (constructed) partly of open work and partly of tight stitching; on these are strewn rosebuds framed with a golden border. . . . It would be best, however, to choose this one if it was meant to be offered as a gift for a bride). And later, in an August 1892 description from the "Bulletin de la mode" column of the same journal of the wedding of the Russian ambassador's daughter to a prominent Frenchman, the *corbeille* contains, along with a wealth of jewels, laces, and a carved parasol handle, a golden *châtelaine* and a silver *aumônière* in the Renaissance style (186). The entire *corbeille*, and not just the purse of gold coins, refers, indirectly, as we have seen, to the outmoded practice of brideprice, the money paid for the bride in Frankish times, and its later inverted incarnation, the dowry.[17] Economy and sexuality are implicitly joined through this ceremonial object, a combination that Zola (and his protaganist Mouret) would fully exploit in *Au Bonheur des Dames*. It thus also refers to the underlying financial exchange that marriage rituals both concealed and revealed.

As we saw above, the *bourse de la mariée*, contained within the *corbeille*, signaled the bride's purity and therefore her value, indeed a remnant of the ancient ritual of brideprice, and could even be construed (again looking ahead to Freud's symbolism) metaphorically as her virginity—the value of which was undeniable. Martin-Fugier explains: "La virginité peut servir d'appât. C'est un capital, au même titre que la dot. Elle ne la remplace pas et ne suffit pas, en général, à attirer un mari. Sa perte, en revanche, se monnaie" (52) (Virginity could serve as a lure. It is capital, like the dowry. It doesn't replace the dowry, and isn't enough, generally speaking, to attract a husband. Its loss, on the other hand, leads to various types of financial negotiations). But by the nineteenth century, the purse also initiated the young bride into the two most important vocations (outside of motherhood) of the proper bourgeois married lady: charity work and needlework; the story of the *sac* uncovers the confluence of these two types of women's work.

The *aumônière*, or alms purse, originated in the Middle Ages and was carried by both men and women. By the nineteenth century, *aumônières* were often embroidered by leisure-class ladies and carried coins offered in charity to the poor and, because of their presumed function, were closely linked to the *bourse de la mariée*. Some were attached to a *châtelaine*, a term for the medieval chain belt with hooks from which women hung keys, scissors, bags, and other small items and which was in vogue

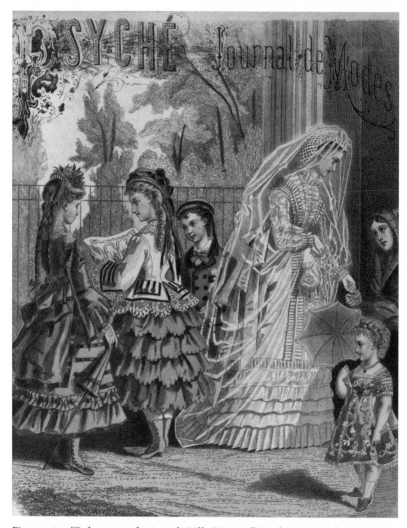

Figure 26.   "Robes et confections de Mlle Régnier," *Psyché: Journal de modes*, May 1873, Bibliothèque nationale de France.

in the second half of the nineteenth century. We see such accessories in Flaubert's *Madame Bovary*, for example. Among Emma's illicit convent readings are the prized and fetishized *keepsakes*, illustrated sentimental stories of passion involving fashionable young ladies and dashing men. Emma studies and cherishes these and eventually constructs her own fashionability in part from these early models: "Elle frémissait, en soulevant de son haleine le papier de soie des gravures, qui se levait à demi plié et retombait doucement contre la page. C'était, derrière la balustrade d'un balcon, un jeune homme en court manteau qui serrait dans ses bras une jeune fille en robe blanche, portant une aumônière à sa ceinture" (64) (She thrilled as she blew back the tissue paper over the prints. It rose in a half-fold and sank gently down on the opposite page. Behind a balcony railing a young man in a short cloak would be pressing to his heart a girl in white with an alms-purse at her waist [51]). For Emma, the keepsake girl's *aumônière* belongs to the sign system of stylish romanticism, equivalent to the golden curls and greyhounds of other such images she admires and tries to appropriate in her quest for a fashionable identity.[18]

It is odd to conceive of the *aumônière*, given its purpose, as a fashion accessory—but this was how it was regarded, signaling a lady's involvement in charitable activity, which, like other aspects of her virtue, as we have seen throughout this study, was readable in her dress. Indeed, the fashion press consistently merged behavior and fashion advice, and charity was foremost among the prescribed behaviors for young ladies and respectable wives.[19] Antonin Rondelet, a frequent contributor to the *Journal des demoiselles* on matters of etiquette and manners for young ladies from the 1840s to the 1870s, explains to his niece Nathalie that upper-class ladies have an obligation to visit the poor in their homes. To this author, such visits are crucial, because with her person the lady transforms the indigent domestic space, bestowing upon it "the dignity, the moral value, the interior charm that had been lacking."[20] In other words, she transposes her own domestic values into those spaces she visits, almost as if she has brought her own *foyer* along with her, in effect, civilizing the poor.

As historians and sociologists have pointed out, respectable bourgeois women's work consisted more of reproducing the symbols of leisure, such as an embroidered *aumônière*, than of engaging in wage-earning activities.[21] As Martin-Fugier remarks in her essay on the *bourgeoise*, building on Veblen's *Theory of the Leisure Class*, "Vivre bourgeoisement, pour une femme, c'est mener une existence de loisir ... les femmes sont chargées d'une multitude de devoirs pratiques, pour faire fonctionner la maison et la sociabilité. De ces petits devoirs, on passe au Devoir" (11) (To live in a bourgeois way, for a woman, is to lead a life of leisure ... women are charged with a multitude of practical duties to make the household and sociability function. From these small tasks, one passes to Duty). The respectable wife proved her family's status by adhering to a code of duty centered in the care of the domestic space, and that included visiting the poor as an extension of domestic work. Through her charity work, the respectable woman could bring the values of one *foyer* to a less fortunate one:

> Philanthropie, sociabilité et direction de l'Intérieur sont les activités obligatoires de la maîtresse de maison, elles forment son Devoir. . . . La vraie vocation de la femme ne s'exerce pas sur la scène publique mais dans le nid, au foyer. Les œuvres philanthropiques ne sont qu'une extension du foyer, la maternité sociale qu'un élargissement de la maternité réelle. (16)

> [Philanthropy, sociability and the management of the domestic space are the obligatory activities of the mistress of the house, they form her Duty. . . . The true vocation of woman is not exercised on the public stage but in the nest at home. Philanthropic works are nothing but an extension of the *foyer*, and social maternity a broadening of actual maternity.]

The embodied object of the alms purse made visible as evidence the invisible work of charity visits she performed. Both charitable visits and sewing occurred primarily within the enclosed domestic space, but these activities could be represented to the broader public through the display of the aestheticized alms purse. While the alms purse did indeed serve the practical function of carrying coins to be given to the poor, its real function, a symbolic one, was to advertise that activity, which would otherwise remain invisible.

Some historians have suggested that nineteenth-century philanthropy was a forerunner of consumption, in that both activities were gendered female and involved women emerging from the domestic sphere into the modern city.[22] In his 1892 historical panorama of nineteenth-century feminine fashion *La Femme et la mode*, Octave Uzanne adds shopping in the *grands magasins* to the very restricted list of activities permitted bourgeois women:

> On les voit, le jour, vêtues d'une grâce exquise, se promener dans ces grands bazars de nouveautés, chercheuses, fureteuses, inventoriant les soieries, les lainages, les lingeries, toutes les menues futilités de la toilette. . . . Le malheur pour elle est qu'en dehors de la famille et des œuvres de charité qu'elle soutient si souvent, la vie ne lui offre que des buts vagues et aléatoires pour la dépense de ses facultés agissantes. (237–38)

> [We see them by day, dressed with exquisite grace, strolling in the big department stores, searchers, questers, examining the silks, the wools,

the sheets, all the little futilities of the *toilette*. . . . The misfortune for her is that outside of the family and charity work that she engages in so often, life only offers her vague and random goals as outlets for her active abilities.]

Uzanne's comments confirm the linking of shopping with charity work, even as he acknowledges, in an unusual flash of understanding, the restrictiveness of bourgeois women's lives. Both activities—philanthropy and shopping in the great department stores of the mid-nineteenth century—can be seen as occurring within a reproduced domestic sphere, which perhaps softens the shock of the inevitable new mobility of modern women. "Department stores," writes Hannah Thompson, "were the first public spaces where women were free to wander unaccompanied and even take on some of the autonomy hitherto reserved for the male *flâneur*."[23] Thompson's analysis of Zola's *Au Bonheur des Dames* elucidates the many moments in the novel when the department store is constructed and described as an interior, domestic space. The *aumônière*, a visible sign of philanthropy, but also of sociability and even *mondanité*, justified a woman's public appearance in the modern city, with her relation to money, otherwise questionable, clearly marked as charitable.[24]

Like the *aumônière*, the ladies' sewing bag, or *sac à ouvrage*, both contained and referred to the (good) works it produced and was itself a visible marker of status and fashion.[25] For along with charity, the other ubiquitous domestic occupation of upper-class womanhood was, of course, needlework, already visible as a status marker in the embroidered *aumônière*. Although women of all classes were engaged in needlework, for upper-class women it was a moral duty and a mark of leisure and had little to do with the practical management of a household.[26] The fashion press especially devotes a great many pages throughout the century to a wide variety of patterns for ladies to follow in order to crochet or embroider their own bags—be they *aumônières* or *sacs à ouvrage* (Figure 27).

In spite of their ostensible purpose, to refer to and facilitate those virtuous *travaux des femmes* (women's work), *sacs à ouvrage* were starting to look fashionable, that is, like their provocative doubles; they were often described as "élégants" in the fashion press, which would include them in their annual lists of desirable New Year's gifts. In an anonymous January 1824 article from the *Journal des dames et des modes*, "L'Oisiveté des femmes," about the laziness of women, the author suggests that the *sac à ouvrage* may be losing its use value and slipping into

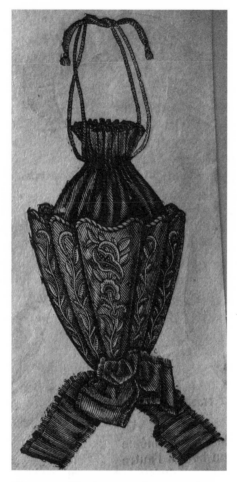

Figure 27. "Sac à ouvrage," nineteenth century, Maciet Collection, Bibliothèque des arts décoratifs.

the realm of fashion, even as fashionable ladies continue to wear it to signal their virtue:

> Aujourd'hui les femmes se croient dispensées de toute occupation sérieuse; tout leur temps est employé à subvenir aux besoins impérieux de la coquetterie, à satisfaire aux lois de la capricieuse déesse, à se rendre dignes enfin de ce qu'on appelle la bonne société; mais elles promènent, en tous lieux, une espèce de sac à ouvrage constamment fermé, qui, sous diverses formes, figure à côté d'elles, en compagnie, au spectacle,

et même à l'église. C'est du moins un hommage qu'elles rendent au travail; c'est un aveu tacite qu'elles le regardent comme un devoir (35).

[Nowadays, women consider themselves absolved of any serious occupations; they spend all their time fulfilling the imperious needs of
coquetry, satisfying the laws of the capricious goddess, making themselves worthy finally of what is called good society; but they carry with
them everywhere a sort of sewing bag, eternally closed, which in di-
verse styles is always with them, in company, at the theater, and even at
church. At least they offer an homage to work; it is a tacit avowal that
they view this work as a duty.]

Given the value placed on a woman's skill with a needle as harbinger
of her domestic prowess, the display of one's craft was tantamount to
advertising one's potential wifely qualities.[27] By mimicking the pro-
ductivity associated with wives, young ladies could present themselves
as capable of contributing to the *économie domestique* of the household, even though, as I have pointed out, any use value of the objects
that were embroidered was superseded by the object's real (symbolic)
function of signifying feminine identity in the fashion social system.
Historian Colette Cosnier, in her study of nineteenth-century girls,
illustrates the great importance of sewing and needlework to a girl's
experience of marriage. Working to collect and embellish her trousseau, "la jeune brodeuse qui marque draps, serviettes et torchons et
rêve à la seconde initiale qui prendra place auprès de la sienne pourrait-
elle penser à autre chose qu'à sa future vie d'épouse et de ménagère?"
(The young embroideress who marks sheets, towels and tea-towels and
dreams of the second initial that will take its place next to her own,
could she be thinking of anything but her future life as wife and housewife?).[28] As Mary Donaldson-Evans argues, giving a contrary example
that nonetheless proves the point, Emma Rouault reveals her incompat-
ibility with the bourgeois ideal of wife when she pricks her fingers while
sewing ineptly on her first encounter with Charles, and her implicit
rejection of sewing indexes the gulf in understanding between Emma
and her husband, who loves to watch her sew (258).[29] In fact, pushing
the argument still further, Emma's repeated performances of sewing
for the men in her life (for Charles initially, for Rodolphe, and for Léon)
expose the constructedness of the nineteenth-century feminine ideal
centered on domesticity and submissiveness, which Emma, arguably,
tries to defy.

Skill with the needle could also prove useful should a woman find
herself without means, as Cosnier explains: "Les travaux d'aiguille sont

une assurance sur l'avenir: à ces adolescentes qui n'ont d'autre horizon que le mariage et qui n'apprennent pas de métier on démontre que la couture pourra subvenir à leurs besoins si elles se retrouvent sans ressources" (215) (Needlework is insurance for the future: these adolescents with no other prospects than marriage and who do not learn a trade are shown that sewing will take care of their needs should they find themselves without resources). No fashionable young bourgeois girl would ever wish to need to sew for the sake of real labor, however; that is the province of poor girls, who are outside of fashionability. And indeed, as Donaldson-Evans points out, Berthe Bovary, Emma's daughter, becomes the victim of her mother's financial ruin when "flung to the bottom of the social scale . . . she will be forced to sew in order to live" (260). Likewise, Edmond de Goncourt's Elisa, from the 1877 novel *La Fille Elisa*, turns to prostitution as the only alternative to the difficult and poorly paid labor of "la couture ou de la broderie" (sewing or embroidery).[30] In an opposite trajectory, Zola's innocent and motherless shopgirl, Denise Baudu of *Au Bonheur des Dames*, who, unlike Berthe Bovary, begins in poverty, struggles in her relationship to fashion and consumption and not only sews and mends her own clothing but makes ends meet by sewing for others before entering into bourgeois femininity and financial security through her marriage to Mouret.[31] She struggles not to choose Elisa's trajectory, although prostitution is never far from the surface of Denise's potential fate; and indeed, like the other shopgirls of the *Bonheur*, she is presumed by many to be engaged in that form of commerce—the iniquitous form of women's work.

More significant still, especially for upper-class women, was the imbrication of womanly virtue with needlework. Madame de Genlis, the tutor of the future king Louis-Philippe and the author of many works on the subject of etiquette and education, insists on the importance of needlework in the maintenance of proper femininity: "L'adresse de doigts, ce travail domestique, constitue véritablement une femme. . . . Une femme assise et dans une totale oisiveté prend l'attitude d'un homme, et c'est perdre la grâce qui la caractérise. C'est pourquoi jadis on avait inventé les navettes, afin que les femmes, même dans un grand cercle, parussent être occupées d'un petit ouvrage et qu'elles eussent le maintien qui convient" (Skill with the fingers, this domestic work, is what truly constitutes a woman. . . . A woman seated in total idleness takes on the attitude of a man, and loses the grace that characterizes her. This is why long ago the shuttle (*navette*) was invented, so that women, even in a crowd, would seem occupied with a small piece of work and that they would have the proper bearing).[32] Woe unto her who does not enjoy or excel at needlework, for she is less than feminine, as Baronne Staffe also suggests in her *Secrets pour plaire et pour être aimée*, proclaiming, "Il sied à la femme de travailler à l'aiguille. . . . Mais la femme qui n'aime pas les travaux à l'aiguille n'est pas de son sexe" (It suits a woman to do needlework. . . . But the woman who does not enjoy needlework is not a woman).[33] Cosnier devotes a chapter of her study entitled "Sainte Aiguille" (Saint Needle) to the supposed virtues of educating young girls in the art of needlework. While the secondary goal may well have been to produce beautiful objects and display one's accomplishments, the primary goal was to combat "oisiveté"—idleness, the "mother of all vices"—with busywork (214).

Many conduct manuals and treatises on the education of young women promoted the moral value of embroidery and other needle-work. And the *sac à ouvrage*, the ubiquitous companion of the proper lady, contained the very tools—scissors, shuttle, thimble, needle—required to create the *bourses* and other fashionable articles that women produced either to become their own fashionable accoutrements or to be offered as gifts (Figure 28).[34] The closed world of female production offered in this picture of woman's work was a circular and self-engendering project; yet women producing fashion in this way and thus making themselves desirable would gain access to the other fashions that were permitted married ladies.

The *Journal des demoiselles* (which ran from 1833 to 1896) and *La Mode illustrée* (which ran from 1859 to 1937) are but two ladies' periodicals containing patterns and detailed descriptions of *bourses*, *aumônières*, and *sacs à ouvrage*. The same Antonin Rondelet from the *Journal des demoiselles* offers an encomium of embroidery as a suitable occupation for ladies, stating its value for each class of woman: according to Rondelet, in economic terms, for the worker, it offers healthy employment; in moral terms, for upper-class women, it offers one of the best occupations to pass leisure time and prevent idleness; and from the artistic perspective, also for the leisure class, it offers a sure way to maintain and perfect taste (97).[35] He also insists that it is the one type of needlework permitted in salons, thus reinforcing its social value and status as well as its relation to female virtue. The *sac à ouvrage* therefore points to needlework as a virtuous, tasteful, and social activity, just as the *aumônière* signified women's appropriate engagement with money in the form of charity. Both types of women's work, and the bags that symbolized these activities, indicated propriety and thereby marriage-

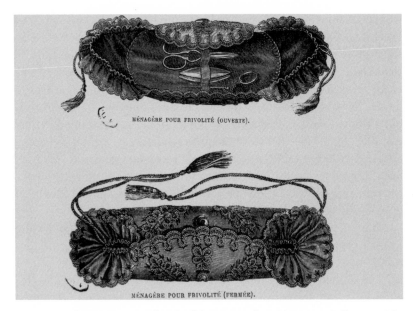

MÉNAGÈRE POUR FRIVOLITÉ (OUVERTE).

MÉNAGÈRE POUR FRIVOLITÉ (FERMÉE).

Figure 28.   "Ménagère pour frivolité" (ouverte et fermée). Maciet Collection, Bibliothèque des arts décoratifs.

ability—the indispensable quality of a young lady cultivated in the pages of a publication such as the *Journal des demoiselles*, or in the state of marriage itself.

FROM GOOD INTENTIONS TO ULTERIOR MOTIVES

Feminine virtue was interwoven with the activities of needlework and charity and was signaled through the objects associated with those activities. The *sac à ouvrage*, containing the tools of bourgeois wifeliness, and the *aumônière* and its cousin, the *bourse de la mariée*, very often the products of women's needlework, were intimately linked, as I have demonstrated. In the pages that follow, I argue that the good intentions implicit in and advertised by certain bags often concealed a different intentionality—one that did not necessarily square with acceptable norms of female respectability in nineteenth-century France, one that indeed pointed to some of the behaviors hinted at by the scandalous reticule. For the good intentions of embroidered alms purses and sewing bags concealed the ulterior motive that must remain hidden of every well-bred young lady—bagging a husband—and thus expressed the unspoken economy of courtship and marriage. By looking at two episodes from Balzac, I tease out the tensions between the social expectations and the intentions of nineteenth-century bourgeois women. In the two readings from Balzac that follow, a *bourse* becomes a troubling fashion object and is used to demonstrate women's growing independence in matters of marriage. While the *bourse de la mariée* is indeed implied by Balzac's two purses, in both cases, a *bourse* is offered to a prospective husband by a marriageable young lady, thus disrupting the script of bourgeois marriage and reversing the gendered agency of the marriage arrangement.

In both texts, *La Cousine Bette* (1846), which I have already considered in some detail, and a less-known short novel, *La Bourse* (1832), a purse serves a crucial dramatic function in the plot and also in the march toward marriage of a beautiful but impoverished *jeune fille*. Given the marriage imperative looming over both heroines and the relative stability of the tradition of the *bourse de la mariée* throughout the nineteenth century in France, the embroidered purses in these texts participate in the web of cultural traditions around marriage that I have been exploring. The realist novelist's inclusion of the detail of the *bourse* acknowledges a financial truth about marriage otherwise so willfully occluded by the romance and trappings surrounding it that were promoted by fashion journals and other organs of bourgeois culture. It also suggests a potentially disturbing agency on the part of the *jeune fille*, who in legal and social terms was entirely dependent on the men in her life but who makes use of a *bourse* in these examples to determine her own destiny.

With the cashmere shawl, the other exotic object that circulates through the various economies of *La Cousine Bette* is Hortense's "pretty Algerian purse." Like the shawl, it is an imperial souvenir but this time of the conquest of Algeria in 1830; it is also linked to marriage, as it figures the absent dowry and procures Hortense a husband. Armed with the name of Bette's lover, we recall, Hortense sees the handsome young sculptor at an antique shop. She invites him home and announces to her father that she has used all of her allowance—usually spent on fashionable *nouveautés*—on a husband, having purchased one of his sculptures. "Un mari, ma fille, dans cette boutique?" (119) ("A husband! In that shop, my child?" [84]), exclaims Hulot, stupefied by his daughter's shopping practices. In the next scene, the deal is enacted: "Hortense tendit au jeune homme en rougissant une jolie bourse algérienne qui contenait soixante pièces d'or" (125) (Hortense, with a blush, held out to the young man a pretty Algerine [sic] purse containing sixty gold pieces [89]), and she promises an equally blushing Wenceslas commissions through her father. They marry shortly thereafter.

Hortense's purse displays not her own needlework, however, but rather that of Algerian craftswomen. Algerian embroidery, handcrafted by women in traditionally floral patterns, was famous and coveted, and it would have been readily available for consumption by French women in the 1840s.[36] By using the *bourse algérienne* to showcase the girl's purchase of a husband, Balzac juxtaposes the debacle of Hulot's involvement in the colonial enterprise with the disruption of traditional codes of feminine respectability. Given this context, the analogy of Hortense's *jolie bourse algérienne* to the traditional *bourse de la mariée* offered by the groom to the bride as part of her *corbeille* becomes legible. The dowryless Hortense reverses the normal sequence of exchanges. The novel elicits the question: is there a problem with Hortense's housewifely skills? Her bag attests that she too is profiting from empire. Bette embroidered uniforms for Napoléon's army, Hortense sports souvenirs of a lesser North African campaign in her purse embroidered by Algerian women—and not by herself—thus throwing her own virtue into question. Balzac repeatedly demonstrates that marriage is a commercial transaction and, through this detail of women's fashion, proposes a link between a domestic scandal—a girl's autonomous decision regarding her own marriage—and the political scandal that ultimately exposes the corruption of the French colonial government offstage in Algeria and nearly brings down the Hulot family.[37]

In this novel, Algeria is the offstage space of chaos and scandal, as this is where Baron Hulot (Hortense's father) sends his Alsatian brother-in-law, ostensibly to manage food stores for French troops but in fact to embezzle money on his behalf so that he may fund the courtesan Valerie Marneffe's extravagant tastes. In the scandal of a dowryless girl buying her own husband, we find foreshadowed the double public/private scandal of the novel's dénouement: Hulot's Algerian financial betrayal doubles the destruction of his family as he funnels government funds into his love nest with Valérie Marneffe. The *jolie bourse algérienne* becomes the matrix of this novel's system of scandal—both offstage and on.

Both types of women's work I have been discussing (charity and sewing) signaled propriety's good intentions and thus indicated marriageability, but they also clearly participated in fashion, which brings us to the disavowed intentionality embedded in the various forms of this accessory we have been exploring. Balzac's earlier short novel, *La Bourse*, showcases this object even more explicitly and in an ironic way—the example may at first seem incongruous because here we are dealing with a man's purse, but it nonetheless fits into the same discourse. The bag figures explicitly and implicitly in this text, which exploits the discourse of virtuous needlework to reward a *jeune fille* with a happily married destiny, but it also raises difficult questions of intentional indeterminacy. The young painter Hippolyte Schinner falls instantly in love with the beautiful Adelaïde, who strikes him as the ideal of virginal purity, when she rushes to his aid after hearing him fall in his upstairs studio. The painter becomes a frequent guest at the shabby apartment of Adelaïde and her widowed mother, along with two elderly gentlemen, and together they play cards—the older men always losing to the ladies by design. One evening, the painter's *bourse* containing fifteen gold pieces vanishes from the card table, and he begins to suspect his beloved of unsavory behavior—she had in fact been eyeing the silk *bourse* that evening. In the end, Adelaïde is vindicated and her unblemished virtue restored and even enhanced when she presents Schinner with a beautiful new *bourse* embroidered with gold beads, whose jeweled details and exquisite needlework attest to the girl's good taste (a prerequisite for propriety)—so much so that the painter proposes marriage on the spot! Her gesture nods at both charity in the form of the disinterested gift and domesticity, sewing a beautiful object, thus reinforcing the social expectations of young girls and women.

But before this happy resolution, in despair over the presumed corruption of his true love, Schinner discusses his dilemma with several of his painter friends. They confirm his worst fears and disparage the reputations of both mother and daughter, claiming to have seen them out and trotting about on the street: "Nous voyons ici, dans cette allée, la vieille mère tous les jours; mais elle a une figure, une tournure qui disent tout. Comment! tu n'as pas deviné ce qu'elle est à la manière dont elle tient son sac?" ("We see the old mother here, in this avenue, every day; why, her face, her appearance, tell everything. What, have you not known her for what she is by the way she holds her bag?").[38] The woman is maligned through references to her style and fashion accessories— her shawl, her gray dress, her way of walking—and the way in which she holds her bag refers to her visible display of a relationship to money, with the implication of the insult, of course, that the mother is pimping the daughter. But the reference also implies the inappropriate sway of the *sac* as the woman walks. An early term for the reticule was in fact *ballantine*, which suggested the swaying motion it produced when held by a woman in motion. The comments of Balzac's characters bring us back to the moral injunctions against the eroticized *ridicule* we saw at the beginning of the century with the "Dialogue" and muddle the lines between "good" intentions and ulterior motives. The *sac* is too closely linked to female sexuality and to money, thus raising the specter of prostitution.

In both of these novels, Balzac seems to support what is known as a *mariage d'inclination* (a love match), as opposed to the *mariage de raison* (arranged marriage) or the *mariage d'intérêt* (marriage for money), which had prevailed until the nineteenth century, even as he also suggests serious dangers associated with such unions.[39] In spite of their auspicious beginning, for example, Wenceslas and Hortense suffer through adultery; and although *La Bourse* ends with a happy marriage looming, the suspicions cast by Schinner's friends over his bride's virtue remain unsettling and unexplained. In the economy of sexuality that Balzac's novels are working through, *corbeille* and dowry, as we have already seen in earlier chapters, are thinly disguised transactional fees; the *bourse* now too becomes central to these narratives structured around marriage and sexuality. The question of the *bourse* in plots of marriage can indeed hardly be innocent in the era of rapidly rising fortunes and increased social mobility, and the mention of a *sac* in a context such as the one just described creates an uneasy link between the financial transactions inherent in prostitution and those lying just under the surface in the marriage bargain.

Balzac's story weaves together the various threads related to the genealogy of the bag I have been discussing, but it also insists on the difficulty of interpreting intention, especially of those who are consigned to performing innocence and submission. His text thus invites the reader to think on a broader cultural level about how gender limits the scope, the expression, and the knowability of one's intention. As both Balzac's story and the fashion press illustrate, bags ended up mediating or expressing a number of different potential intentionalities either concealed under the surface or proudly displayed in nineteenth-century French bourgeois culture. On the one hand, women's bags were construed as emblems of disinterested virtue: linked to charity as alms purses, they signified pure disinterest; linked to industry or aesthetics as sewing bags, they signified domestic virtue. Both of these "virtuous" bags were, however, not too distant from their promiscuous cousin, the reticule, belonging, as we have seen, to fashion, eroticism, and consumption. For the disingenuous "good intentions" referenced by the bags of virtue also work systematically and intentionally in an interested way—to secure a husband or consolidate respectability. While this object expresses, then, a discourse of good intentions tied to the appropriate social conventions befitting a young girl, it also conceals intentions that cannot be stated. In this way, marriage disavows its own self-interested structures, hiding them behind a veil of virtue.

The pretense of romance surrounding the bourgeois marriage transaction would be stripped bare in Zola's 1882 novel *Pot-Bouille*, the precursor to *Au Bonheur des Dames*.[40] Here Berthe Vaque (Josserand), the recently married daughter of a petit-bourgeois family, brings this unspoken truth to the surface when, having been caught in an adulterous liaison with the young Octave Mouret, she blames her mother's mercenary tactics for her own moral lapse: "L'histoire entière de son mariage revenait, dans ses phrases courtes, lâchées par lambeaux: les trois hivers de chasse à l'homme, les garçons de tous poils aux bras desquels on le jetait, les insuccès de cette offre de son corps, sur les trottoirs autorisés des salons bourgeois; puis, ce que les mères enseignent aux filles sans fortune, tout un cours de prostitution décente et permise" (409–10) (And it all came out; in fragments and then suddenly in a rush of words: the story of her marriage; the three winters devoted to man-hunting; the various youths at which she'd been hurled; these failed attempts to sell her body on the streets of middle-class drawing-rooms; what mothers taught their penniless daughters, a complete course in polite and acceptable prostitution [329]). *Pot-Bouille*, which introduces some of the characters of *Au Bonheur des Dames*, most notably Octave Mouret, who will become the founder of Zola's fictional department store, reveals, as Hannah Thompson has shown, what lies "underneath the veil of bourgeois respectability."[41] Not only is the bourgeois apartment house of *Pot-Bouille* teeming with illicit carnal relations (homosexual, adulterous, across classes), exposing the lie of the respectable marriages it supposedly houses, but those marriages themselves are also quite starkly revealed to be held together or orchestrated only through brutal financial transactions. Even the one apparent love match—between the shop clerk Octave Mouret and the store owner, the widow Madame Hédouin—is predicated on financial gain. The widow "a le sac" (337) ("she's loaded" [266]), Octave overhears the servants saying when they learn of Monsieur Hédouin's death; he subsequently plots his next move up the commercial and social ladder of Paris. Her "sac" will be converted into Mouret's commercial and erotic success—the department store Au Bonheur des Dames.[42]

THE BOTTOMLESS BAG OF FEMALE DESIRE

The accessory of the *sac* and its genealogy through the *aumônière* and the *sac à ouvrage* functioned to define and express the feminine, as we have seen. Both objects pertained to the largely invisible domestic work of bourgeois women; and the *bourse de la mariée* signaled the crucial rite of passage to married femininity and was intimately tied to the quest for a husband. But the *sac* and its variants ultimately would indicate a third and increasingly important type of "work" of nineteenth-century bourgeois women—the work of consumption.[43]

The transition from the various forms of the *sac* discussed above to the *sac à main*—what we know today as the truly indispensable woman's accessory—must be understood in conjunction with the emergence of the woman consumer. Zola's department store novel, *Au Bonheur des Dames (The Ladies' Paradise)*, was published in 1883, at about the time that the *sac à main* was becoming popular and widespread, but set in the late 1860s, when the department store as we know it was born.[44] An 1885 fashion plate from the *Journal des demoiselles* illustrates the new public dimension of women's activities, as two women stroll with a child, one of them carrying what would soon become the ubiquitous *sac à main* (Figure 29). Indeed, by the 1880s, the color plates of some of the most widely read journals, such as *La Mode illustrée*, contained many images of small handbags, some of which are called "ridicules," as is the case for the image in Figure 30, while just a decade or so earlier one could only find *sacs à ouvrage* and the occasional handbag usually associated with travel but not yet a fashionable accessory.

Zola's novel follows the literal and figurative rise of the department store, at the expense of the specialty boutiques that are decimated in its wake, and the ascent of its owner Octave Mouret, the engineer of publicity, consumption, and sexual conquest targeted at women. As we watch the store devour its competitors and its clients in a symbiotic relationship of desire and destruction, we should also consider the detail of the *sac*—for this is now the word employed in Zola's novel, a novel that both celebrates and decries women's entry into the marketplace. Not as yet the desirable *nouveauté* it would soon become, in the 1860s of Zola's novel there are no *sacs* yet for sale at the Paradise, although virtually every other accessory appears to be available for purchase. As we shall

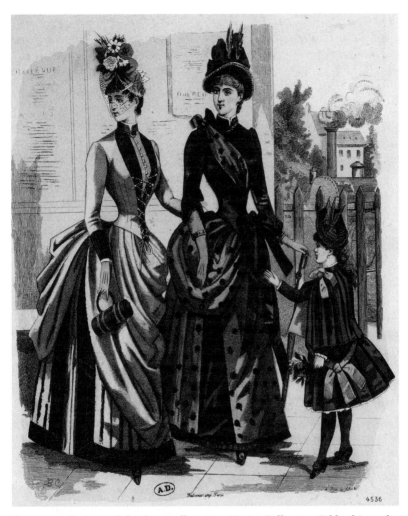

Figure 29. *Le Journal des demoiselles*, 1885, Maciet Collection, Bibliothèque des arts décoratifs.

see, however, Zola's store itself becomes metaphorically linked to the one handbag that does figure in the novel—Madame Marty's little red bag. This bag combines the functionality of the *sac à ouvrage*, as it contains a multitude of items, with the secretive allure of the scandalous reticule, which advertises its existence even as it conceals its contents.

Mouret has inherited the small shop of his wife, who between the end of *Pot-Bouille* and the beginning of *Au Bonheur des Dames*, has died tragically. She had all the money, as we recall from the quip of *Pot-Bouille* cited above—"[elle] *a le sac*," the sack of gold, that is. Mouret decides to transform it into an ever-expanding *grand magasin* that appeals to women from all social classes because it offers a vast selection ranging in quality and price. My focus here will be on Madame Marty, a secondary character but frequent and obsessive shopper at the Ladies' Paradise, who carries a small red leather handbag in her right hand as she enters the salon of Madame Desforges, the wealthy widow with designs on Mouret.[45] Like Anna Karenina's red leather purse, Madame Marty's bag is highly sexualized through its color, its size, and its material—the erotic connection of handbag to female sexuality is posited by these details and developed by Madame Marty's behavior in the scene, which portrays her fever for consumption in sexualized terms.[46]

Madame Marty is the wife of a teacher, whom she is ruining with her devotion to the latest fashions and, as Zola puts it, the weakness of her flesh before "le moindre bout de chiffon" (68) (the slightest piece of finery [62]). The figure of Madame Marty and her little red handbag frames the very important chapter 3 of Zola's novel, in which Mouret lays out his plan for the conquest of women through commercial seduction to Parisian banker Hartmann. With her sensual abandon to all things fashionable, the all-desiring Madame Marty and her eligible daughter come to incarnate the consummate victims of Mouret's scheme: Madame Marty is consumer desire made flesh, exhibiting a false subjecthood through her consumption, while her daughter—the frequent recipient of Madame Marty's purchases—figures the woman as consumable object of desire.[47]

In Madame Desforges's salon are gathered a sampling of Mouret's female clientele, and Madame Marty arrives desperate to open her bag and reveal the ravishing *nouveautés* she has purchased. "Elle se décida enfin à ouvrir le sac. Des dames allongeaient le cou, lorsque, dans le silence, on entendit le timbre de l'antichambre. -C'est mon mari" (69) (She finally decided to open the bag. The ladies were craning their necks forward when, in the silence, the ante-room bell was heard. "It's my husband" [63]). Collective female desire is projected through the ladies' stretching to see the contents of Madame Marty's bag. A comic scene unfolds in which she clutches and opens her bag, then quickly snaps it shut and hides it under her chair when she hears her husband approach, then opens it again to reveal to her friends some lace, unable to contain her "besoin sensuel" (sensual urge), then closes it again "comme pour y cacher des choses qu'on ne montre pas" (88) (as if to hide things in it

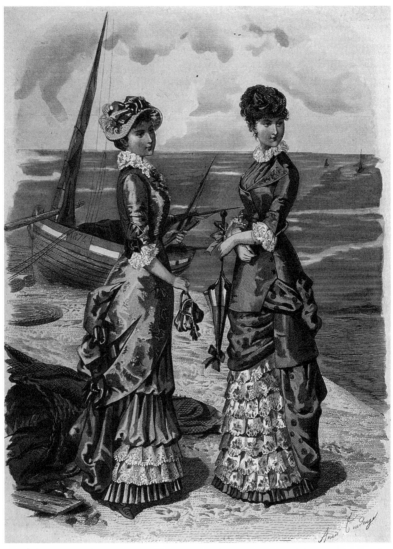

Figure 30.   *La Mode illustrée*, 1880, Maciet Collection, Bibliothèque des arts décoratifs.

that must not be shown [82]), only to open it yet again, unable to resist showing off the *mouchoir* (handkerchief) she has just purchased at the Paradise. The sexualization of Madame Marty's bag is hard to overstate in this scene. After this, the little bag becomes bottomless, and from it emerge a veil and a lady's tie, among other small items, each of which is described according to the price paid for it, and each contributing bit by bit to the financial disaster of the hapless Monsieur Marty.[48] "Elle rougissait de plaisir, une pudeur de femme qui se déshabille la rendait charmante et embarrassée, à chaque article nouveau qu'elle sortait" (89) (As she took out each fresh article she blushed with pleasure, with the modesty of a woman undressing [82]). This game of hide and seek (*cache-cache*) repeats with an important difference the similar games of seduction inherent in the *cachemire*, the *ombrelle*, and the *éventail*. Here, the handbag does *not* perform seduction the way these other accessories did: instead, it allows her to hide (*cacher*) from the husband those objects purchased with his money. This purse thus signifies a certain interference with the domestic space and economy of marriage, a perturbation of the wifely role, and suggests finally the separation of woman from the domestic sphere. For Madame Marty's bag portrays her libidinous displacement into the pseudodomestic space of the consumer's paradise, often constructed by Mouret as a boudoir or a *sérail* (harem).

Madame Marty's bag becomes figuratively overstuffed in the gendered economy of this novel—it stands for the Ladies' Paradise in miniature, its irresistible contents driving women to folly and men to ruin.[49] Small and portable, it ambulates with Madame Marty, allowing her to take possession on the spot of whatever fashionable item strikes her fancy. And, like the pockets of the last century, it also allows her to conceal her intimacies, which are not the secret portraits or *billets doux* of lovers but rather the material goods of fashion that Zola quite explicitly shows to inspire her lust. The bag thus doubles the Bonheur itself, which also contains plots of lust, adultery, crime, and passion. The bag also simultaneously refers to the diabolical financial scheme concocted by Mouret; merging the erotic and the economic in a perfect Pandora's box, a seemingly endless array of accessories and luxury fashion items continuously stream from the bag-Bonheur, leading, unchecked, to financial disaster. Like the reticule, too, however, it is a visible sign of women's mobility, purchasing power (if by proxy), and fashionability. Madame Marty may have no real economic power, however, and her purchases, and dissimulation of them, both facilitated by the handbag, may serve ultimately to reveal her dependency on her husband's meager salary; but the question of female agency through the vehicle of the handbag nonetheless lays claim to a new, if dangerous, potency in this text.

Madame Marty's little red handbag has its masculine counterpart in the actual male economy in the huge sacks of money that Mouret's staff drag up to his office after each sale—from one bag to another, money and goods pass hands, and women are irrevocably implicated in the commerce of things. The dangers to the ideology of the feminine of women's visible entry into production and consumption are tied to Madame Marty's little purse; her husband is helpless since, to appear generous before his friends, he has said she is "free" to spend as she pleases.[50] The heroine, Denise Baudu, who represents productive femininity in this novel and is thus potentially dangerous, worries about whether to be fashionable. She is elevated because she exercises self-control, is not profligate with her money, and is not blind to fashion's power; and yet her dangerous "equality" with her male counterparts is ultimately counterbalanced when she is subsumed into bourgeois marriage, becoming, as Naomi Schor has observed, the vehicle for the reestablishment of family within the capitalist structure of the department store: "Octave doit se soumettre à Denise afin que la lignée se perpétue, que l'affaire reste dans la famille, que la famille soit restaurée, mais sur un mode ou un modèle mieux adaptés au capitalisme triomphant" (182) (Octave must bow to Denise so that they produce an heir, the business remains in the family, the family is restored, but according to a mode or a model better suited to triumphant capitalism). Madame Marty's profligacy is likened to promiscuity, leading ultimately to the subversion of the family, that precious ideal that comes asunder when women leave the *foyer* and assume a masculine role. Madame Marty emblematizes the potential dangers of being too loose with money—no longer embroidering quietly at home, she is separated from the domestic space, out shopping and engaging in unproductive expenditure.[51] This fashion accessory in its many incarnations, once a metonymy for the *foyer* in the *sac à ouvrage* and in the *aumônière*, here becomes a metonymy for the *grand magasin*, and this metonymic slippage emblematizes modernity.

SANS DESSUS DESSOUS: FROM *CORBEILLE* TO *SAC À MAIN*

Madame Marty's bag itself is not yet the fashionable status marker that it would become and that the cashmere shawl, for example, had been. This transformation would occur in the early twentieth century, once the handbag became universal, the word *réticule* and its referent came back into vogue, and fashion itself invented new markers of status. The handbag became fashionable beginning in the 1880s, and by the early

1900s it was visible everywhere. Shopgirls, working girls, and society
ladies alike wore bags, marking at once the handbag's entry into fashionability and the lower classes' increased access to fashionable objects.
In 1901, an article in the women's magazine *Fémina* announces the new
universality of the handbag:

> Quant aux sacs à main, les voilà entrés dans le domaine usuel. Long-
> temps on a résisté, laissant cette mode aux étrangères, les Parisiennes
> n'aimant guère à s'embarrasser les mains d'accessoires. Mais on a eu
> tant de déplaisirs par l'absence de poche aux jupes trop ajustées, tant
> d'objets souvent précieux ont été perdus: bourses, carnets, mouchoirs,
> que l'on s'est résigné à recourir, jour et soir, au sac à main.

> [As for handbags, they have now entered the common domain. Parisi-
> ennes have long resisted them, leaving this fashion to foreigners, for
> they do not like to encumber their hands with accessories. But we have
> had such displeasure caused by the absence of pockets and the close
> fit of dresses, so many precious objects have been lost: change purses,
> notebooks, handkerchiefs, that we have resigned ourselves to turn, day
> and night, to the handbag.][52]

Until 1907, working women could not legally have use of their salary
without the authorization of their husbands.[53] It is perhaps a coincidence worth noting, then, that in 1908, *Fémina* offers a two-page illustrated spread entitled "Du réticule à la trousse" (from the reticule to
the case), with an article by Camille Duguet on the new fashion of the
handbag, "un des plus charmant compléments de notre toilette" (one
of the most charming complements to our toilette).[54] After outlining
the history of the reticule and explaining its disappearance and recent
revival, Duguet launches into a full description of the many varieties
of contemporary fashionable bags and their advantages. Her detailed
description empties out the bag, divulging all the secrets a lady's *sac à
main* might conceal:

> Comme il sont loin de leurs devanciers, nos sacs en peau de daim, en
> peau de chagrin, ou en tout autre cuir souple! Pour se faire plus com-
> modes ils se divisent en compartiments; l'un pour le porte-carte et la
> tablette d'ivoire pour inscrire les commissions, les adresses, les choses
> à ne pas oublier; l'autre pour la bonbonnière, la glace où l'on répare
> le désordre de ses cheveux; un troisième pour la houppette à poudre
> de riz. Compartiments aussi pour l'or et pour l'argent, afin d'éviter
> les familiarités de ces deux métaux, de valeur si différente. Les plus
> privilégiées de nos élégantes portent des bourses en mailles d'or, dont

l'intérieur est également divisé en trois ou quatre compartiments, avec une toute petite bourse pour les louis d'or, qui s'adapte intérieurement. Elles ont aussi leur place pour le mouchoir que son inutilité a réduit à un petit rien de linon et de dentelle, pour l'étui à rouge. (149)

[How distant from their precursors, our bags of buckskin, of shagreen, or of any other supple leather! To be more convenient, they are divided into compartments; one for the card holder and the ivory pad to write notes, addresses, thing not to forget; the other for the candy box, the mirror in which one fixes disorderly hair; a third for the rice powder puff. There are also compartments for gold and silver, in order to avoid mixing these two metals, of such different values. The most privileged of our elegant ladies carry golden mesh purses, whose interiors are also divided into three or four compartments, with a tiny purse for gold *louis*, that fits inside. They also have a place for the handkerchief whose uselessness has reduced it to a tiny piece of linen and lace to make room for rouge.]

The fashion journal not only describes in great detail the styles and materials used for the exterior of the bag but also offers a minute description of the bags' interiors, making visible, once and for all, the feminine accessories indispensable to the production of femininity and thus signaling the opening of the door to a fuller exploration of female sexuality. Fabricated from the softest of skins, or from precious metal, the *sac* opens up to reveal multiple secret compartments—hierarchized and internalized spaces for the various props of modern femininity: useful notepads, referring to the social business of bourgeois ladies; candy, to satisfy one appetite and equating woman with child; mirror and powder, referring to the artful technologies of the self that femininity in the public sphere requires. The new purses also have separate compartments for different coins, and the description classes the coins even as it classes women of differing social milieux who carry different styles of bags. The handkerchief, once a ubiquitous fashion accessory and necessary emblem of female virtue, has made way for lipstick, the very element of artifice once reserved for actresses.[55] The ubiquity of the handbag thus proves at last the visible coexistence, and perhaps the false moral hierarchy, of the *femme comme il faut* and her seamy double, the *femme comme il en faut*, so anxiously separated earlier in the century.

The *sac à main* serves as a foil to the *corbeille de mariage*, the containing and hierarchizing object that initiated this study. I have shown how the *corbeille* was idealized by the fashion press and used to sweeten a perhaps unsavory marriage with its promise of a life of luxury.

The fashion correspondent for the periodical *La Corbeille* writes: "Que de promesses de coquetterie contenues dans ce mot magique: une corbeille de mariage! C'est la boîte de Pandore de la mode et de l'industrie" (*La Corbeille*, August 1853, 162) (So many promises of coquetry contained in this magic word: a *corbeille de mariage*! It's the Pandora's box of fashion and of industry). But surely the *corbeille*'s more modern double, the *sac*, more closely reflects both the feminine power of seduction and the perturbing and potentially destructive agency associated with the ancient myth of Pandora. Both objects are receptacles for the accessories deemed essential to the production and performance of the feminine—whether items associated with a woman's role as wife, with her social function as the artfully embellished inscription of her husband's wealth, or with her position as eroticized body in the gendered economy of modern nineteenth-century France. But the *sac*, as we have seen, is portable and ventures away from home and family to accompany women in their move toward greater visible agency in the public sphere. I have explored here the emergence of the *sac à main* as portable *foyer*, as scandalous instrument of female pleasure, and as ultimate luxury accessory. Tracing the *sac à main* in this way from the early nineteenth century through the fin de siècle allows us to see how the object's use value, originally linked to women's independence and practicality, is ultimately co-opted by consumerist fashion.[56]

The handbag potentially turns the hidden pockets of previous generations inside out (*sans dessus dessous*), displaying publicly what once had been carefully guarded under the skirts of women. Perhaps more than any of the other accessories I have discussed, the *sac à main* engages in the seductive game of hiding and revealing a woman's secrets. Certainly, of all the fashion accessories I analyze here, the handbag is the only one with real staying power, and so it is fitting to conclude my analysis of women's fashion accessories with this one object that still survives, and indeed thrives, in today's fashion world.

Epilogue

The Feminine Accessory

"Je pense que la femme a la mission d'être belle pour idéaliser la vie de l'homme, et que le besoin de se parer lui est un sentiment inspiré par la nature. Toutefois, je n'ai pas écrit ce livre pour développer chez elle un goût qui n'est déjà que trop accusé, et qu'elle devrait savoir enrayer dans certaines conditions de vie, et aussi par compréhension de la véritable élégance, qui n'existe pas sans une simplicité relative" (I believe that woman's mission is to be beautiful in order to idealize man's life, and that the need to accessorize is inspired in her by nature. All the same, I did not write this book to develop in her a taste that is already very much ingrained in her, and that she should know how to curb in certain situations, through her understanding of true elegance, which only exists in relation to simplicity).[1] So announces Baronne Staffe in the opening lines of the preface to her turn-of-the-century work on women's fashion accessories—*Les Hochets féminins*—rehearsing the definitions of *élégance* made popular by Balzac some seventy years earlier, repeating the clichés of woman's dangerous penchant for luxury, and reiterating female object status that is as old as time.

While Staffe's title may seem to reduce the accessory to the infantile and the superfluous (*hochet* means "baby's rattle"), her preface deploys a vocabulary decipherable to the social and political elite of modern France. And although she does not qualify woman's *mission* by the all too familiar adjective *civilisatrice*, she nonetheless ascribes to women the duty not only to embellish but also to *idealize* the lives of men, thus suggesting that women's "natural" role is to better a man's world through her achievement of a higher ideal of beauty.[2] The implicit "civilizing" women are admonished here to perform, however, assumes an agency where there is in fact only self-objectification. For according to the wildly popular arbiter of *savoir vivre* and journalist, whose real name was Blanche Soyer, and who in actuality did not frequent the brilliant salons of Paris but lived quietly in the country with her two spinster aunts, women's agency should be directed toward becoming the reconstructed object of male desire.[3] This idealization was to be accomplished, naturally, through the material objects on which women depended to produce their feminine identities—their accessories.

Yet in those same material things, as we have seen, some women found ways to contest, or redirect, the role Staffe prescribes, if sometimes only unintentionally. Marguerite Durand, a contemporary of Baronne Staffe and the editor of the woman's paper *La Fronde* (1897–1905), offers a counterpoint to the etiquette writer.[4] Mary Louise Roberts queries, "How did women such as Durand, sometimes called 'new women,' break free of the nineteenth century 'real woman' ideal considered 'natural' to female identity? How did they extricate themselves from this ideal, which defined woman as nothing more than a decorative creature and a domestic housewife?" (172). The example of Durand is compelling, for the beautiful blonde actress turned journalist proposes a "feminist aesthetics" that would rely on a thoughtful deployment of feminine charms to advance a feminist agenda. Her stealthy acknowledgment of her own performance of the feminine and her very careful appropriation of feminine agency, relying on all the props that fashion and the beauty industry had to offer, earned her scorn from many contemporary feminists, who rejected ornamentation in order to challenge "an aesthetic economy that had historically trivialized them" (184). But in her "Confession" published in *La Fronde* of 1903, Durand traces the contours of her feminism and in it presents a rebuttal to the kind of "duty" imposed on women by the discourse of Baronne Staffe: "the extreme care of one's person and a studied sense of elegance are not always a diversion, a pleasure, but rather often excess work, a duty that she must nevertheless impose upon herself, if only to deprive shortsighted men of the argument that feminism is the enemy of beauty and of a feminine aesthetic."[5] Durand indeed championed the signifying power of femininity and channeled it into a feminist conception of woman's duty in the form of her women's paper, the first of its kind, staffed entirely by women. As Durand claims in her 1902 explanation of the origins and the goals of *La Fronde*:

Méditer sur la justesse de ces revendications, en reconnaître le bien
fondé et considérer comme un devoir social d'aider à leur triomphe par
leur divulgation, voilà ce qui m'amena à concevoir l'idée d'un grand
journal féministe où, quotidiennement, des femmes défendraient les
intérêts des femmes.
   Dans mon écrin étaient vingt-deux perles patiemment collectées
une à une pendant des années. Perles sans défaut, perles parfaites de
forme et d'orient et destinées à composer un collier rare. Leur prix fut
le capital de *la Fronde*.

[To meditate on the validity of these claims, to recognize their legitimacy and to consider as a social duty to help their triumph by their
disclosure, this is what led me to conceive of the idea of an important
feminist paper, where on a daily basis, women would defend the interests of women.
   In my jewelry box there were twenty-two pearls, patiently collected
one by one for many years. Flawless pearls, perfect pearls in form and
luster and destined for an exquisite necklace. Their value provided the
capital for *La Fronde*].[6]

Imagining the stuffy and supercilious Baronne Staffe in conversation
with the vivacious former actress turned feminist Marguerite Durand
plots the feminine accessory in productive ways, and I can only suggest
here what that exchange might have sounded like. In the image of a be-
jeweled and boa-clad Durand, the objects of feminine construction—
les hochets féminins, as Staffe had termed them—would serve a purpose
rather more subversive of the prevailing gender hierarchy than the baronne had envisioned. Indeed, they would be willfully and outspokenly
recast as powerful tools of the twentieth-century feminine.
   Women's fashion accessories of the nineteenth century are embedded in histories that both reinscribe women in traditional gendered social identities and point to fissures or subversions of those identities.
Unearthing the cultural history of these objects begins to open up the
crevices of a new gender order already imagined in the early years of
the nineteenth century, in spite of the repressive regression of the *Code
Civil* and the sexual politics that emerged from the Revolution of 1789.[7]
In this book, I have mapped out the cultural, social, and literary values of women's fashion accessories and their relation to women's roles
within French modernity. *Accessories to Modernity* plays precisely on
the duplicity of intention that I believe becomes rooted in certain objects. Objects like fashion accessories work within structures of visible
intentions that conceal other sets of intentions, which, in nineteenth-

century France, propriety demanded remain concealed. Each of the objects I have examined here participates in this seductive game of *cache-cache*, performing the apparently frivolous function of beautification, as Staffe would have it, alternately disclosing the feminine as seductive and wrapping it in a veil of modesty.

The *cachemire*, the *ombrelle*, the *éventail*, and the *sac* each participated in this double gesture in different ways, but they also, I have argued, contributed to a broader form of concealment. They are tied to French modernity in unexpected ways—in their imbrication with the stories of imperialism, with class dominance, with industry and commerce— in short, in those stories of modernity that were gendered male and from which bourgeois women were ostensibly excluded. But as I have shown, from the *corbeille de mariage* to the *sac à main*, these accessories to feminine performance were indeed intimately connected to the processes of modernity. What appeared to be only frivolous and beautiful accoutrements, the objects of desire of a classed presentation of the fairer sex, turn out to be objects of conquest, objects of oppression, objects of transgression, objects of liberation. As Gyp's staging of the voiceless bride surrounded by the animate and talking luxuries of her *corbeille* demonstrates, there was an uncanny operation of exchange between subject and object at work in the material culture of modernity. When a discursive power is accorded to the object, the girl's silence is both amplified and displaced—as voice—onto the material stuff of her life. My study of objects has thus also been a study of women as readable objects, as luxury ornaments themselves in the gendered economy of nineteenth-century France. At the same time, and conversely, my analysis also postulates a potential agency of the most material of goods and of the women who possessed them. For there are ideas in things that can be uncovered to reveal treasures of cultural knowledge, remarkable histories, as yet unconstituted, lingering on the margins of dominant discourses, if we can but listen to their stories and grasp their materialization.[8] As both objects and signifiers, but potentially also as subjects and agents, these things, and the women who wielded them in nineteenth-century France, were also ideas taking shape in an unstable cultural landscape, and they were indeed powerful accessories to modernity.

PROLOGUE

1. Elaine Freedgood's work on the things of Victorian novels has been particularly helpful in my approach to reevaluating objects in French realist novels. See Elaine Freedgood, *The Ideas in Things: Fugitive Meaning in the Victorian Novel* (Chicago: University of Chicago Press, 2006). Other important studies on the importance of objects and/or the detail in their relation to literature and, in particular, concepts of the feminine, include Naomi Schor, *Reading in Detail: Aesthetics and the Feminine* (1987; reprint, New York: Routledge, 1989), Emily S. Apter, *Feminizing the Fetish: Psychoanalysis and Narrative Obsession in Turn-of-the-Century France* (Ithaca, N.Y.: Cornell University Press, 1991), and Rae Beth Gordon, *Ornament, Fantasy, and Desire in Nineteenth-Century French Literature* (Princeton, N.J.: Princeton University Press, 1992). Marni Reva Kessler's *Sheer Presence: The Veil in Manet's Paris* (Minneapolis: University of Minnesota Press, 2006) offers not only a wealth of valuable material to the project of fashion and the feminine in nineteenth-century France but also a model of scholarship linking the things of fashion to their social and gendered contexts. See also Arjun Appadurai, "Commodities and the Politics of Value," introduction to *The Social Life of Things: Commodities in a Cultural Perspective* (Cambridge: Cambridge University Press, 1986), and W. David Kingery, introduction to *Learning from Things: Method and Theory of Material Culture Studies* (Washington, D.C.: Smithsonian Institution Press, 1996).

2. Works that have in particular informed my understanding of the status of bourgeois and elite women in nineteenth-century France include Anne Martin-Fugier, *La Vie élégante, ou, la formation du Tout-Paris, 1815–1848* (Paris: Fayard, 1990), Bonnie Smith, *Ladies of the Leisure Class: The Bourgeoises of Northern France in the Nineteenth Century* (Princeton, N.J.: Princeton University Press, 1981), and Mary Louise Roberts, *Disruptive Acts: The New Woman in Fin-de-Siècle France* (Chicago: University of Chicago Press, 2002). See also Claire Goldberg Moses, *French Feminism in the Nineteenth Century* (Albany: State University of New

York Press, 1984), and James F. McMillan, *France and Women, 1789–1914: Gender, Society, and Politics* (New York: Routledge, 2000).

3. *Modernity* is a fluid and unstable term. While I acknowledge its reach back through capitalism to the early modern period and its reach forward into the present, I wish here to situate a particularly fraught period within the long history of modernity in the time beginning in the First Empire through the fin de siècle. The primary focus of this book is from the July Monarchy (1830) through the Second Empire (1870) with some consideration of the margins on either end. For important discussions of modernity that have shaped my thinking, see in particular David Harvey, *Paris: Capital of Modernity* (New York: Routledge, 2003), Rosalind Williams, *Dream Worlds: Mass Consumption in Late Nineteenth-Century France* (Berkeley: University of California Press, 1982), Rita Felski, *The Gender of Modernity* (Cambridge, Mass.: Harvard University Press, 1995), Ulrich Lehmann, *Tigersprung: Fashion in Modernity* (Cambrige, Mass.: MIT Press, 2000), Elizabeth Wilson, *Adorned in Dreams: Fashion and Modernity* (1985; reprint, New Brunswick, N.J.: Rutgers University Press, 2003), and Barbara Vinken, *Fashion Zeitgeist*, trans. Mark Hewson (New York: Berg, 2005).

CHAPTER 1

1. Alexandre Dumas *fils*, *La Dame aux camélias* (Paris: Pocket, 1994), 38–39. Translation from Project Gutenberg (http://www.gutenberg.org/wiki/Main_Page). All other translations are mine unless otherwise indicated.

2. Balzac's pun also appears in "La Femme comme il faut," an earlier essay included in the panoramic collection of social types published from 1840 to 1843 entitled *Les Français peints par eux-mêmes: encyclopédie morale du dix-neuvième siècle*, ed. Léon Curmer and Pierre Bouttier, 2 vols. (Paris: Omnibus, 2003); Balzac's piece was also published in an expanded form as *Autre étude de femme* in 1842. Honoré de Balzac, *Autre étude de femme* (Paris: Gallimard, 1970), 69. All references are to this edition. This text is discussed at length below. Translation from Honoré de Balzac, *At the Sign of the Cat and Racket and La grande Breteche and Other Stories*, vol. 8 of *Balzac's Novels*, ed. George Saintsbury, trans. Clara Bell (London: Dent, 1898), 37 (translation modified).

3. This scene was modeled on the real auction of the historical "Dame aux Camélias," Marie Duplessis. The auction was described by journalist and critic Jules Janin in 1851. This scene serves as a pendant to the auction scene in Flaubert's *L'Education sentimentale*, in which Marie Arnoux's personal effects are sold due to bankruptcy, discussed in greater detail in Chapter 3.

4. See Martin-Fugier, *La Vie élégante*.

5. The key text here is Pierre Bourdieu's *Distinction: A Social Critique of the Judgement of Taste*, trans. Richard Nice (Cambridge, Mass.: Harvard University Press, 1984).

6. Obviously, there were other social groups, in particular lower-class groups,

which I do not have space to consider here. I recognize that to reduce the social landscape to *monde* and *demi-monde* is a simplification, a by-product in part of the very texts under consideration in this chapter.

7. Aubrey Cannon, "The Cultural and Historical Contexts of Fashion" in *Consuming Fashion: Adorning the Transnational Body*, ed. Anne Brydon and Sandra Niessen (New York: Berg, 1998), 26. See also Norbert Elias, *The Civilizing Process: Sociogenetic and Psychogenetic Investigations*, rev. ed., ed. Eric Dunning, Johan Goudsblom, and Stephen Mennell, trans. Edmund Jephcott (Malden, Mass.: Blackwell, 2000).

8. See Madame de Girardin's *Lettres parisiennes* for a panoramic look at *le monde* also as style and behavior. Madame de Girardin, *Lettres parisiennes du vicomte de Launay*, 2 vols., ed. Anne Martin-Fugier, Le Temps retrouvé series (Paris: Mercure de France, 1986).

9. See Elias.

10. Alexandre Dumas *fils*, *Le Demi-monde, comédie en cinq actes, en prose* in *Théâtre complet d'Alexandre Dumas*, vol. 2 (Paris: Calmann Lévy, 1896), 10. Balzac would surely disagree with Dumas's suggestion that the *demi-monde* was new territory: one has only to examine his chapter entitled "Un Paysage Parisien" from the opening pages of *Splendeurs* (published between 1838 and 1847) to situate both literally and figuratively this "monde à l'envers" where "les conditions atmosphériques y sont changées; on y a chaud en hiver et froid en été. . . . En y passant pendant la journée, on ne peut se figurer ce que toutes ces rues deviennent à la nuit; elles sont sillonnées par des êtres bizarres qui ne sont d'aucun monde; des formes à demi-nues et blanches meublent les murs, l'ombre est animée. Il se coule entre la muraille et le passant des toilettes qui marchent et qui parlent." Honoré de Balzac, *Splendeurs et Misères des courtisanes*, ed. Pierre Barbéris (Paris: Gallimard, 1973), 57 (atmospheric conditions are reversed there: there it is hot in winter and cold in summer. . . . Passing through in the daytime, one could never imagine what these streets become by night; they are furrowed with strange creatures belonging to no world; half-naked white forms furnish the walls, the shadows are animated. Between the wall and the passerby, walking and talking outfits creep by).

11. Most scholars who work on this problem focus on the period of the Second Empire, a particularly rich period for the study of social mobility and modernity in France, but I want to locate the problem much earlier in conjunction with social practices of the early nineteenth century and the July Monarchy as much as in the Second Empire. For a rich and thorough treatment of fashion's gendering social power in the Second Empire, see, in particular, Kessler; see also Arden Reed, *Manet, Flaubert, and the Emergence of Modernism: Blurring Genre Boundaries* (Cambridge: Cambridge University Press, 2003).

12. Maurice Alhoy was a journalist and playwright of the first half of the nineteenth century. For a new treatment through the prism of gender of panoramic literature in nineteenth-century France, see Catherine Nesci, *Le Flâneur et les flâneuses: les femmes et la ville à l'époque romantique* (Grenoble: ELLUG, Université Stendhal, 2007).

13. Catherine Nesci, *La Femme mode d'emploi: Balzac de "La Physiologie du mariage" à "La Comédie humaine"* French Forum Monographs (Lexington, Ky.: French Forum, 1993), 81.

14. See Bonnie Smith for a full discussion of the shifting position of bourgeois women during the period of French industrialization.

15. The *lorette* was a particular variation on Balzac's *femme comme il en faut*, a figure discussed in greater length below. Maurice Alhoy, *Physiologie de la lorette*, ill. Paul Gavarni (Paris: Aubert, 1841), Edmond and Jules de Goncourt, *La lorette*, ed. Alain Barbier Sainte Marie (Tusson: du Lérot, n.d.).

16. The *corbeille de mariage* traditionally included cashmere shawls, fans, laces, ribbons, purses of money, and jewels.

17. Roland Barthes, "Le Dandysme et la mode," in *Le Bleu est à la mode cette année* (1962; reprint, Paris: Editions de l'Institut Français de la Mode, 2001), 98. Also published as "Dandyism and Fashion," trans. Andy Stafford, in *The Language of Fashion*, ed. Stafford and Michael Carter (New York: Berg, 2006), 66.

18. Jukka Gronow, *The Sociology of Taste* (New York: Routledge, 1997), 11.

19. See Georg Simmel, "On Fashion," in *On Individuality and Social Forms*, ed. Donald Levine (1904; reprint, Chicago: University of Chicago Press, 1971), 294–323, and Thorstein Veblen, *The Theory of the Leisure Class*, ed. Robert Lekachman (New York: Penguin Classics, 1994).

20. See Peter Wollen, "The Concept of Fashion in *The Arcades Project*," *boundary 2* 30:1 (Spring 2003): 131–42, quote on 138–39.

21. Charles Baudelaire, "A Une Passante," in *Les Fleurs du mal, Oeuvres complètes* (Paris: Laffont, 1980), 68; for translation, Charles Baudelaire, *Les Fleurs du mal*, trans. Richard Howard (Boston: Godine, 1983), 97. See also Baudelaire's "Le Peintre de la vie moderne," in which he defines the modern as transitory.

22. Philippe Perrot, *Fashioning the Bourgeoisie: A History of Clothing in the Nineteenth Century*, trans. Richard Bienvenu (Princeton, N.J.: Princeton University Press, 1994), 20.

23. Cissie Fairchilds, "Fashion and Freedom in the French Revolution," *Continuity and Change* 15:3 (2000): 419. See also Richard Wrigley, *The Politics of Appearances: Representations of Dress in Revolutionary France* (Oxford: Berg, 2002).

24. See also Henri Baudrillart, *Histoire du luxe privé et public depuis l'antiquité jusqu'à nos jours*, vol. 4 (1880) (Paris: Hachette, 1878–80), Gilles Lipovetsky and Elyette Roux, *Le Luxe éternel* (Paris: Gallimard, 2003), and Philippe Perrot, "Du Luxe et du bien-être au dix-neuvième siècle en France," in *Le Luxe: essais sur la fabrique de l'ostentation*, ed. Olivier Assouly (Paris: Éditions de l'Institut français de la mode-regard, 2005), 101-15.

25. See Daniel Roche, *La Culture des apparences: une histoire du vêtement (XVIIe-XVIIIe siècle)*(Paris: Fayard, 1991), Aileen Ribeiro, *The Art of Dress: Fashion in England and France 1750-1820* (New Haven, Conn.: Yale University Press, 1995), and Jennifer Jones, *Sexing la Mode: Gender, Fashion and Commercial Culture in Old Regime France* (Oxford: Berg, 2004), for detailed and

groundbreaking discussions of the consumer revolution of the eighteenth century.

26. The term *élégance* and other terminology associated with respectability and fashion are crucial to Balzac's work. See, for example, Balzac, *Traité de la vie élégante*, published in 1830 in the fashion journal *La Mode*. For a detailed study of the importance of this vocabulary, see also Algirdas Julien Greimas, *La Mode en 1830: essai de description du vocabulaire vestimentaire d'après les journaux de mode de l'époque*, Langage et société: écrits de jeunesse series, ed. Thomas F. Broden and Françoise Ravaux-Kirkpatrick (Paris: Presses Universitaires de France, 2000).

27. I refer here to Judith Butler's theorization of the performative in her inquiry into the genealogy of the subject. Her notion of the performative disrupts the category of essential (gender) identity by proposing that we *perform* those identities rather than are those identities. See Judith Butler, *Gender Trouble: Feminism and the Subversion of Identity* (New York: Routledge, 1989), and *Bodies That Matter: On the Discursive Limits of "Sex"* (New York: Routledge, 1993).

28. The *marchande des modes* embodied a feminine tradition (Rose Bertin, who dressed Marie-Antoinette, is the most famous example) of embellishment and accessorizing women's fashion and can be contrasted to the male *couturier* (tailor), who gained prominence especially during the Second Empire (the most notable being Charles Frederick Worth). Women were excluded from the tailoring guilds but were legally permitted to work in the area of millinery, though not dressmaking. See Jones, *Sexing la mode*.

29. Authenticity, as Vinken and others before her have pointed out, becomes a new key value, and it, too, is gendered: "The all-determining opposition that constitutes sexual difference is now that of authentic and inauthentic. Men 'are'—they are someone, they are authentic, real; women on the other hand lack essence and are sheer appearance, artificial, inauthentic" (13).

30. Lucienne Frappier-Mazur, "Lecture d'un texte illisible: *Autre étude de femme* et le modèle de la conversation," *Modern Language Notes* 98:4 (1983): 712.

31. See V. Marcadé, *Explication théorique et pratique du Code Napoléon* (Paris:Garnier, 1869). See also Patricia Mainardi, *Husbands, Wives, and Lovers: Marriage and Its Discontents in Nineteenth-Century France* (New Haven, Conn.: Yale University Press, 2003), for a lucid examination of the effects of the *Code Civil* on the cultural practices surrounding marriage.

32. Alexandre Dumas *père*, *Filles, lorettes, et courtisanes* (Paris: Flammarion, 2000), 14. Parent-Duchâtelet, a government-commissioned Parisian hygienist, wrote *De la Prostitution dans la ville de Paris* in 1836. See also Alain Corbin, *Les Filles de noces: Misère sexuelle et prostitution aux dix-neuvième et vingtième siècles* (Paris: Aubier Montaigne, 1978), and Jann Matlock, *Scenes of Seduction: Prostitution, Hysteria, and Reading Difference in Nineteenth-Century France* (New York: Columbia University Press, 1994).

33. Balzac might indeed have taken exception to this remark, since *La Torpille* (the prequel to *Splendeurs et misères des courtisanes*) was published in 1838.

34. *Lorette* was a term coined by Nestor Roqueplan, man-about-town and director of the Théâtre des Variétés. Martin-Fugier explains that he "inventa en 1841 le terme de 'lorettes' à cause de l'abondance des prostituées dans le quartier neuf autour de Notre-Dame-de-Lorette" (341) (coined in 1841 the term "*lorettes*" because of the abundance of prostitutes in the new neighborhood around Notre-Dame-de-Lorette).

35. Michel Butor, *Scènes de la vie féminine: Improvisations sur Balzac III* (Paris: Éditions de la Différence, 1998), 77.

36. Baudelaire does something similar, although from a divergent moral perspective, in his "Éloge du Maquillage," contained in "Le Peintre de la vie moderne," (809–11). It is useful here to note the origins of the pejorative adjective *seamy*, a word that, in English, refers specifically to the negative moral implications of the visibility of seams. Their invisibility, by contrast, points to the notion of naturalized social identities that hierarchies depend on to maintain power. My thanks to Jeffrey Schneider for deepening my understanding of this important detail.

37. Honoré de Balzac, *Ferragus*, in *Histoire des Treize*, ed. Gérard Gengembre (Paris: Presses Pocket, 1992), 37. All references are to this edition. Translation from Honoré de Balzac, *Balzac's Works*, ed. George Saintsbury, vol. 14, trans. Clara Bell (Freeport, N.Y.: Books for Libraries, 1971), 12–13. All subsequent translations are from this edition.

38. Translation modified.

39. According to the *Dictionnaire de l'Académie française* of 1835 the term *grisette* first signified an article of clothing made of cheap grey cloth and worn by common women. But the term entered into popular usage and came to mean a young woman of little means, and more specifically, a flirty young working girl, and particularly those "young shop girls . . . who tended the counter and stitched the elaborate creations of the marchandes de modes." Jennifer Jones, "Coquettes and Grisettes: Women Buying and Selling in Ancien Régime France," in *The Sex of Things: Gender and Consumption in Historical Perspective*, ed. Victoria de Grazia (Berkeley: University of California Press, 1996), 29.

40. Translation modified.

41. Walter Benjamin, "The Work of Art in the Age of Mechanical Reproduction," in *Illuminations* (New York: Harcourt Brace and World, 1968), 221. Nancy L. Green makes the coexistence of art and industry in the emerging garment business in nineteenth-century France the subject of her very thorough article. In it, she cites Benjamin's concept of "aura," arguing that "both uniqueness and reproducibility have shaped the trade, ultimately forming two distinct branches within it, *haute couture* and ready-to-wear." Nancy L. Green, "Art and Industry: The Language of Modernization in the Production of Fashion," *French Historical Studies* 18:3 (Spring 1994): 723. This problem of compatibility, which she situates toward the end of the century, is arguably already present in the debates over cashmere shawls in the earlier part of the century.

42. See especially Corbin, *Les Filles de noces*.

43. This too is a fiction, as courtesans did not exist as such in antiquity, but only prostitutes. The courtesan is a phenomenon of Renaissance Italy. See Lisa Rengo George, "Reading the Plautine Meretrix" (Ph.D. diss., Bryn Mawr College, 1997).

44. Matlock, 107.

45. Along with the *physiologies* treated here, the *lorette* was the subject of several series of lithographs by Gavarni, in particular, "La Lorette" and "Les Lorettes vieillies."

46. See Gabrielle Houbre, *La Discipline de l'amour: L'éducation des filles et des garçons à l'âge du romantisme* (Paris: Plon, 1997), 360–70.

47. See Perrot. See Zola's *La Curée* and *Nana* for literary examples of this.

48. Quoted in Victoria Thompson, *The Virtuous Marketplace: Women and Men, Money and Politics 1830–1870* (Baltimore: Johns Hopkins University Press, 2000), 134. Thompson offers a rich analysis of the social function of the *lorette* and her symbolism in the modernizing of Paris, arguing that the *lorette* "was created to discuss the impact of big capital and finance on French society . . . a transitional figure, used to discuss the shift from older networks of credit and investment (in which women could participate) to newer, more formalized (and excessively masculine) institutions" (131). Her arguments about the *lorette*'s engagement in speculation are compelling; she draws heavily on Alhoy's *Physiologie de la lorette*, and her readings of this and other texts surrounding the *lorette* have been central to my understanding of this figure. While Thompson focuses primarily on the economic metaphors surrounding the *lorette*'s presence in the Paris of the Second Empire, I am interested in how the *lorette*'s particular use of fashion signs emphasizes her social hybridity and connects her to her presumed foil—the *femme comme il faut*.

49. Lucette Czyba, "Paris et la lorette," in *Paris au XIXe siècle: aspects d'un mythe littéraire*, ed. Roger Bellet (Lyon: Presses universitaires de Lyon, 1984), 110.

50. Henry Murger, *Scenes de la vie de bohème*, ed. Loïc Chotard (Paris: Gallimard, 1988), 311.

51. See, in particular, Corbin, *Les Filles de noces*, who carefully breaks down the various gradations among types of prostitutes and explains that *fille* was the common term for a low class prostitute.

52. See Alhoy.

53. Colette Guillemard, *Les Mots du costume* (Paris: Belin, 1991), 247.

54. This relationship echoes the most important such literary example in the French tradition of Emma Bovary and Lheureux.

55. *Crispin* is a term most frequently used for a small coat for ladies and children. It may also indicate, however, an embellishment to a glove originating in fencing. Because the word is plural, and the subject is singular, the meaning of *crispin* here must refer to the glove style and not to the coat. I acknowledge some ambiguity here over the translation of this term.

56. See Victoria Thompson in particular.

57. While a discussion of male fashion is beyond the scope of this project, a great deal of scholarship has been devoted to this subject, and it would be fruit-

ful to pursue this subject in conversation with my own discussion of femininity and the fashion accessory. Gloves, as Rastignac learns early on in Balzac's *Le Père Goriot*, are the indispensable male accessory without which social dominance is impossible; Rastignac's education is complete when Madame de Beauséant gives him her glove box, a token of thanks for his loyalty, symbolically bequeathing him with the weapons of the social duel he will need to possess in order to succeed. The dandy, as Barthes reminds us in his 1962 essay "Dandyism and Fashion," relies on the fashion detail, much like the women treated in this study, for distinction in the world of nineteenth-century male fashion that tends toward greater and greater uniformity. For some of the classic discussions of male fashion, and in particular of the dandy and the flâneur, see Rhonda Garelick, *Rising Star: Dandyism, Gender and Performance in the Fin de Siècle* (Princeton, N.J.: Princeton University Press, 1998), Jessica Feldman, *Gender on the Divide: The Dandy in Modernist Literature* (Ithaca, N.Y.: Cornell University Press, 1993), Colin Campbell, *The Romantic Ethic and the Spirit of Modern Consumerism* (New York: Blackwell, 1987), Ellen Moers, *The Dandy: Brummell to Beerbohm* (New York: Viking, 1960).

58. Alain Barbier Sainte Marie, the editor and annotator of the Goncourt text defines the "corset à la paresseuse" in his note to page 39:

> Sorte de corset qui, contrairement aux modèles courants, n'avait pas besoin d'être lacé par derrière, soit par un mari, soit par la femme de chambre. Dans son poème "L'Amour à Paris" (février 1846) inclus dans ses *Odes funambulesques*, Théodore de Banville remercie la Muse de Paris d'avoir inventé les "corsets à la minute"; et dans un commentaire de 1873, le poète explique qu'il s'agit de corsets "qu'on détache en tirant une baleine" et qu'ils "passaient, en 1846, pour des engins pernicieux, réservés seulement aux *belles et honnestes dames* qui ne sont jamais sans amours, comme le samedi n'est jamais sans soleil. Aujourd'hui, il n'y a plus d'autres corsets que ceux-là; aussi faut-il une explication historique au joli dessin de Gavarni, dans lequel un mari délaçant sa femme murmure avec inquiétude: 'C'est drôle, ce matin j'ai fait un nœud à ce lacet-là, et ce soir il y a une rosette!'" (67)

> [Type of corset, which, contrary to the usual type, did not need to be laced from behind, either by a husband or by a maid. In his poem "L'Amour à Paris" (February 1846), included in his *Odes funambulesques*, Théodore de Banville thanks the Muse of Paris for having invented the "one-minute corset." In an 1873 note, the poet explains that such corsets "are undone by pulling one bone" and that they were "in 1846, taken for dangerous machineries, to be used exclusively by beautiful and honest ladies who are never without lovers, much like Saturdays are never without sunny weather. Today, only such corsets are in use; therefore one needs to provide a historical explanation for Gavarni's pretty drawing, in which a puzzled husband undoing his wife's corset notes 'how peculiar, this morning I tied this ribbon with a knot, and tonight there is a bow!'."]

59. See Valerie Steele, *The Corset: A Cultural History* (New Haven, Conn.: Yale University Press, 2001), and Leigh Summers, *Bound to Please: A History of the Victorian Corset* (New York: Berg, 2001).

60. Thompson writes, "Associated with modernization, masculinity, and speculation, the *lorette* seemed to embody, for good or for bad, the new mores and attitudes of a society in search of easy money" (133).

61. The fetish and its structure are the focus of Chapter 5, which deals with the fan.

62. See Margaret Waller, "Disembodiment as a Masquerade: Fashion Journalists and Other 'Realist' Observers in Directory Paris," *Esprit Créateur* 37:1 (1997): 44–54.

63. See Perrot, *Fashioning the Bourgeoisie*. See also Zola, *La Curée*, for the thematization of this phenomenon.

CHAPTER 2

1. Stéphane Mallarmé. *La Dernière Mode* in *Œuvres complètes*, ed. H. Mondor and G. J. Aubry (Paris: Gallimard, 1965), September 1874, issue 1, 713–14, quote on 714.

2. P. N. Furbank and A. M. Cain, "*La Dernière Mode* and Its Pre-History," in *Mallarmé on Fashion: A Translation of the Fashion Magazine* La Dernière Mode *with Commentary*, ed. and trans. Furbank and Cain (New York: Berg, 2004), 23–24.

3. A growing body of scholarship is emerging surrounding Mallarmé's fashion writing. See in particular Claire Lyu, "Stéphane Mallarmé as Miss Satin: The Texture of Fashion and Poetry," *Esprit Créateur* 40:3 (Fall 2000): 61–71, Barbara Bohac, "*La Dernière Mode* de Mallarmé sous les feux du drame solaire," *Romantisme* 132 (2006): 129–39, Françoise Grauby, "Le Parfum de l'homme en noir: Mallarmé et *La Dernière Mode* (1874)," *Australian Journal of French Studies* 41:1 (2004): 102–20.

4. I refer to the principal conceit of Diderot's first novel *Les Bijoux indiscrets* (1748), which portrays Louis XV as a sultan with a magic ring that has the power to make women's genitals ("jewels") talk. Denis Diderot, *Les Bijoux indiscrets*, ed. Jacques Rustin (Paris: Gallimard, 1981).

5. For a historical discussion of the *corbeille*, see See Isabelle Bricard, "La Corbeille," in *Saintes ou pouliches: l'éducation des jeunes filles au XIXe siècle* (Paris: Albin Michel, 1985), 310–11.

6. Bricard explains: "Selon un usage établi, le fiancé doit dépenser pour l'achat de la corbeille une somme équivalant à 5% de la dot, au début du siècle, et à 10% à la fin du Second Empire" (311) (According to custom, the fiancé should spend on the *corbeille* a sum equivalent to 5% of the dowry at the beginning of the century, and 10% at the end of the Second Empire). Marie de Saverny, writing in 1876, suggests that *corbeilles* had become, in her day, disproportionally opulent: "Les cadeaux doivent être proportionnés à la fortune des époux. Autrefois la corbeille représentait une année des revenus du jeune ménage, mais de nos jours cette somme est bien souvent dépassé" (Gifts should be proportionate to the wealth of the couple. Before, the *corbeille* represented one year of the young household's revenue, but these days this amount is very often

surpassed). *La Femme chez elle et dans le monde* (Paris: Au Bureau du journal *La Revue de la Mode,* 1876), 209.

7. Étienne de Jouy, *L'Hermite de la Chaussée d'Antin ou observations sur les mœurs et les usages parisiens au commencement du XIXe siècle,* 6th ed., vol. 2 (Paris: Pillet, 1815), 117.

8. The relevant clause in the *Code* is title 3, article 1124, which states that those who are not allowed to enter into contracts are "les mineurs, les interdits, les femmes mariées" (minors, *interdits,* and married women). "Interdits" refers to people who have lost all civil, family, and judicial rights. This clause essentially indicates that married women remain minors, retaining the legal status of the *demoiselle.* V. Marcadé, 383.

9. See Mainardi.

10. Edmond Duranty, *Le Malheur d'Henriette Gérard,* pref. by Jean Paulhan (1860; reprint, Paris: Gallimard, 1981). The novel, little read in its day and still relatively unknown, is considered a precursor to naturalism. According to Paulhan, Duranty was one of the first champions of Manet and Degas (6).

11. On the commonplace of violence on the wedding night, see Laure Adler, *Secrets d'alcove: histoire du couple, 1830–1930* (Paris: Éditions Complexes, 1990). See in particular ch. 2, "La Nuit de noces ou l'horreur du viol legal," 31–65.

12. La Baronne Staffe, "La Jeune Fille," in *Usages du monde: règles du savoir-vivre dans la société moderne* (Paris: Victor Havard, 1891), 273.

13. Marie Emery, "Une Corbeille," in *Le Journal des demoiselles* 37:3 (1869): 79–85.

14. A similar fate befalls Cécile Camusot in Balzac's *Le Cousin Pons,* whose engagement falls through ostensibly for reasons of the opulent tastes of spoiled only daughters. I discuss this novel at length in Chapter 4.

15. See Jane Schneider, "Trousseau as Treasure: Some Contradictions of Late Nineteenth-Century Change in Sicily," in *The Marriage Bargain: Women and Dowries in European History,* ed. Marion Kaplan (New York: Harrington Park, 1985), 81–119.

16. Laurel Bossen explains the three basic models of marriage transactions, decrying their terminology as "archaic and misleading": brideservice, bridewealth, and dowry systems. "Towards a Theory of Marriage: The Economic Anthropology of Marriage Transactions," *Ethnology* 27:2 (April 1988): 127–44, quote on 127.

17. Diane Owen-Hughes, "From Brideprice to Dowry in Mediterranean Europe," in *The Marriage Bargain: Women and Dowries in European History,* ed. Marion Kaplan (New York: Harrington Park, 1985), 13–58.

18. Bricard, note 68, 346. See also Jack Goody and S. J. Tambiah, *Bridewealth and Dowry* (Cambridge: Cambridge University Press, 1973), for a discussion of the anthropology of marriage transactions. Goody and Tambiah show that dowry and bridewealth should not necessarily be considered opposites, and in fact, that they could be interchangeable. The essential point is that both forms of transaction involved property and its consolidation.

19. Honoré de Balzac, *Une Double Famille suivi du Contrat de mariage et de l'Interdiction,* ed. Jean-Louis Bory (Paris: Gallimard, 1973), 143–44. All references

are to this edition unless otherwise indicated. All translations of this text, unless otherwise indicated, are from the edition translated by Project Gutenburg (http://www.gutenberg.org/files/1556/1556.txt).

20. Many of Balzac's novels and essays focused on the question of marriage and the complexity of making a good marriage. The *corbeille* figures in several of his novels.

21. The Pléiade edition of *Le Contrat de mariage* offers the following explanation of the *majorat*:

> Sur l'histoire du majorat, voir l'article de P.A. Perrod "Balzac et les majorats" dans *AB 1968*. Le majorat est une "dotation de titre héréditaire", "une combinaison de la *substitution* et du *droit de l'aînesse*". Balzac a été fortement intéressé par les problèmes relatifs aux successions, à l'hérédité et au majorat. Il déplore, sans varier d'opinion, "le partage égal des biens, décrété par la Révolution, qui produit l'émiettement des fortunes à l'infini et la diminution de leur rendement, l'envie générale de posséder ou d'accéder à une position supérieure." Cette opinion, émise dès 1824 dans la brochure *Du droit de l'aînesse*, se retrouve dans la lettre de Louis Lambert à son oncle (1835), dans l'article sur "La Femme comme il faut" des *Français peints par eux-mêmes* (1840), dans *Le Curé de village* (éd. Souverain, 1841): "la cause du mal gît dans le Titre des Successions du Code Civil qui ordonne le partage égal des biens." Ce titre des successions, Balzac l'a étudié dans des ouvrages de droit.... Balzac défend le droit de l'aînesse ou ses substituts, l'hérédité de la pairie et la constitution d'un majorat. (1458–59, n. 1)

[On the history of the *majorat*, see P.A. Perrod's article "Balzac et les majorats" in *AB* [*l'Année balzacienne*] 1968. The *majorat* is an "endowment of hereditary title," "a combination of the *substitution* and the *birthright*." Balzac was extremely interested in the problems relating to succession, heredity, and *majorat*. He deplores, without ever changing his opinion, "the equal sharing of goods, decreed by the Revolution, which produces the infinite frittering away of fortunes and the diminishment of their yield, the general desire to possess or obtain a higher position." This opinion, expressed as early as 1824 in the pamphlet *Du droit de l'aînesse*, is found again in Louis Lambert's letter to his uncle (1835), in the article "La Femme comme il faut" in *Les Français peints par eux-mêmes* (1840), in *Le Curé de village* (ed. Souverain, 1841): "the cause of the evil lies in the Title of Successions of the Civil Code which orders the equal sharing of goods." This title of successions Balzac studied in works on law ... Balzac defends the law of birthright or its substitutes, the heredity of peerage and the constitution of a *majorat*.]

22. Louis M. Verardi, *Manuel du bon ton et de la politesse française: nouveau guide pour se conduire dans le monde* (Paris: Passard, 1850–59), 100–101.

23. Madame Évangélista continually deplores the French customs surrounding marriage that demand legal and financial transactions, claiming that her own marriage was purely for love alone.

24. Or, a love match, as opposed to an arranged marriage. See Mainardi. This midnight torch-lit ceremony may have inspired Emma Bovary's wedding fantasies.

25. These were usually family heirlooms reset (made new) for the bride by her fiancé.

26. Alice Granger, "Le Contrat de mariage, Honoré de Balzac" (http://www.e-literature.net/publier/spip/article.php3?id_article=147).

27. For a history of diamond commerce, see Adrienne Munich, "Jews and Jewels on the South African Diamond Fields," in *The Jew in Late-Victorian and Edwardian Culture: Between the East End and East Africa*, ed. Eitan Bar-Yosef and Nadia Valman (New York: Palgrave-Macmillan, 2009), 28–44.

28. The Pléiade note assists in understanding the "comédie des diamants":

Les diamants de Mme Évangélista jouent un rôle important non seulement pour l'établissement du contrat, mais dans l'évolution du drame conjugal dont la belle-mère manie les ressorts.... Le vocabulaire est imprécis. Le terme "diamants" désigne parfois des perles. Ainsi le collier que Mme Évangélista a reçu de son mari est dit à plusieurs reprises "collier de perles"; or Magus le décrit, ainsi que les boucles d'oreilles, comme "entièrement composé de diamants asiatiques". Le diamant de famille que Mme Évangélista portait agrafé à son collier est, en manuscrit, attribué à un héritage de sa mère; sur épreuves, il est dénommé "le Carlos" et vient du Roi; enfin, sur nouvelles épreuves, il s'appellera "le Discreto", remis par Philippe II au duc d'Albe, et que Mme Évangélista a hérité de sa tante. Malgré ces imprécisions entraînées par les remaniements du texte, qui omettent parfois les renseignements donnés sur épreuves antérieures, ce sont bien ces trois pièces (boucles d'oreilles, collier de perles et Discreto) que Mme Évangélista se réserve d'abord, puis qu'elle échange avec le lot attribué à Paul." (1474–75, n. 2)

[Madame Évangélista's diamonds play an important role not only in the establishment of the contract, but also in the evolution of the conjugal drama, which the mother-in-law orchestrates.... The language is imprecise. The term "diamonds" sometimes designates pearls. Thus the necklace that Madame Évangélista received from her husband is described several times as a "pearl necklace"; and yet Magus describes it, along with the earrings, as "entirely composed of Asian diamonds." The family diamond that Madame Évangélista wore fastened to her necklace is, in the manuscript, attributed to an inheritance from her mother; in the advance sheets, it is called "the Carlos" and comes from the king; finally, in later proofs, it will be called "le Discreto," given by Philip II to the Duke of Alba, and which Madame Évangélista inherited from her aunt. In spite of these inconsistencies brought on by revisions to the text, which sometimes omit information given in anterior proofs, it is precisely these three pieces (earrings, pearl necklace and Discreto) that Madame Évangélista keeps for herself at first, which she then exchanges with the set given to Paul.]

29. We have to assume that Madame Évangélista instructs Natalie in the art of

birth control, for the only way to elude the *majorat*, and for Natalie to gain control of Paul's fortune, is not to produce an heir. Her mother's advice to Natalie on her wedding night: "Songe, ma chère enfant, à mes dernières recommandations, et tu seras heureuse. Sois toujours sa femme et non sa maîtresse" (227) (Think, my dear child, about my last bit of advice, and you will be happy. Be always his wife and not his mistress). This is precisely what unfolds.

30. Graham Robb, *Balzac: A Biography* (New York: Norton, 1996), 253.

31. Woodruff D. Smith, *Consumption and the Making of Respectability 1600–1800* (New York: Routledge, 2002), 23–24. Smith's book is devoted primarily to the period leading up to the nineteenth century, and his focus is England, not France. But his arguments can be convincingly applied to a French culture of respectability that takes shape in the wake of the Revolution and in the shadow of earlier social transformations in England. Smith makes the point, in fact, that the French term "respectabilité" does not really enter the French lexicon until the early nineteenth century, and he argues that it is surely a linguistic borrowing from English. Consumption habits in France too shifted more slowly than in England, in large part because of the slower development of modern industrialism in France and the culture of luxury artisanship that stalled industry.

32. See "L'Histoire d'un schall" in Jouy, 304–16.

33. For a full discussion of "la reine en gaulle" and the relationship of Marie-Antoinette to fashion and politics, see Caroline Weber, *Queen of Fashion: What Marie Antoinette Wore to the Revolution* (New York: Holt, 2006). See also Chantal Thomas, *La Reine scélérate: Marie-Antoinette dans les pamphlets* (Paris: Seuil, 1989).

34. We can contrast the idealized Indian "true" wife, the childbearing one, to Natalie Évangélista, who refuses intimacy with her husband so as *not* to produce an heir.

35. Gyp (pseudonym of Sibylle Aimée Marie Antoinette Gabrielle de Riquetti de Mirabeau, Comtesse de Martel de Janville), *Pauvres petites femmes* (Paris: Calmann Lévy, 1888).

CHAPTER 3

1. "Monologue du Cachemire," in *La Silhouette* 3 (1830): 12. The *Circassienne* refers to the favorite slave of the Turkish sultans during the nineteenth century. Hailing from the northern Caucasus, and expelled into diaspora by a sustained invasion by Russia that picked up in 1821 and concluded in genocide in the 1860s, the *Circassienne* was considered the "purest" of the white race and she was thus prized for her beauty in the nineteenth century. Not only was the term *Circassienne* shorthand for white female slave, it was also indicative of rare beauty. The *Circassienne* became a sideshow phenomenon in nineteenth-century circuses and in popular culture. See Marc Hartzman, *American Sideshow: An Encyclopedia of History's Most Wondrous and Curiously Strange Performers* (New York: Penguin, 2005), and Linda Frost, "The Circassian Beauty and the Circassian Slave: Gender,

Imperialism, and American Popular Entertainment," in *Freakery: Cultural Spectacles of the Extraordinary Body*, ed. Rosemary Garland Thomson (New York: New York University Press, 1996), 248–64.

2. I.e., spinsterhood and prostitution. "Bourre-de-soie" has a slang meaning— "Prostituée, prostituée de bas étage; femme richement entretenue," http://www.languefrancaise.net/bob/detail.php?id=12062.

3. It is impossible to know whether she slept with these suitors or not, but it certainly seems likely given her caricatured portrayal as a mercenary young lady. If so, in spite of her possession of the cashmere, her respectability is compromised.

4. See Edward Said, *Culture and Imperialism* (New York: Knopf, 1993). See also Ruth Yeazell, *Harems of the Mind: Passages of Western Art and Literature* (New Haven, Conn.: Yale University Press, 2000).

5. Michelle Maskiell, "Consuming Kashmir: Shawls and Empires, 1500–2000," *Journal of World History* 13:1 (2002): 27–65, quote on 32.

6. Walter Benjamin, *The Arcades Project*, trans. Howard Eiland and Kevin McLaughlin (Cambridge, Mass.: Belknap Press, 1999), 55.

7. This is not the subject of my work. See, however, for example, Mary Louise Pratt, *Imperial Eyes* (New York: Routledge, 1992), and Lisa Lowe, *Critical Terrains: French and British Orientalisms* (Ithaca, N.Y.: Cornell University Press, 1991), for discussions of this question.

8. One recent exception is Marni Kessler's approach in *Sheer Presence*. See especially ch. 5, "The Other Side of the Veil," 94–141.

9. Maskiell offers a full and fresh consideration of the historical trade in cashmeres from a global perspective. Her concern is primarily with British reception of cashmere, and she wishes to redress a Eurocentric perspective that she claims has given undue weight to the European consumption of cashmere at the expense of the Eastern history of production and trade. For a recent and fascinating discussion of the history of the production and consumption of the Kashmiri shawl and its relation to British empire, see also Chitralekha Zutshi, "'Designed for Eternity': Kashmiri Shawls, Empire, and Cultures of Production and Consumption in Mid-Victorian Britain," *Journal of British Studies* 48 (April 2009): 420–40.

10. Frank Ames, *The Kashmir Shawl and Its Indo-French Influence* (Woodbridge, England: Antique Collectors' Club,1997), 135. Earlier still, French traders to India in the seventeenth and eighteenth centuries had discovered the valuable *cachemire*.

11. Another pertinent understanding of the term *domestication* would involve the appropriation of Eastern textiles and fabrication techniques by French manufacturers. These manufacturers imported Tibetan goats, studied Eastern weaving practices, and called their shawls *cachemires*, a word identical to the place name of the origin of the shawls—Kashmir. Michelle Maskiell writes, "This appropriation, a naturalization of the violence enabling colonial possession of shawl design as well as the earlier possession of Kashmiri shawls, continues today in Europe and in America" (29).

12. Woodruff D. Smith, 76.

13. The word itself, borrowed in French from the place of origin, combines two French words suggestive of seductive play: *cacher* (to hide) and *mirer* (to reflect). My thanks to Patricia Célérier for pointing this out to me.

14. With its Napoleonic origins, already the cashmere shawl falls within the purview of the "noblesse d'Empire," but, as Sarah Maza argues, for Balzac, this was nonetheless a legitimate aristocracy, for "he believed that social hierarchy - though not necessarily of a traditional sort - was a natural and desirable source of order and stability." Sarah Maza, "Uniforms: The Social Imaginary in Balzac's *La Cousine Bette*," *French Politics, Culture and Society* 19 (Summer 2001): 23. What is coded as "aristocracy" in many of Balzac's novels is in fact this other aristocracy, created by Napoléon. Camille Laparra develops the notion of the "two aristocracies" of pre–July Monarchy France as represented in Balzac's work in her article "L'Aristocratie dans *La Comédie humaine* de Balzac: ses pluralismes," *French Review* 68:4 (March 1995): 602–14.

15. Betty Werther, "Paisley in Perspective: The Cashmere Shawl in France," *American Craft* 58 (February–March 1983): 6–8, 88, quote on 88.

16. For a complete discussion, see Monique Lévi-Strauss, *Cachemires parisiens 1810–1880 à l'école de l'Asie* (Paris: Éditions des Musées de la Ville de Paris, 1998).

17. See, for example, MM. Gabriel and Armand, *La Féerie des arts, ou le sultan de cachemire (folie féerique, vaudeville en un acte)* (Paris: Huet-Masson, 1819), Henri Dupin, *Le Cachemire, comédie en un acte et en prose* (Paris: Masson, 1810), and J.-B. Dubois, *Le Cachemire, ou l'étrenne à la mode, comédie anécdotique, en un acte et en prose* (Paris: Barba, 1811).

18. Deportment manual of 1863 cited by Philippe Perrot and quoted in Maskiell, 39.

19. Nathalie Aubert proposes that *La Cousine Bette* illustrates the emergence of women as a social class: "Si la subversion, à la veille de 1848, est féminine, c'est parce que ce sont les femmes du peuple qui émergent après le triomphe total, mais de brève durée, de la petite bourgeoisie" (If subversion, on the eve of 1848, is feminine, it is because it is women of the people who emerge after the total, if brief, triumph, of the petty bourgesoisie). Nathalie Aubert, "En attendant les barbares: *La Cousine Bette*, le moment populaire et féminin de *La Comédie humaine*," *Women in French Studies* 8 (2000): 136.

20. Julien Hayem, Licencié ès-lettres, Avocat à la Cour impériale, *M. X*** contre Mlle Z***, Plaidoyer prononcé à la chambre du tribunal civil de la Seine pour un Cachemire des Indes* (Paris: Chaix, 1868). The case is fascinating because it addresses not only the question of the impropriety of unmarried ladies wearing shawls but also the problem of a shawl's authenticity. One reason Mlle Z*** apparently doesn't want to pay the remainder of the bill is that she has determined that the shawl is *français* and not *des Indes* as was claimed. Another fascinating digression that this court transcript invites is an examination of the Parisian used-clothing market in the nineteenth century. Mlle Z*** obtained the

shawl from a consignment merchant, and its original owner, an elderly lady, had pawned it at the Mont-de Piété.

21. See Simmel, "Fashion," who defines fashion through this paradox.

22. John Irwin, *Shawls: A Study of Indo-European Influences* (London: Her Majesty's Stationery Office, 1955), 27.

23. I refer here to the Lyon silk riots of 1831, 1833, and 1848, violent uprisings by the Canuts (the silk workers of Lyon) in protest over worker exploitation. Both men and women worked in the silk workshops.

24. Honoré de Balzac, *La Cousine Bette*, ed. André Lorant (Paris: Garnier-Flammarion, 1977), 82. All references are to this edition unless otherwise indicated. All translations are from *The Works of Honoré de Balzac*, vol. 11, ed. George Saintsbury (Freeport, N.Y.: Books for Libraries, 1971), 31–32.

25. See, for example, in reference to *La Cousine Bette*, Peter Hulme, "Balzac's Parisian Mystery: *La Cousine Bette* and the Writing of Historical Criticism," *Literature and History* 11:1 (Spring 1985): 47–64, and Aubert; and in reference to *L'Éducation sentimentale*, among others, Michel Crouzet "Passion et politique dans *L'Éducation sentimentale*," in *Flaubert, la femme, la ville*, ed. Marie-Claire Bancquart (Paris: Presses Universitaires de France, 1982), 39–71.

26. Hulme addresses this theme at some length, asserting that the primary axis of interpretation of the novel is the trope of "civilisation and barbarism. These terms entered the political debate in response to the incident that Marx would later refer to as marking the beginning of class conflict in France: the 1831 Lyons silk riots." He goes on to quote a contemporary journalist who, focusing on the vocabulary of possession, writes, "The uprising at Lyons has brought to light a grave secret, the civil strife that is taking place in society between the possessing class and the class that does not possess" (56).

27. It is curious that Bette is repeatedly assimilated to Napoléon both in the novel's insistence on her "imperialist" thirst for power and in the adjective frequently used to describe her character—Corsican.

28. Flaubert never explicitly indicates that this particular shawl is a *cachemire*; however, as I show below, there are sufficient signs in the text to support this assumption, notably, its value, its links to exoticism, and its quality of warmth. My thanks to Anna-Lisa Dieter for raising this question.

29. Gustave Flaubert, *L'Éducation sentimentale*, ed. Pierre-Louis Rey (Paris: Pocket, 1998), 24. All references are to this edition unless otherwise indicated. Translations from Gustave Flaubert, *Sentimental Education*, ed. and trans. Robert Baldick (New York: Penguin, 1964), 19.

30. For a very suggestive discussion of Arnoux's relationship to kitsch, see Juliette Frølich, *Des hommes, des femmes et des choses: Langages de l'objet dans le roman de Balzac à Proust* (Vincennes: Presse Universitaires de Vincennes, 1997): "tout en étant un formidable consommateur d'objets kitsch, Arnoux est d'abord, dans ce Paris capitale du XIXe siècle flaubertien, un fabricant d'objets d'art et de kitsch. En effet, au moment de son incontestable succès, il 'fabrique' et vend tout

ce qui relève du savoir-vivre de son époque; c'est lui qui octroie à la classe bourgeoise les objets qui meublent ses intérieurs; c'est son commerce qui 'donne le ton' socio-esthétique. C'est lui qui est la Mode: son commerce d'objets marque de son cachet particulier l'esprit bourgeois de son temps" (65) (All the while an extraordinary consumer of kitsch, Arnoux is first, in Flaubert's Parisian capital of the nineteenth century, a maker of kitsch art objects. Indeed, at the height of his success, he "makes" and sells everything pertaining to the manners of his time; he is the one who distributes to the bourgeoisie the objects that will decorate their homes; his business determines socioaesthetic tone. He is Fashion: his trade in objects gives an identifiable cachet to the bourgeois mindset of his time).

31. See in particular Georges Zaragoza, "Le Coffret de Madame Arnoux ou l'achèvement d'une éducation," *Revue d'histoire littéraire française* 89:4 (July–August 1989): 674–88. The author does some very fine readings of this key scene, but it should be noted that he incorrectly places it at "ce premier décembre 1848," an error that empties out the political punch of Flaubert's juxtaposition of the scene of the "vente aux enchères" and the immenent coup d'état of Louis-Napoléon of December 2, 1851. Surely Flaubert wished to connect the humiliation and desecration of the idealized Marie Arnoux with the failed Republic.

32. This scene also offers an ironic intertextual inversion of the famous opening scene of Alexandre Dumas fils's 1848 novel *La Dame aux camélias*, discussed in Chapter 1. As we recall, this novel opens with the scandalous auctioning of the courtesan Marguerite Gautier's effects, among them *cachemires*, and present for purchase and ogling are both high society women and prostitutes.

33. Eugène Labiche, *Le Cachemire X.B.T.*, in *Théâtre complet*, vol. 6 (Paris: Calmann Lévy, 1885), 415–63.

34. Marcel Proust, *À la recherche du temps perdu*, vol. 1 (Paris: Gallimard, Bibliothèque de la Pléiade, 1954), 36. All references are to this edition unless otherwise indicated. Translations from Marcel Proust, *Swann's Way,* trans. C. K. Scott Moncrieff and Terence Kilmartin (New York: Vintage, 1989), 39.

35. Marcel Proust, *À la recherche du temps perdu*, vol. 8, 724. Translation from Marcel Proust, *Time Regained*, trans. Andreas Mayor and Terence Kilmartin (New York: Random House, 1993), 48.

CHAPTER 4

1. Gustave Flaubert, *Madame Bovary*, ed. Pierre-Marc de Biasi (Paris: Seuil, l'école des lettres, 1992), 33. All references unless otherwise indicated are to this edition. All translations are from Gustave Flaubert, *Madame Bovary*, ed. and trans. Geoffrey Wall (New York: Penguin, 1992), 13.

2. Quote from anonymous author. "Bulletin des modes," *La Mode*, 26 March 1847: 584 ("dômes portatifs" in original).

3. Bonnie Smith documents women's shift in status and role during the nineteenth century through case studies of bourgeois industrialists' families in north-

eastern France, the region perhaps best known for Valenciennes lace and other textiles. She traces the emergence of a gendered division of space, in which women became the caretakers of the domestic and men focused on the capitalist enterprises of their industries. Thorstein Veblen, *Conspicuous Consumption* (New York: Penguin Books, 2006), explains that leisure emerges alongside consumption, as a signifier of status and even honor in a society that prizes wealth and abstinence from physical labor. Women, and wives in particular, become the decorative ornaments displaying a family's status and decency through their persons, their attire, and their domestic and leisure activities.

4. Veblen defines leisure as "non-productive consumption of time" and links it to domesticity by characterizing many of the domestic duties of the household as "vicarious leisure." He explains, "There supervenes a division of labour among the servants or dependents whose life is spent in maintaining the honour of the gentleman of leisure. So that, while one group produces goods for him, another group, usually headed up by the wife, or chief wife, consumes for him in conspicuous leisure, thereby putting in evidence his ability to sustain large pecuniary damage without impairing his superior opulence" (*Conspicuous Consumption*, 35, 40).

5. *Dictionnaire de l'Académie française*, 6th ed., 1835 (ARTFL), http://artflx.uchicago.edu.libproxy.vassar.edu/cgi-bin/dicos/pubdico1look.pl?strippedhw=ombrelle. The *parapluie*, which evolves after the *ombrelle*, also derives from the parasol: "L'origine du parasol, ancêtre commun de l'ombrelle et du parapluie, reste obscure" (the origins of the parasol, the common ancestor of the *ombrelle* and the umbrella, remains obscure), recounts Annie Sagalow in her essay on the honorific origins of the parasol, "L'Ombrelle," in *Les Accessoires du temps: ombrelles et parapluies*, exhibition catalogue, ed. Catherine Join-Diérterle (Paris: Paris Galliéra, 1989–90), 16–45.

6. See the Musée de la Mode et du Costume's exhibition catalogue *Indispensables accessoires: XVI–XXe siècle* (Paris: Galliéra, 1983–84).

7. Gloves also function in this way: recall that Ourika, the title chararacter of Claire de Duras's 1823 novel, on realizing she is not white, wears gloves constantly.

8. See Richard Dyer, *White* (New York: Routledge, 1997).

9. See Pauline Schloesser, *The Fair Sex: White Women and Racial Patriarchy in the Early American Republic* (New York: New York University Press, 2002). While Schloesser limits her analysis of the linkage between whiteness and ideal femininity to the English context, as she is interested in the Anglo-Saxon origins of the articulations of whiteness in early America, Dyer's study, and more recently, Elsa Dorlin's *La Matrice de la race*, make similar claims more broadly about Western European culture. Elsa Dorlin, *La Matrice de la race* (Paris: Éditions la Découverte, 2006).

10. Dorlin, 216. The classic work on the subject of France's evolving theories of race is William Cohen, *The French Encounter with Africans: White Response to Black, 1530–1880* (Bloomington: Indiana University Press, 1980).

11. Cohen writes, "Frenchmen saw the blackness of Africans as symbolic of

some inner depravity, since they thought the color aesthetically unappealing. They followed a tradition rooted in the classical doctrine of *physiognomos*, which held that what was not beautiful was somehow depraved" (14).

12. *Dictionnaire de l'Académie française*, http://artflx.uchicago.edu.libproxy. vassar.edu/cgi-bin/dicos/pubdico1look.pl?strippedhw=blanc. "'Propre par opposition à Sale'; Fig. et fam., Sortir d'une accusation, d'une affaire, blanc comme neige, Être déclaré innocent, être acquitté par un arrêt ou un jugement, en matière criminelle ou correctionnelle. BLANC, ANCHE se dit en outre, substantivement, Des races d'hommes qui ont le teint blanc, ou même olivâtre, à la différence de celles qui l'ont noir. Cet enfant est fils d'un blanc et d'une négresse. Il est né d'une blanche et d'un nègre. Il y a, dans cette colonie, moins de blancs que d'hommes de couleur" ("Clean by contrast to dirty"; figurative and familiar. To get out of an accusation, a situation, white like snow, To be declared innocent, to be acquitted by a stay or a judgment, in a criminal or correctional matter. WHITE is used as well as a substantive, Human races of white complexion, or even olive, as opposed to those of dark complexion. This child is the son of a white and a negress. He is born of a white and a Negro. In this colony, there are fewer whites than men of color). The *Dictionnaire de la langue française* of Émile Littré of 1872 repeats the same definitions.

13. Octave Uzanne, *La Femme et la mode: métamorphoses de la Parisienne de 1792 à 1892* (Paris: May, 1892), iii. Article 213 of the *Code Civil* mandates that "Le mari doit protection à sa femme, la femme obéissance à son mari" (30) (The husband owes protection to his wife, the wife obedience to her husband).

14. A similar gendering can be seen in consumption practices of men and women. Colin Campbell's 1993 study reveals that male shoppers were guided by a principle of utility, whereas female shoppers were driven by pleasure. These gendered practices and observations regarding consumption emerge with the advent of shopping as a leisure activity. See Colin Campbell, "Shopping, Pleasure, and the Sex War," in *The Shopping Experience*, ed. Pasi Falk and Colin Campbell, 166–76 (London: Sage, 1997).

15. Maurice Gardot, "Parasol et parapluie," *Journal des demoiselles* 54:12 (1883): 317–20. The etymology of the word *riflard* instructs: "Dû à la vogue d'une pièce de Picard (*La Petite ville*, 1801), où l'acteur chargé du rôle ridicule de Riflard paraît armé d'un énorme parapluie" (Result of the fad of a play by Picard (*La Petite ville*, 1801), in which the actor in the ridiculous role of Riflard appears armed with an enormous umbrella). Émile Littré, *Dictionnaire de la langue française*, 1872–77, ARTFL Project, http://artflx.uchicago.edu.libproxy.vassar.edu/cgi-bin/dicos/pub-dico1look.pl?strippedhw=riflard.

16. An *en-cas* was a dainty lady's umbrella; "en cas" means "in case," presumably, of rain.

17. See Danielle Dupuis, "La Mode féminine dans les romans de mœurs d'Honoré de Balzac," Ph.D. diss. (Université de Paris IV, Sorbonne, 1988).

18. Anonymous, "Modes," *Le Journal des demoiselles* 37:4 (1869): 123.

19. Jeremy Farrell, *Umbrellas and Parasols* (London: Batsford, 1985), 62–63.

20. Émile Zola, *Au Bonheur des Dames*, ed. Robert Sctrick and Claude Aziza (Paris: Pocket, 1990), 252. All references hereinafter to this text are to this edition. Translations from Émile Zola, *The Ladies' Paradise*, ed. and trans. Brian Nelson (New York: Oxford University Press, 2008), 241–42. All references unless otherwise indicated are to this translation.

21. In her article on Victorian fashion plates, Sharon Marcus discusses the paradoxical role of nineteenth-century fashion iconography on many levels. She makes the point here that in spite of a great deal of caricature of women's fashions in the press which targeted women and trivialized fashion, fashion plates and images and advertisements in fashion journals were publicizing for consumption and broadly proclaiming the desirability of those same fashions. Sharon Marcus, "Reflections on Victorian Fashion Plates," *Differences: A Journal of Feminist Cultural Studies* 14:3 (Fall 2003): 4–33.

22. MM. Arsène and Eugène Trouvé, *Une Ombrelle compromise par un parapluie: Vaudeville en un acte*, in *Théâtre contemporain illustré*, vol. 5, no. 41 (Paris: Michel Lévy frères, 1861), 1–6.

23. For a fresh analysis of the pervasiveness of jealousy in nineteenth-century literature, see Masha Belenky, *The Anxiety of Dispossession: Jealousy in Nineteenth-Century French Culture* (Lewisburg, Pa.: Bucknell University Press, 2008).

24. See Summers for a history of the corset.

25. Farrell provides a rich history of the accessory, drawing on both British and French sources. In an article on the *parapluie* in her recent encyclopedia of clothing, entitled *Les Habits*, Claire d'Harcourt writes of the importance of the *canne* and its aristocratic symbolic value: "C'est la canne, adoptée par les hommes comme par les femmes, qui soutient les pas et complète la toilette des gentilshommes, qui la préfèrent désormais à l'épée" (203) (it's the cane, adopted by men as well as women, which supports the step and completes the look of gentlemen, who prefer it now to the sword); and of the *parapluie* and its more humble associations: "Brevets d'invention se multiplient pour perfectionner cet abri portatif qui devient, sous le règne de Louis-Philippe, le symbole de la bourgeoisie—le roi lui-même se promène fréquemment parapluie à la main. Acteurs de théâtre, caricaturistes et pamphlétaires ridiculisent alors le parapluie, synonyme des vertus domestiques de ce petit-bourgeois ventripotent, rangé, médiocre et solennel. Dans les campagnes, seules quelques riches paysannes possèdent un parapluie, dont l'usage ne se généralisera qu'à la fin du XIXe siècle, comme en atteste le portrait de Bécassine" (205) (Patents multiply to perfect this portable shelter which becomes, under Louis-Philippe's reign, the symbol of the bourgeoisie—the king himself frequently strolls umbrella in hand. Theater actors, caricaturists, and pamphleteers ridicule the umbrella, a synonym of the domestic virtues of this portly, uptight, mediocre and somber petty-bourgeois. In the country, only a few rich peasants own an umbrella, the use of which becomes common only at the end of the nineteenth century, as the portrait of Becassine attests). Claire d'Harcourt, *Les Habits* (Paris: Seuil, 2001).

26. Evelyne Woestelandt, "Système de la mode dans *L'Éducation sentimentale*," *French Review* 58:2 (December 1984): 245.

27. Horace Raisson, *Le Code de la toilette: manuel complet d'élégance et d'hygiène, contenant les lois, règles, applications et exemples de l'art de soiger sa personne et de s'habiller avec goût et méthode* (Paris: Roret, 1828), 28.

28. Philippe Perrot, *Le Travail des apparences, ou, les transformations du corps feminine, VIII–XIXe siècle* (Paris: Éditions du Seuil, 1984).

29. See d'Harcourt, 205–6.

30. Anonymous, "Bulletin des modes," *La Mode* (26 March 1847): 584.

31. See Alain Corbin, *L'Avènement des loisirs, 1850–1960* (Paris: Aubier, 1995).

32. For an overview of the cosmetics and makeup industries in nineteenth-century America, which drew on the same traditions as those in France, see in particular ch. 1, "Masks and Faces," in Kathy Peiss, *Hope in a Jar: The Making of America's Beauty Culture* (New York: Holt, 1998). According to Peiss, the use of makeup was not meant to be noticeable for ladies, and a strict division was insisted upon between cosmetics, or reparative products, and makeup, considered paints and therefore artificial. Peiss offers examples of how the concealment of one's use of deadly makeup products often led to death.

33. See also Peiss.

34. François-René de Chateaubriand, *Atala*, ed. Pierre Moreau (Paris: Gallimard, 1971), 69. All references are to this edition unless otherwise indicated. Translations are from François-René de Chateaubriand, *Atala*, trans. Irving Putter (Berkeley: University of California Press, 1952), 37. On the popularization of images of Atala, Naomi Schor writes, "The publication of *Atala* was by all accounts (and not just Chateaubriand's, that master of self-promotion) a major literary event. The exotic tale of doomed love between a Europeanized noble savage and a Christianized Indian maiden made Chateaubriand a celebrity and gave rise to a veritable industry of popular iconography and artifacts" (136). Naomi Schor, "*Triste Amérique*: *Atala* and the Construction of Post-Revolutionary Femininity," in *Bad Objects: Essays Popular and Unpopular*, 132–48 (Durham, N.C.: Duke University Press, 1995). And Susan Delaney, in her study of *Atala*'s reception in popular culture, documents how Chateaubriand's heroine was the subject of classical painters and printmakers alike. She writes, "*Atala* also provided subjects for decorative artists: scenes from the novel appeared on vases, plates, upholstery fabrics and clocks. And the theme was common in popular graphic arts. Printmakers stamped Atala's image on cheap, garishly-colored engravings meant for unsophisticated people who had nothing in common with the aristocratic Chateaubriand but their pleasure in the love story he wrote" (209). Susan Delaney, "*Atala* in the Arts," in *The Wolf and the Lamb: Popular Culture in France from the Old Regime to the Twentieth Century*, ed. Jacques Beauroy, Marc Bertrand, and Edward T. Gargan, 209–31 (Satatoga, Calif.: Amna Libri, 1977).

35. Atala's virginity is one of her most appealing qualities to the unlettered public, according to Delaney. The visual iconography of virginity, of which white-

ness is key, becomes essential to an unreading public. "Atala becomes a *vedette*, an example of the virtuous female. For over five decades her image is carried throughout the provinces and printers add multilingual captions in response to her widespread popularity" (218).

36. Honoré de Balzac, *Le Lys dans la vallée*, ed. Roger Pierrot (Paris: Librairie Générale, 1984). All references to this novel are from this edition unless otherwise indicated. Translations from Balzac, *Balzac's Works*, vol. 9.

37. See Sagalow, who cites Dupuis's dissertation, "La Mode féminine."

38. As she languishes in the knowledge that Félix has slept with Lady Dudley and thus betrayed her, she begs him to love her "saintement," "comme une vierge Marie, qui doit rester dans ses voiles et sous sa couronne blanche" (182) (like the virgin Mary, who must remain veiled and under her white crown).

39. The theme of whiteness in this novel is everywhere, especially with respect to Madame de Mortsauf's *toilettes*. Seemingly always dressed in white and referred to constantly as "ma blanche Henriette," "Blanche," or metaphorically as "le lys dans la vallée," she is the fictional hyperbole of female marital virtue and maternal sacrifice. Peter Brooks's article "Virtue-Tripping: Notes on *Le Lys dans la vallée*," in *Yale French Studies* 50 (1974): 150–62, is particularly useful in contextualizing the notion of virtue and establishing this novel as its "deconstruction."

40. See Peter Brooks, "Storied Bodies, or Nana at Last Unveil'd," *Critical Inquiry* 16:1 (1989): 1–32, for a rich analysis of this opening scene and of the novel's relationship to contemporary painting. See also two other important pieces that discuss the problematics of Nana's nudity: Janet Beizer, *Ventriloquized Bodies: Narratives of Hysteria in Nineteenth-Century France* (Ithaca, N.Y.: Cornell University Press, 1993), 174–87, and Therese Dolan, "Guise and Dolls: Dis/covering Power, Re/Covering Nana," *Nineteenth-Century French Studies* 26:3–4 (1998): 368–86.

41. Émile Zola, *Nana*, ed. Marie-Ange Voisin-Fougère (Paris: Flammarion, 2000), 39. All further references will be to this edition. All translations of this novel refer to the following edition: Émile Zola, *Nana*, trans. Burton Rascoe, ed. Luc Sante (New York: Barnes and Noble Classics, 2006), 7.

42. See Kessler on *maquillage*; see also Philippe Perrot, *Le Travail des apparences*.

43. Sander Gilman, *Difference and Pathology: Stereotypes of Sexuality, Race, and Madness* (Ithaca, N.Y.: Cornell University Press, 1985).

44. Gilman's argument is complex and dense. He draws a parallel between the discursive and visual representations of the black woman and the prostitute in nineteenth-century Europe (mostly France and England) by considering scientific documents, paintings, and novelistic discourse of the period. He concludes that the black woman and the prostitute, through their discursive and visual assimilation, reveal the pathologizing of female sexuality in the nineteenth century. For an important and insightful reexamination of Gilman's pathbreaking article, see Zine Magubane, "Which Bodies Matter? Feminism, Poststructuralism, Race, and the Curious Theoretical Odyssey of the 'Hottentot Venus,'" *Gender and Society* 15:6 (2001): 816–34.

45. Beizer, 181. Beizer offers a compelling reading of Nana's nudity and the veiling processes of discourse that the novel performs.

46. See Dolan and Gilman.

47. Charles Bernheimer writes, "Nana's bisexuality participates in both the currents of male fantasy that I am analyzing. As same-sex love, it has obvious analogies with Nana's auto-seduction in the mirror. Its premise is 'open contempt for the male' (N, 1368), and Nana and Satin together emasculate an entire assembly of aristocratic men, smearing them with the ordure of their working-class origin (this origin is, in Zola's bourgeois fantasy, the social equivalent of castration). Futhermore, Nana's lesbianism constitutes a breach within her desire that erodes and decomposes the biological model of sexuality, the vital basis of the patriarchal social order" (226). Charles Bernheimer, *Figures of Ill Repute: Representing Prostitution in Nineteenth-Century France* (1989; reprint, Durham, N.C.: Duke University Press, 1997).

48. The pairing of *Le Lys* and *Nana* has been brilliantly orchestrated in Colette Becker's illuminating article "Dire la femme en régime réaliste/naturaliste: du lys à la chienne en chaleur," in, *Europäische Realismen: Facetten, Konvergenzen, Differenzen: Internationales Symposium der Fachrichtung Romanistik an der Universität des Saarlande*, ed. Uwe Dethloff, 263–75 (Röhrig Universitätsverlag, St. Ingbert, Germany: Annales Universitatis Saraviensis, Philosophische Fakultät, 2001).

49. See in particular Hannah Thompson, *Naturalism Undressed: Identity and Clothing in the Novels of Émile Zola* (Oxford: Legenda, 2004) for lively and informed discussions of Nana's unstable identity.

50. See Bernheimer, *Figures of Ill Repute*.

51. Louis Chollet, *Monsieur Parapluie et Mademoiselle Ombrelle* (Tours: Maison Mame et Fils, 1912), 12.

CHAPTER 5

1. For a fascinating look at this object, especially in the context of women's embroidery, see Mary Donaldson-Evans, "Pricking the Male Ego: Pins and Needles in Flaubert, Maupassant and Zola," *Nineteenth-Century French Studies* 30:3-4 (2002): 254–65. For some of the best discussions of the scene of the Vaubyessard ball in *Madame Bovary*, see Mary Orr, "Reflections on 'Bovarysme': The Bovarys at Vaubyessard," *French Studies Bulletin: A Quarterly Supplement* 61 (Winter 1996): 6–8, and Jorge Pedraza, "Le Shopping d'Emma," in *Emma Bovary*, ed. Alain Buisine, 100–121 (Paris: Éditions Autrement, 1997). The gallant romance that Emma imagines as she gazes upon the cigar case's embroidery work is comparable to the visual stories typically painted on ladies' fans.

2. I am thinking in particular of her emotional use of the keepsakes and of the broader cultural phenomenon of historical fetishism that the novel illustrates in objects such as the plates from which Emma and her father eat at the *auberge* on their way to the convent, painted with scenes of the life of Mademoiselle de La

Vallière. Emma's attachment to things has been well documented. See in particular Carol Rifelj, "'Ces Tableaux du Monde': Keepsakes in Madame Bovary," *Nineteenth-Century French Studies* 25:3–4 (1997): 360–85, and Pedraza.

3. See Edward J. Ahearn, "The Magic Cigar Case: Emma Bovary and Karl Marx," in *Women's Voices and Figures, from Marie de France to Marie Cardinal*, ed. Michel Guggenheim, 181–86 (Palo Alto, Calif.: Stanford French and Italian Studies, 1989).

4. Fans were routinely painted with scenes of gallantry. As Avril Hart and Emma Taylor maintain, "The scenes of quiet flirtation and summer walks in the country which are characteristic of eighteenth-century Pastoral fans might be seen to echo the activities of the ladies carrying them. . . . The French artist who most influenced the painters of pastoral fans throughout Europe was Antoine Watteau (1684–1721)" (28–29). Avril Hart and Emma Taylor, *Fans* (London: V&A Publications, 1998). See also Françoise de Perthuis and Vincent Meylan, *Éventails* (Paris: Éditions Hermé, 1989), in particular "La Vie sociale au XVIIIe siècle dans les décors d'éventails," in which the authors discuss the influence of Mme de Pompadour and the artist François Boucher on the reproduction of "scènes galantes" on fans.

5. "Le Lac," published in 1820 in Alphonse de Lamartine's *Méditations poétiques*. Along with a romantic meditation on the theme of time's passage, the poem recounts the autobiographical story of the poet's emotional response upon returning to the lake where he first knew his now dead lover. The poem was well known in its day, an anthem of French romanticism and lost love.

6. See Tony Tanner, *Adultery and the Novel: Contract and Transgression* (Baltimore: Johns Hopkins University Press, 1981), for an authoritative analysis of the place of *Madame Bovary* in the literary history of adultery. The concept of the fetish has been widely studied, most frequently in relation to its anthropological and psychoanalytic origins. More recently, fashion historians have taken up the notion of fetish in connection with fetishistic fashion, e.g., corsets and certain fabrics. Valerie Steele's *Fetish: Fashion, Sex and Power* (New York: Oxford University Press, 1996) brings together a broad range of cultural discourses on the fetish and offers a helpful overview of the critical uses of the term. I am using the term to suggest the intense power and value of a particular fashion accessory—the fan—in nineteenth-century France to connote both female sexuality and nostalgic worship for a bygone era. In both circumstances, Freud's understanding of the fetish object as standing in for something that is apparently absent does apply. See also E. L. McCallum, *Object Lessons: How to Do Things with Fetishism* (Albany: State University of New York Press, 1999), Emily Apter and William Pietz, *Fetishism as Cultural Discourse* (Ithaca, N.Y.: Cornell University Press, 1993), and Slavlov Zizek, *The Plague of Fantasies* (New York: Verso, 1997), ch. 3, for more developed analyses of the concept of fetishism.

7. See Valerie Steele, *The Fan* (New York: Rizzoli International Publications, 2002), and Hart and Taylor in particular.

8. Steele, *The Fan*, 14.

9. Henry Vesseron, *Études et souvenirs* (Sedan: Tellier, 1870).

10. Steele, *The Fan*, 14.

11. Elizabeth Outka, *Consuming Traditions: Modernity, Modernism, and the Commodified Authentic* (New York: Oxford University Press, 2009). What Outka observes in relation to late nineteenth-century Britain is already at work in mid-nineteenth-century France and is in plain view throughout Flaubert's novel. As Outka proposes, "the commodified authentic emerged as an appealing and dexterous tool, one uniquely designed to satisfy both a longing for tradition and a rapidly modernizing future" (7).

12. Ali Coffignon, "Accessoires féminins," *Paris-vivant: les coulisses de la mode* (Paris: Librairie illustrée, 1888), 231–38, quote from 236.

13. Baronne Staffe in a treatise on feminine accessories called *Les Hochets féminins* offers further insight into the "langage de l'éventail": "Ailleurs, quand un gentleman présente à une femme, de la main gauche, l'éventail qu'elle a laissé tombé et qu'il vient de lui ramasser, c'est un aveu de l'impression que la dame a faite sur lui. Si elle reçoit l'objet de la main gauche aussi, c'est qu'elle accueille favorablement l'offre de cette sympathie. Si elle prend l'éventail de la main droite au contraire, elle refuse ce cœur qui voulait se donner à elle" (Moreover, when a gentleman presents to a women, with his left hand, a fan that she has dropped and that he has just retrieved for her, it is an admission of the impression that the lady has made on him. If she receives the object with her left hand also, it means that she welcomes with favor the offer of this sentiment. If she takes the fan with her right hand, on the contrary, she refuses this heart, which wanted to give itself to her). Baronne Staffe, *Les Hochets féminins: les pierres précieuses, les bijoux, la dentelle, la broderie, l'éventail, quelques autres superfluités* (Paris: Flammarion, 1902), 295. On the language of the fan and its relation to kitsch, see Noël Valis, *The Culture of Cursilería: Bad Taste, Kitsch, and Class in Modern Spain* (Durham, N.C.: Duke University Press, 2002).

14. Duvelleroy was perhaps the best known *éventailliste* of the Second Empire, famous for his luxury fans representing imitations of famous paintings by eighteenth-century masters, such as Watteau. He was a good publicist and understood the evolving market for women's fashions. See Perthuis and Meylan.

15. Quoted in Coffignon, who in turn claims to be repeating "les indications véridiques d'un initié" (237) (the true instructions of an initiate).

16. Gustave Droz, "Sous l'éventail," in *Entre nous* (Paris: Havard, 1883).

17. See Michel Maignan, *L'Éventail à tous vents: du XVI au XXe siècle* (Paris: Le Louvre des Antiquaires, 1989), for an overview of the history of the fan.

18. "Sur la requête à lui présentée par 'les maîtres doreurs sur cuir et autres ouvriers exerçans le métier d'éventailliste,' au nombre de soixante, Louis XIV les constitua en corporation par un édit du 23 mars 1673" (On the request presented to him by "the master painters of gold on leather and other workers in the fan-making profession," in the number of sixty, Louis XIV constituted them as a guild by the edict of March 23, 1673). Exposition internationale, *Travaux de la commission française sur l'industrie des nations*, 12 vols. (Paris: Imprimerie impériale, 1854–67),

vol. 7, *Exposition universelle de 1851*, intro. by M. le baron Charles Dupin, 74. See also Joan DeJean, *The Essence of Style: How the French Invented High Fashion, Fine Food, Chic Cafés, Style, Sophistication, and Glamour* (New York: Free Press, 2005).

19. Edmond and Jules de Goncourt, *La Femme du dix-huitième siècle*, Elibron Classics Series (1862; facsimile ed., Adamant Media Corporation, 2006). See also Uzanne.

20. Exposition internationale, 75.

21. J.-B. Fonssagriues, *Dictionnaire de la santé ou répertoire d'hygiène pratique à l'usage des familles et des écoles* (Paris: Librairie Charles Delagrave, 1876), 364.

22. Hart and Taylor, 49.

23. See Carmen Martin Gaite's *Love Customs of Eighteenth-Century Spain*, trans. Maria G. Tomsich (Berkeley: University of California Press, 1991). It was in Spain that this "language" was perfected. "Dans un pays où la Sainte Inquisition règne en maîtresse et où les mœurs sont particulièrement rigides, il est parfois dangereux de s'aventurer inconsidérément sur la 'Carte du Tendre.'. . . . [L]es Espagnols vont-ils mettre au point un code très perfectionné dont l'instrument principal sera l'éventail" (Perthuis and Meylan, 25) (In a country where the Holy Inquisition dominates and where the customs are particularly rigid, it is sometimes dangerous to wander thoughtlessly on the "Carte du Tendre.". . . . [T]he Spanish would develop and perfect a code whose main tool would be the fan).

24. Quoted in Lady Morgan, *Le Livre du boudoir*, vol. 2, trans. A.-J.-B. Defauconpret (Paris: Gosselin, 1829), 3–4.

25. These smaller fans became conflated during the Restoration with another indispensable object of ballroom behavior—the *carnet de bal*. The small fan would open to reveal vellum sheets on which a lady would inscribe her dance partner's name, the type of dance, etc. See, for example, Balzac's *Le Père Goriot*, which features this object; Honoré de Balzac, *Le Père Goriot*, edited by Félicien Marceau (Paris: Gallimard, 1999).

26. Gabriel Marc, "L'Éventail," in *Sonnets parisiens* (Paris: Lemerre, 1875).

27. From the *Journal des dames et des modes*, (April or May) 1798, we find "L'éventail de Juliette" (15–16):

Combien j'aime à voir voltiger
Cet éventail léger!
Sur la rose et le lys il erre et se promène;
Il rafraîchit ta douce haleine;
Soulève ton fichu, permet qu'un demi-jour
Eclaire d'un beau sein le ravissant contour.
Quand je suis d'un regard avide
Son mouvement rapide,
Mon cœur est agité des plus brûlants désirs . . .
J'écarte l'importun, j'applique sur ta bouche
Tendre baiser qui s'exhale en soupirs.
Juliette devient farouche,

Et le coup d'éventail vient chasser les plaisirs;
Mais pourquoi te cédé-je, aimable Juliette?
L'amour me prête un de ses traits;
Vite au combat, et serrons-nous de près.
Tu n'oses pas . . . ; Tu fuis . . . ; craindrais-tu ta défaite?

[How I love to see it fly
This lightweight fan!
On the rose and lily it wanders and strolls;
It refreshes your sweet breath;
Lifts your fichu, allows a little peek
Reveals a ravishingly curvy bosom.
When I follow with a hungry eye
Its quick movements,
My heart beats with the most burning desires . . .
I remove the intruder, and give your lips
A tender kiss filled with sighs
Juliette becomes unsociable,
And the smack of the fan comes to chase away pleasure;
But why would I give you up, lovable Juliette?
Love lends me one of its traits;
Quick to combat, and let us embrace tightly.
You don't dare . . . ; you flee . . . ; would you fear your defeat?]

28. Fashion descriptions in the *Journal des demoiselles*, for example, a journal that ran from 1833 through 1896, along with numerous fashion plates from the era, confirm the popularity of the fan. Many of the most well-known painters (Degas, Manet, Caillebotte, etc.) not only included fans in the composition of their paintings but also, according to Maignan, painted fans themselves. See Maignan, 35.

29. See Orr, and Rannveig Yeatman, "Le Château de la Vaubyessard: L'Enchantement d'Emma Bovary," *Dalhousie French Studies* 29 (1994): 169–80.

30. Mlle Ermance Dufaux de la Jonchère, *Le Savoir-vivre dans la vie ordinaire et dans les cérémonies civiles et religieuses*, 6th ed. (Paris: Garnier frères, 1883), 264. Emmeline Raymond, novelist and frequent contributor to *La Mode illustrée*, and Baronne Staffe, among others, offer similar injunctions.

31. This is Larry Riggs's expression (48). For one of the most stimulating readings of the Vaubyessard ball scene, see Riggs's article, "Semiotics, Simulacra and Consumerist Rhetoric of Status in Molière's Cérémonie Turque and Flaubert's Château de la Vaubyessard," *Cincinnati Romance Review* 14 (1995): 44–50.

32. See Outka for an exploration of the links between consumption and nostalgia.

33. This is Caroline Weber's expression.

34. For my analysis of the first three, see Chapter 1. Octave Uzanne engages in the same kind of nostalgic lament in many of his luxury books, among them

L'Éventail, illustrated by Paul Avril (Paris: Quantin, 1882). For a thorough analysis of Uzanne's work, see Willa K. Silverman, *The New Bibliopolis: French Book Collectors and the Culture of Print, 1880–1914* (Toronto: University of Toronto Press, 2008). See in particular "Books Worthy of Our Era? Octave Uzanne, Technology and the Luxury Book," 21–60.

35. Leora Auslander, "The Gendering of Consumer Practices in Nineteenth-Century France," in *The Sex of Things: Gender and Consumption in Historical Perspective*, ed. Victoria de Grazia, 79–112, quote on 86 (Berkeley: University of California Press, 1996).

36. Janelle Watson, *Literature and Material Culture from Balzac to Proust* (New York: Cambridge University Press, 1999), 60.

37. The theme of legitimacy, both social and political, haunts nearly all of Balzac's work, from novels to nonfictional texts. Benjamin's classic work on the question of authenticity, "The Work of Art in the Age of Mechanical Reproduction," while written with photography and cinema in mind, is often cited with reference to nineteenth-century industrialization. See Walter Benjamin, *Illuminations*.

38. This dialectical understanding of fashion originates with the still pertinent theory set forth by German sociologist Georg Simmel in his seminal article of 1901, which argues that fashion operates in a dialectical movement between conformity and individualism, tradition and modernity. Simmel understands fashion to evolve through two competing "social tendencies . . . namely, the need of union on the one hand and the need of isolation on the other" (294). Georg Simmel, "Fashion," in *The Rise of Fashion: A Reader*, ed. Daniel L. Purdy, 294–323 (Minneapolis: University of Minnesota Press, 2004). From his position of proximity to the nineteenth century, Simmel asserts that women are particularly attached to fashion as a kind of compensation for their weak social position, that is, not determined by their participation in a professional class. "The fact that fashion expresses and at the same time emphasizes the tendency towards equalization and individualization, and the desire for imitation and conspicuousness, perhaps explains why it is that women, broadly speaking, are its staunchest adherents" (299).

39. *Prêt-à-porter* and *haute couture* eventually emerge as fashion's equivalents to the collector's mass-produced copy and the connoisseur's *objet d'art*.

40. Uzanne, 7. A fin-de-siècle fashion writer, editor, and ardent bibliophile, Uzanne charts the illustrious history and symbolic function of the fan in his 1882 *L'Éventail* showcasing drawings by celebrated illustrator Paul Avril, published on the eve of the fan's great revival during the Belle Époque (roughly from 1890 to 1913). Long before Uzanne's promotion of the fan to a feminine readership anxious to be fashionable, along with his art book to a male coterie of book collectors, the fan was already an indispensable lady's fashion accessory.

41. As Felski writes, "Whereas female sexuality remained a problematic notion throughout the century . . . women's desire for commodities could be publicly acknowledged as a legitimate, if often trivialized, form of wanting. . . . . [W]oman, it seemed, could only attain the status of an active object in relation to other objects.

The circuit of desire thus flowed from man to women, from woman to the commodity" (65).

42. Pierre Barbéris, *Mythes balzaciens* (Paris: Armand Colin, 1972).

43. See especially Eric Bordas, "Le Rôle de la peinture dans *Le Cousin Pons*," *Australian Journal of French Studies* 32:1 (1995): 19–37.

44. See Henry Majewski, *Transposing Art into Texts in French Romantic Literature* (Chapel Hill: University of North Carolina Press, 2002).

45. Barbéris, 259–60. See also Bordas.

46. During the Second Empire, with Charles Frederick Worth, the male couturier and *haute couture* as we know it emerged. Fin-de-siècle designers like Paul Poiret, following Worth's lead, conceived of themselves as artists, and began to collaborate with artists in their creations. See Valerie Steele, *Paris Fashion: A Cultural History* (New York: Berg, 1999).

47. Honoré de Balzac, *Le Cousin Pons*, ed. André Lorant (Paris: Gallimard, 1973). All references are to this edition. Translations are from Honoré de Balzac, *Cousin Pons*, in *Balzac's Works*, vol 11.

48. The fan in *Le Cousin Pons* doubles the yellow cashmere shawl of *La Cousine Bette* in its polyvalent use value in the former novel's economy discussed in Chapter 2. This is also the subject of my article entitled "Lust for *Luxe*: Cashmere Fever in Nineteenth-Century France," *Journal of Early Modern Cultural Studies* 5:1 (2005): 76–98. See also John Patrick Greene, "Balzac's Most Helpless Heroine: The Art Collection in *Le Cousin Pons*," *French Review* 69:1 (October1995): 13–23.

49. See Pierre-Marc de Biasi, "La Collection Pons comme figure du problématique," *Balzac et les parents pauvres: Le Cousin Pons, La Cousine Bette*, ed. Françoise van Rossum-Guyon and Michiel van Brederode, 61–73 (Paris: SEDES, 1981).

50. For a reading of the personification of Pons's collection as his mistress, see Greene.

51. See Bordas.

52. The history of the recuperation of Antoine Watteau, rediscovered by the Goncourts in the mid-nineteenth century, is fascinating and worth exploring in relation to fan popularity especially during the Second Empire. This inquiry is, however, beyond the scope of this project.

53. In German, *Schmucke* means treasure, jewel, and thus his friendship offers a nonmaterial corollary to the material treasures so coveted in the novel. See Lorant's postface to the Gallimard edition of *Le Cousin Pons*.

54. This is Balzac's witticism, merging the terms *gastronomie* and *idolâtrie*. For a groundbreaking study of gastronomy and its relation to other nineteenth-century cultural activities, see Priscilla Parkhurst Ferguson's *Accounting for Taste: The Triumph of French Cuisine* (Chicago: University of Chicago Press, 2004).

55. In *The Function of Gift Exchange in Stendhal and Balzac* (New York: Peter Lang, 2000), Doreen Thesen omits a discussion of *Le Cousin Pons*, although she acknowledges that with its gift scene at the incipit and its thematic preoccupation with the corrupting influence of a utilitarian, market-based economy encroach-

ing on the hallowed territory of art, this novel seems ideal for inclusion in such a study. While he certainly advocates the idealism of preeconomic cultures, Mauss also determined ultimately that the notion of the "pure gift" is a nostalgic fiction. This makes a nice parallel to Balzac here, where the gift is indeed tainted by Pons's expectation of compensation. Marcel Mauss, *The Gift: Forms and Functions of Exchange in Archaic Societies*, trans. Ian Cunnison, intro. E. E. Evans Pritchard (New York: Norton, 1967).

56. The Camusot family is in a tenuous financial situation, having overextended their finances to appear wealthier than they are. They are struggling to get by in the social spectacle of Paris and are thus anxious to acquire Pons's collection.

57. The nexus Pons-Schmucke-Brunner, each implicated in the protection of Pons's treasure, suggests a homosocial plot revolving around the circulation of lust among men. The representation of that desire, the fan, while ostensibly serving to broker a marriage, ends up alienating the bachelor and reminding us all of Pons's family jewels.

58. The fan's link to marriage is already ironic in that it belonged to the favorite *mistress* of the king.

59. Maignan, 29.

60. "Il s'agit évidemment d'une pièce fictive, Mme de Pompadour pouvait posséder un éventail décoré par Watteau, mais le peintre de *l'Embarquement pour Cythère*, mort en 1721, année de la naissance d'Antoinette Poisson, ne put travailler pour elle" (We are obviously dealing with a fictitious piece, Mme de Pompadour could have possessed a fan decorated by Watteau, but the painter of *l'Embarquement pour Cythère*, dead in 1721 the year of Antoinette Poisson's [Madame de Pompadour's] birth, could not have worked for her). Honoré de Balzac, *La Comédie humaine*, vol. 7, ed. Pierre-Georges Castex and André Lorant (Paris: Gallimard-Pléiade, 1977), 1407 (n. 3).

61. Some fans may have been painted by Watteau, perhaps in his early days, and at the end of the nineteenth century and into the early twentieth century, couturiers who wanted to be construed as artists began to design fans—Paul Poiret is the most obvious example. At the same time, artists such as Paul Iribe and Edgar Degas were also painting fans. The *éventaillistes* of the seventeenth century, however, had a strict guild. "[L]es maîtres-éventaillistes, protégés depuis 1678 par un statut très strict, étaient particulièrement jaloux de leurs privilèges. Ils n'auraient sans doute jamais accepté qu'un peintre, aussi célèbre soit-il, s'immisçât dans le domaine de la peinture sur éventails, une de leurs activités réservées" (Perthuis and Meylan, 27) (The master fan makers, protected since 1678 by a very strict statute, were particularly protective of their privileges. They would probably have never accepted that a painter, no matter how famous, interfere in the domain of fan painting, one of their reserved activities). In Eugène Sue's *Les Mystères de Paris* (Paris: Éditions Robert Laffont, 1989), Rodolphe the aristocrat goes undercover as an *éventailliste*.

62. Hart and Taylor, 30.

63. Watteau was apparently quite taken by the world of commerce, as Stephen Bayley explains in *Commerce and Culture*, where he recounts the origins of the famous painting "L'Enseigne de Gersaint" as a shop sign: "Watteau (1684–1721) was a painter of languor and grandeur, of poetic scenes from the Commedia dell'arte ... but throughout his brief career, he became increasingly sensitive to the commercial opportunities of a new age, particularly after a visit to England in 1719" (8). Stephen Bayley, *Commerce and Culture: From Pre-industrial Art to Post-industrial Value* (London: Fourth Estate, 1989).

64. See Greene.

65. Zola's novel, like Uzanne's *L'Éventail*, was published on the eve of the fan's major comeback as high luxury accessory during the Belle Époque. On Uzanne and his link to the deeper content of this chapter, the relation of the commodity to the aesthetic, and woman's place within that relationship, Willa Z. Silverman's evaluation in her chapter "Books Worthy of our Era? Octave Uzanne, Technology, and the Luxury Book in *Fin-de-siècle* France" is useful. Here, she characterizes Uzanne as a "reactionary modernist," arguing that he "helped advance an elitist aesthetic of the book based on originality, novelty, and fantasy. He disparaged technology's potential to replicate, leading to overproduction and (worse, in his view) democratization of the type of *livre d'amateur* he envisioned" (240). Uzanne's interest in the fan is predicated on his bibliomania: in many ways, in their material presence, fans resemble illustrated books (i.e., albums). Uzanne's project combines fashion and collecting.

66. *Au Bonheur des Dames*, 67/61.

67. See especially Rose Fortassier's chapter on Proust in which she points out that Proust's overarching metaphor for the production of his novel is that of the couturier: "il bâtira son œuvre, dit-il, en cousant patiemment, avec l'aide de Françoise ... , les *paperolles* ... 'comme une robe'" (167) (he built his work, he said, through patiently sewing together, with Françoise's help ... , little bits of paper ... "like a dress"). Rose Fortassier, *Les Écrivains français et la mode* (Paris: Presses Universitaires de France, 1988).

68. See Michael Angelo Tata, from whom I borrow the phrase "social miscegenation" in relation to Proust and whose reading of fashion's importance in Proust has strongly informed my own reading. Michael Angelo Tata, "Post-Proustian Glamour," *Rhizomes: Cultural Studies in Emerging Knowledge* 5 (2002), http://www.rhizomes.net/issue5/tata.html#1.

69. Madeleine Delpierre, *L'Éventail, miroir de la Belle Époque* (Paris: Musée de la Mode et du Costume, 1985).

70. We have come a long way from Eugène Sue's *Mystères de Paris*, in which the blue-blooded Rodolphe disguises himself as a fan painter in order to pass as a man of the people. Now, fan painting is not only an aristocratic pastime, but recognized painters engaged in fan painting, and, as mentioned above, couturiers such as Paul Poiret sought artists such as Paul Iribe to paint fans for their collections.

71. "This forgotten figure in the history of art, a painter of minor importance,

but whose talent was classical and varied, is not widely known except for the illustrations, not just of flowers, that she did for *Les Plaisirs et les Jours*. Proust used her as his model for Mme Verdurin; she was referred to as 'the Mistress' (*la Patronne*) by her followers, she dubbed those she disliked 'bores'. But her creativity was stolen from her, to be conferred on Elstir, an artist inspired by painters on a different scale." Jean-Yves Tadié, *Marcel Proust*, trans. Euan Cameron (New York: Viking Penguin, 2000), 154.

72. Fortassier, 166.

73. Marcel Proust, *La Prisonnière*, ed. Pierre-Edmond Robert (Paris: Gallimard, 1989), 262. Translations from Marcel Proust, *Remembrance of Things Past*, vol. 3, trans. C. K. Scott Moncrieff and Terence Kilmartin (New York: Vintage Books, 1982), 277.

74. See Tata, note 25. Pauline de Metternich famously broke her fan at the opening performance of *Tannhäuser* by Wagner in an angry response to the booing of the Parisian crowd. Jules Janin in the *Almanach de la littérature, du théâtre, et des beaux-arts* (1853–69) (Paris: Pagnerre, 1862) composed something of a prose poem in her honor, entitled "l'Éventail," in which he elaborates on the grandness of her gesture and of the magnitude of her sacrifice of such a beautiful object, which doubles as a weapon: "Il est brisé, le bel éventail. . . . Autour de ses branches nacrées circulaient, dans un meandre enchanté, l'humble lotus, le lierre jaunissant, la pâle violette, et le lis mêlé à la rose, et la flûte du berger" (90) (It is broken, the beautiful fan. . . . Around its pearly branches circulated in an enchanted meandering, the humble lotus, the yellowing ivy, the pale violet, and the lily mixed with the rose, and the shepherd's flute).

75. Fortassier, 167.

76. See Felski and also Andreas Huyssen, *After the Great Divide: Modernism, Mass Culture, Postmodernism* (Bloomington: Indiana University Press, 1986).

77. Hart and Taylor, 117. Publicity fans existed before the nineteenth century, but became ubiquitous at the fin de siècle.

78. The term *nouveauté*, along with its literal meaning of that which pertains to the new, within fashion discourse refers specifically to the latest fashion trend. The term derived from those flounces, frills, and detail work that dressed up hats and dresses. *Nouveautés* also designated, quite simply, fashion trends and accessories.

CHAPTER 6

1. See John Westbrook, "Digesting Godard Filming Bataille: Expenditure in 'Week-end,'" *Contemporary French and Francophone Studies* 9:4 (December 2006) 345–52, and Kaja Silverman and Harun Farocki, *Speaking About Godard*, who sets up the film in the following way: "*Weekend* (1967) opens on a sunny day in a luxurious Parisian apartment. The inhabitants of that apartment, Roland (Jean Yanne) and Corinne (Mireille Darc), are having drinks on the balcony with a friend. Roland is called to the phone, and the fiction of bourgeois propriety is quickly shat-

tered. Within seconds, we learn that the friend is in fact Corinne's lover, and that she and Roland are both scheming to kill each other. At the same time, the couple is working together to dispose of Corinne's father, who stands between them and a substantial fortune" (83). Kaja Silverman and Harun Farocki, *Speaking About Godard* (New York: New York University Press, 1998). For "serial consumption," see also Silverman and Farocki, 91.

2. My thanks to Rebecca Colesworthy for reminding me that Hermes was (among other things) the god of commerce.

3. Consumption is not necessarily all bad, however, as Mary Louise Roberts reminds us in her excellent biographical essay on Marguerite Durand, founder and chief editor of the fin-de-siècle feminist journal *La Fronde*: "With foresight, Durand sensed that power in the twentieth century would rest as much with the newspaper and the department store as with Parliament and suffrage" (196). Mary Louise Roberts, "Acting Up: The Feminist Theatrics of Marguerite Durand," in *The New Biography: Performing Femininity in Nineteenth-Century France*, ed. Jo Burr Margadant, 171–217 (Berkeley: University of California Press, 2000).

4. See, for example, the proliferation of websites such as bagborroworsteal. com, which offers rentals of "it" bags to those who are devoted to luxury display.

5. See Dana Thomas, *Deluxe: How Luxury Lost Its Luster* (New York: Penguin, 2007).

6. See Roberts, *Disruptive Acts*.

7. Farid Chenoune, ed., *Le Cas du sac: histoires d'une utopie portative* (Paris: Hermès, 2004), 21. This exposition catalog was an extremely valuable resource for this chapter.

8. The *châtelaine*, which, like the alms purse, was a medieval vestige and attached to a lady's belt to hold small personal items on little chains, also became popular again in the nineteenth century. Of all these bags, the reticule is the one most closely related to what is understood today as the "sac de mode," the handbag as fashion object. Olivier Saillard, "A Bout portant: modernités du sac," in Chenoune, 35.

9. For an authoritative account of consumption in France especially in the second half of the nineteenth century, see Williams; for the woman consumer see Rita Felski's chapter "Imagined Pleasures: The Erotics and Aesthetics of Consumption" in *The Gender of Modernity*, 61–90. Felski writes, "The *grand magasin* brought about a number of significant innovations in merchandising: fixed prices, which made bargaining unnecessary; 'free entry,' which allowed customers to examine goods on display without any obligation to buy; and a dramatic expansion of the range and diversity of goods offered for sale under one roof. As a result, shopping came to be seen for the first time as a leisure activity; the department store sold not just commodities but the very act of consumption, transforming the mundane activity of shopping into a sensuous and enjoyable experience for a bourgeois public" (67).

10. In all the major department stores as well as in small high-end boutiques

today, handbags occupy a prominent spot in the visual field of consumption just as
they are today the uncontested status objects of feminine fashion.

11. For a succinct summary of the Dora case, see Sharon Heller, *Freud A to Z*
(Hoboken, N.J.: Wiley and Sons, 2005), 83–89.

12. See especially Charles Bernheimer and Claire Kahane, eds., *In Dora's Case:
Freud—Hysteria— Feminism* (New York: Columbia University Press, 1985), for a
critique of Freud's approach to Dora.

13. On the significance of the *gaulle*, see Weber, especially pages 150–53;
164–92. Weber writes, "certain observers remarked that the loose cut of gowns
like the *lévite* and the *gaulle* allowed for easier access to women's breasts and
genitals, and thus enabled hasty dressing after covert rendezvous" (152). On
the "ridiculousness" of the reticule, see Saillard: "De même il faut revenir sur
le terme de 'réticule' ainsi dérivé de *reticulum*, en souvenir du petit filet que
portaient les dames romaines et que s'empressent de déformer en 'ridicule' tous
ceux pour qui porter ses poches à la main est comble de ridicule" (35) (At the
same time we must reexamine the term "reticule" derived from *reticulum*, recalling the little net that Roman women carried and that hastens to distort
as "ridiculous" all those for whom carrying one's pockets in one's hand is the
height of ridiculousness).

14. The rhyming "bon mot" corresponding to the title "ridicule" in the *Almanach des ridicules* from which the frontispice image is reproduced reads as follows:
"Une femme avait perdu son ridicule, elle voulait le faire afficher.—N'en faites rien,
lui dit son mari, il vous en restera toujours assez" (108) (A woman had lost her
"ridicule" [and] wanted to post a sign.—Don't do a thing, said her husband, you
will always have enough [ridiculousness]). "Le ridicule," *Almanach des ridicules,
pour l'année 1801* (Paris: Imprimerie des Sourds-Muets, 1801), 108. The anecdote
reinforces the association of women with ridiculousness already suggested by the
popular renaming of reticule as ridicule.

15. For a comprehensive study of Mésangère's work in the fashion press, see
Annemarie Kleinart, *Le "Journal des dames et des modes" ou la conquête de l'Europe
féminine, 1797–1839* (Stuttgart: Jan Thorbecke Verlag, 2001). On the fashion press
and its relation to feminism, see Nina Rattner Gelbart, *Feminine and Opposition
Journalism in Old Regime France* (Berkeley: University of California Press, 1987),
and more recently, on the fashion press in France more generally, Vincent Soulier,
Presse féminine: La puissance frivole (Paris: L'Archipel, 2008).

16. For a historical discussion of the origins of the handbag, see Katherine Lester and Bess Viola Oerke, *Accessories of Dress: An Illustrated Encyclopedia* (Mineola, N.Y.: Dover Publications,2004), 415–25. See also Chenoune.

17. For an informative discussion on the history and practice of dowry in
France, see Anne Martin-Fugier, *La Bourgeoise: femme au temps de Paul Bourget*
(Paris: Grasset, 1983), 45–49.

18. See Carol Rifelj, "The Language of Hair in the Nineteenth-Century Novel,"
Nineteenth-Century French Studies 32:1–2 (2003): 83–96. She writes, "curls are as-

sociated with 'jolies femmes,' and that is true in novels as well, where they often appear in conjunction with a form of the adjective 'charmant'" (83).

19. Mica Nava, "Modernity's Disavowal: Women, the City and the Department Store," in *The Shopping Experience*, ed. Pasi Falk and Colin Campbell, 56–91 (London: Sage, 1997). See also Sarah Curtis, "Charitable Ladies: Gender, Class and Religion in Mid Nineteenth-Century Paris," *Past and Present*, 177:1 (2002): 121–56.

20. Antonin Rondelet, "Lettre à Nathalie: Sur l'obligation de visiter les pauvres," *Journal des demoiselles* 44:11 (1876): 327–29, quote on 328.

21. See especially Bonnie Smith.

22. See Nava.

23. Hannah Thompson, 85. And Felski writes, "this public domain presented itself as an extension of the private sphere, providing the visitor with an experience of intimacy and pleasure intended to reflect, in magnified form, the comforts of the bourgeois home" (68).

24. Charity work was indeed linked to *mondanité*, or society life, in part because it afforded women the opportunity to be seen in public and so to participate in the culture of fashion. But also, as Martin-Fugier explains in *La Bourgeoise*, charity work and *mondanité* overlapped in other ways as well: "Les ventes de charité font si bien partie des habitudes mondaines qu'elles sont répertoriées dans les manuels de savoir-vivre" (204) (Charity auctions are so well integrated into high society customs that they are included in etiquette manuals). Citing one such manual by the baronne d'Orval, Martin-Fugier explains that the charity fairs were potentially an occasion for fashionability, even as upper-class women ("les dames de bonnes œuvres") sewed, embroidered or painted little objects to sell in order to raise money for charitable organizations.

25. See Stéphane Laverrière, "Le Sac à ouvrage, accessoire de la femme vertueuse," in Chenoune, 154–63.

26. For the authoritative study on working-class women and the embroidery industry, see Judith Coffin, *The Politics of Women's Work: The Paris Garment Trades, 1750–1915* (Princeton, N.J.: Princeton University Press, 1996).

27. See Martin-Fugier, *La Bourgeoise*: "Il ne faut pas craindre, écrit Adrienne Cambry, de montrer à son futur époux ses talents pratiques. Et d'abord ses talents de couturière" (61) (One should not be afraid, writes Adrienne Cambry, to show one's future husband one's practical talents. And first of all, one's talents as a seamstress).

28. Colette Cosnier, *Le Silence des filles: de l'aiguille à la plume* (Paris: Fayard, 2001), 216.

29. Donaldson-Evans's article makes many brilliant observations about the literary symbolism of sewing and its relation to female subversion in nineteenth-century France.

30. Edmond de Goncourt, *La Fille Elisa* (Paris: Zulma, 2004), 27. In this novel Goncourt explains Elisa's simple fall into prostitution as the only alternative to the other type of work available to poor women in the provinces, service and sewing.

31. See Coffin.

32. Quoted in Laverrière, "Le Sac à ouvrage," 160.

33. Baronne Staffe, *Mes secrets pour plaire et pour être aimée* (Paris: Les Éditions 1900, 1990), 347.

34. "Embroidery had been for centuries the pastime of aristocrats, and women
often embroidered small items—suspenders, slippers, etc.—for their lovers" (Donaldson-Evans, 259).

35. Because embroidery (*broderie*) is more closely linked to the accessory since
it is a form of embellishment and beautification, it is the more appropriate activity
for bourgeois women to be engaged in; sewing, on the other hand, has more practical applications and is more useful and thus is more clearly associated with Berthe,
Elisa, and Denise—that is, working-class girls.

36. See Catherine Amaroso Leslie, *Needlework Through History: An Encyclope-
dia* (Westport, Conn.: Greenwood, 2007), and Margaret Lee Meriwether and Judith
E. Tucker, *Social History of Women and Gender in the Modern Middle East* (Boulder,
Colo.: Westview, 1999). See also the website http://www.auverasoie.com/broderie.htm:

La broderie de soie est née à Alger durant les trois siècles de domination otto-
mane (du XVIème au XIXème siècle). D'une surprenante beauté, ces broderies
s'exécutent d'après un tracé et à fils comtés sur des métiers à bras. Les décors
sont pour la plupart floraux à dominante violette, soit rouge et bleu sur fond
d'étamine de lin de couleur bistre. Elles sont destinées au costume ou à la déco-
ration intérieure et furent longtemps l'apanage des femmes de la haute société.
Le plus bel exemple de broderie d'Alger conservé en France est le voile de la Vierge de la cathédrale de Chartres appelée: Notre-Dame du Pilier.

[Silk embroidery was born in Algiers during the three centuries of Ottoman
domination (from the sixteenth to the nineteenth century). Of surprising beauty, these embroideries were executed from a traced pattern and with threads
on a loom with arms. The patterns are mostly floral with violet as the dominant color, or red and blue on a linen muslin background of yellowish-brown.
They were destined for clothing or for interior decoration and were for a long
time the privilege of high society women. The most beautiful example of Algiers
embroidery preserved in France is the veil of the Virgin at Chartres Cathedral
called Notre-Dame du Pilier.]

37. For a discussion of Bette's relation to *passementerie*, uniforms, and empire,
see Sara Maza's article on uniforms, cited earlier.

38. Honoré de Balzac, *La Bourse*, ed. Anne-Marie Baron (Paris: Garnier-Flammarion, 1993), 257. Translations are from Honoré de Balzac, *The Purse*, in *Balzac's
Works*, vol. 4, 26–27.

39. Mainardi explains these terms: "The idea of marriage based on romantic
love instead of familial ambition, what was called *mariage d'inclination* as opposed
to *mariage d'intérêt* or *mariage de raison* was new in France, for the courtly love
tradition had always regarded love and marriage as mutually exclusive"(5).

40. Émile Zola, *Pot-Bouille*, ed. Marie-Ange Voisin-Fougère (Paris: Librairie Générale Française, 1998). All translations are from Émile Zola, *Pot-Bouille*, trans. Percy Pinkerton, ed. Robert Lethbridge (London: Dent, 2000).

41. Thompson, 139–40. Thompson's excellent discussion of this novel is rich in detailing the lengths to which securing a husband through the seductions of clothing could and must be accomplished. Her likening of Zola's novel of bourgeois mores to his great novel of prostitution (*Nana*) through the "dynamics of the striptease" is illuminating.

42. The slang expression "avoir le sac" is used in *Pot-Bouille* to refer to Madame Hédouin's fortune.

43. Felski and Bonnie Smith both discuss this. See in particular Felski's remarks about the "commodification of the household" (62).

44. Among the many important studies on women and consumption in relation to this novel, see Rosalind Williams, *Dream Worlds*, Rachel Bowlby, *Just Looking: Consumer Culture in Dreiser, Gilling, and Zola* (New York: Methuen, 1985), and Rita Felski, *The Gender of Modernity*.

45. Felski devotes much of her chapter on consumption to Zola's 1883 novel and very briefly considers the figure of Madame Marty:

> Unable to resist the temptations proffered by Mouret, she spends compulsively and recklessly, squandering her husband's meager earnings on the acquisition of ever more feminine luxuries. A weak and ineffectual figure, Marty can only stand by and watch helplessly as his wife gradually brings about his financial ruin; every new piece of lace brings closer the threat of impending economic disaster. The culture of consumerism reaches into and disrupts the sanctity of the private sphere, encouraging women to indulge their own desires in defiance of their husbands and of traditional forms of moral and religious authority (74).

46. I am grateful to Linda Nochlin for reminding me of Anna Karenina's red purse—all that is left on the train platform after her suicide. *Anna Karenina* was published serially from 1873 to 1877.

47. See Naomi Schor, "Devant le château: Femmes, marchandises et modernité dans *Au Bonheur des Dames*," in *Mimesis et semiosis: littérature et représentation*, miscellanées offertes à Henri Mitterand, ed. Philippe Hamon and Jean-Pierre Leduc-Adine, 179–86 (Paris: Nathan, 1992).

48. The eroticized opening and closing of the sac, motivated in part by the anxiety that her husband will discover her expenditures, looks forward to Freud's patient Dora.

49. See Hannah Thompson's smart analysis of the ways in which the erotic and commercial rhetorics overlap in the novel.

50. The clearest example of this danger is to be seen in the transparently named character of Madame Lhomme.

51. She does, however, purchase a dress for her daughter at the Bonheur to copy at home and then return. See Hannah Thompson. According to Veblen's theory

of conspicuous consumption, waste was productive, however, for it illustrated the wealth and power of elites. See Veblen, *Conspicuous Consumption*.

52. I am indebted to Olivier Saillard's article in Chenoune for alerting me to the *Fémina* articles. Fanchon, "Fanfreluches," *Fémina* 1901, 15.

53. See McMillan, Moses, and Roberts, *Disruptive Acts*.

54. Camille Duguet, "Du réticule à la trousse," *Fémina* 1908, 148–49.

55. See Kessler, 41.

56. This explains why handbags function as they do today, as objects of conspicuous consumption that are not always practical. Saillard writes, "Survivant orphelin d'une silhouette qui a vu disparaître tour à tour au XXe siècle les attributs satellites qui dictaient l'apparence d'hier—parmi lesquels on peut citer les ombrelles, les éventails, les gants courts ou longs, de jour comme de soirée, les manchons, les chapeaux, menus ou généreux, autant d'accessoires que la garde-robe contemporaine a supprimés des dressings—, le sac a su se maintenir aux poignets des femmes" (32) (The surviving orphan of a silhouette that witnessed in the twentieth century the disappearance one by one of the satellite attributes that dictated the look of the past—among which one could cite parasols, fans, long or short gloves, for day and for evening, muffs, hats either tiny or generous, all the many accessories that the contemporary wardrobe has suppressed—the handbag understood how to hang on to the wrists of women).

EPILOGUE

1. Staffe, *Les Hochets féminins*, 1.

2. I am referring to Jules Ferry's popularization of the expression of France's "duty" vis-à-vis its colonial territories—the "mission civilisatrice." Ferry was the forty-fourth prime minister of France, serving from 1880 to 1881.

3. While Staffe was prolific and widely read for her seeming inside knowledge of the manners and behaviors appropriate to the Parisian upper classes, ironically, Blanche Soyer lived out her days quietly and modestly with her aunts in Savigny-sur-Orge.

4. Roberts, "Acting Up."

5. Quoted in Roberts, "Acting Up," 184. See also Roberts, *Disruptive Acts*.

6. See the following website: http://www.marievictoirelouis.net/document. php?id=88&auteurid=87.

7. See Moses and McMillan. See also Karen Offen, *European Feminisms, 1700–1950: A Political History* (Palo Alto, Calif.: Stanford University Press, 2000).

8. Here I borrow Elaine Freedgood's marvelously evocative expression, which she develops in rich and rewarding ways in her book *The Ideas in Things*.

Abélès, Luce. "Du Cousin Pons à l'aiguille creuse: les musées privés romanesques au XIXe siècle." *Revue d'histoire littéraire de la France* 95:1 (1995): 27–35.

Adler, Laure. *Secrets d'alcove: histoire du couple, 1830–1930.* Paris: Éditions Complexes, 1990.

Ahearn, Edward J. "The Magic Cigar Case: Emma Bovary and Karl Marx." In *Women's Voices and Figures, from Marie de France to Marie Cardinal,* edited by Michel Guggenheim, 181–86. Palo Alto, Calif.: Stanford French and Italian Studies, 1989.

Alhoy, Maurice, and Paul Gavarni, illus. *Physiologie de la lorette.* Paris: Aubert, 1841.

Allison, Maggie. "Marguerite Durand and *La Fronde*: Voicing Women of the Belle Époque." In *A Belle Époque? Women in French Society and Culture, 1890–1914,* edited by Diana Holmes and Carrie Tarr, 37–49. New York: Berghahn Books, 2006.

Almanach des ridicules, pour l'année 1801. Paris: Imprimerie des Sourds-Muets, 1801.

Ames, Frank. *The Kashmir Shawl and Its Indo-French Influence.* Woodbridge, England: Antique Collectors' Club, 1997.

Amossy, Ruth. "L'Esthétique du grotesque dans *Le Cousin Pons.*" In Rossum-Guyon and Brederode, 135–45.

Appadurai, Arjun. "Introduction: Commodities and the Politics of Value." In *The Social Life of Things: Commodities in Cultural Perspective,* edited by Arjun Appadurai. 3–63. Cambridge: Cambridge University Press, 1986.

Apter, Emily. *Feminizing the Fetish: Psychoanalysis and Narrative Obsession in Turn-of-the-Century France.* Ithaca, N.Y.: Cornell University Press, 1991.

Apter, Emily, and William Pietz. *Fetishism as Cultural Discourse.* Ithaca, N.Y.: Cornell University Press, 1993.

Assouly Olivier, ed. *Le Luxe: essais sur la fabrique de l'ostentation*. Paris: Éditions de l'Institut français de la Mode-Regard, 2005.

Aubert, Nathalie. "En attendant les barbares: *La Cousine Bette*, le moment populaire et féminin de *La Comédie humaine*." *Women in French Studies* 8 (2000): 129–37.

Auslander, Leora. "The Gendering of Consumer Practices in Nineteenth-Century France." In *The Sex of Things: Gender and Consumption in Historical Perspective*, edited by Victoria de Grazia, 79–112. Berkeley: University of California Press, 1996.

Baguley, David. *La Curée de Zola, ou, "La vie à outrance": actes du colloque du 10 janvier 1987*. Colloques de la Société des études romantiques. Paris: SEDES, 1987.

Bailbé, Joseph-Marc. "Autour de *La Dame Aux Camélias*: présence et signification du thème de la courtisane dans le roman français (1830–1850)." In *Aimer en France, 1760–1860*, edited by Paul Villaneix, Jean Ehrard, et al., 1: 227-39. 2 vols. Clermont-Ferrand: Association des publications de la Faculté des lettres et sciences humaines, 1980.

Baker, Deborah Lesko. "*L'Éducation sentimentale*: Figural Dimensions of Madame Arnoux." *Symposium: A Quarterly Journal in Modern Literatures* 44: 1 (1990): 3–14.

Balzac, Honoré de. *Autre étude de femme*. In *Les Secrets de la princesse de Cadignan et autres études de femmes*, edited by Samuel Sacy, 38–114. Paris: Gallimard, 1980.

———. *Balzac's Novels*, edited by George Saintsbury, translated by Clara Bell. 40 vols. London: Dent, 1898.

———. *Balzac's Works*, edited by George Saintsbury. 18 vols. 1901; reprint, Freeport, N.Y.: Books for Libraries, 1971.

———. *La Bourse*, edited by Anne-Marie Baron. Paris: Garnier-Flammarion, 1993.

———. *La Comédie humaine*. Vol. 7. Edited by Pierre-Georges Castex and André Lorant. Paris: Gallimard-Pléiade, 1977.

———. *La Cousine Bette*, edited by André Lorant. Paris: Garnier-Flammarion, 1977.

———. *Le Cousin Pons*, edited by André Lorant. Paris: Gallimard, 1973.

———. "La Femme comme il faut." In *Les Francais peints par eux-mêmes: encyclopédie morale du dix-neuvième siècle*, edited by Léon Curmer and Pierre Bouttier, 1: 55–65. 2 vols. Paris: Omnibus, 2003.

———. *Ferragus, chef des dévorants*. In *Histoire des Treize*, edited by Gérard Gengembre, 21–131. Paris: Pocket, 1992.

———. *Le Lys dans la vallée*, edited by Roger Pierrot. Paris: Librairie Générale, 1984.

———. *Le Père Goriot*, edited by Félicien Marceau. Paris: Gallimard, 1999.

———. *Splendeurs et Misères des courtisanes*, edited by Pierre Barbéris. Paris: Gallimard, 1973.

———. *Théorie de la démarche*, edited by Jacques Bonnet. Paris: Albin Michel, 1994.

———. *Traité de la vie élégante*. Paris: Arléa, 1998.

———. *Une Double Famille suivi du Contrat de mariage et de l'Interdiction*, edited by Jean-Louis Bory. Paris: Gallimard, 1973.

Barbéris, Pierre. *Mythes balzaciens*. Paris: Armand Colin, 1972.

Barthes, Roland. "Le dandysme et la mode." In *Le bleu est à la mode cette année*, 97–103. 1962; reprint, Paris: Éditions de l'Institut français de la Mode, 2001.

———. *The Language of Fashion*, translated by Andy Stafford, edited by Stafford and Michael Carter. New York: Berg, 2006.

Baudelaire, Charles. "A Une Passante." In *Les Fleurs du mal, Œuvres complètes*, 68. Paris: Robert Laffont, 1980.

———. *Les Fleurs du mal*, translated by Richard Howard. Boston: Godine, 1983.

———. "Le Peintre de la vie moderne." In *Œuvres completes*, 790–815. Paris: Laffont, 1990.

Baudrillart, Henri. *Histoire du luxe privé et public depuis l'antiquité jusqu'à nos jours*. Vol. 4. Paris: Hachette, 1878–80.

Bayley, Stephen. *Commerce and Culture: From Pre-industrial Art to Post-industrial Value*. London: Fourth Estate, 1989.

Becker, Colette. "Dire la femme en régime réaliste/naturaliste: du lys à la chienne en chaleur." In *Europäische Realismen: Facetten, Konvergenzen, Differenzen: Internationales Symposium der Fachrichtung Romanistik an der Universität des Saarlandes*, edited by Uwe Dethloff, 263–65. Röhrig Universitätsverlag, St. Ingbert, Germany: Annales Universitatis Saraviensis, Philosophische Fakultät, 2001.

Beizer, Janet. "*Au* (delà du) *Bonheur des dames*: Notes on the Underground." *Australian Journal of French Studies* 38:3 (2001): 393–406.

———. *Ventriloquized Bodies: Narratives of Hysteria in Nineteenth-Century France*. Ithaca, N.Y.: Cornell University Press, 1993.

Belenky, Masha. *The Anxiety of Dispossession: Jealousy in Nineteenth-Century French Culture*. Lewisburg, Pa.: Bucknell University Press, 2008.

Benjamin, Walter. *The Arcades Project*, translated by Howard Eiland and Kevin McLaughlin. Cambridge, Mass.: Belknap Press, 1999.

———. "The Work of Art in the Age of Mechanical Reproduction." In *Illumi-*

nations, translated by Harry Zohn, introduction by Hannah Arendt. New York: Harcourt, 1968.

Bernheimer, Charles. *Figures of Ill Repute: Representing Prostitution in Nineteenth-Century France*. Durham, N.C.: Duke University Press, 1989.

———. "Prostitution and Narrative: Balzac's *Splendeurs et misères des courtisanes*." *L' Esprit Créateur* 25: 2 (1985): 22–31.

Bernheimer, Charles, and Claire Kahane, eds. *In Dora's Case: Freud—Hysteria—Feminism*. New York: Columbia University Press, 1985.

Biasi, Pierre-Marc de. "La Collection Pons comme figure du problématique." In van Rossum-Guyon and van Brederode, 61–73.

Blanc, Charles. *Art in Ornament and Dress*. London: Chapman and Hall, 1877.

Bohac, Barbara. "*La Dernière Mode* de Mallarmé sous les feux du drame solaire." *Romantisme* 132 (2006): 129–39.

Bordas, Eric. "Le Rôle de la peinture dans *Le Cousin Pons*." *Australian Journal of French Studies* 32: 1 (1995): 19–37.

Bossen, Laurel. "Towards a Theory of Marriage: The Economic Anthropology of Marriage Transactions." *Ethnology* 27:2 (April 1988): 127–44.

Bourdieu, Pierre. *Distinction: A Social Critique of the Judgement of Taste*, translated by Richard Nice. Cambridge, Mass.: Harvard University Press, 1984.

Bouvier-Ajam, Maurice. "Zola et les magasins de nouveautés (*Au Bonheur Des Dames*)." *Europe: revue littéraire mensuelle* 468–69 (1968): 47–54.

Bowlby, Rachel. *Just Looking: Consumer Culture in Dreiser, Gilling, and Zola*. New York: Methuen, 1985.

Bricard, Isabelle. *Saintes ou pouliches: l'éducation des jeunes filles au XIXe siècle*. Paris: Albin Michel, 1985.

Brooks, Peter. "Balzac: Epistemophilia and the Collapse of the Restoration." *Yale French Studies* 101 "Fragments of Revolution (2001): 119–31.

———. "Storied Bodies, or Nana at Last Unveil'd." *Critical Inquiry* 16:1 (1989): 1–32.

———. "Virtue-Tripping: Notes on *Le Lys dans la vallée*." *Yale French Studies* 50 (1974): 150–62.

Bruzzi, Stella, and Pamela Church Gibson. *Fashion Cultures: Theories, Explorations, and Analysis*. London: Routledge, 2000.

Butler, Judith. *Bodies That Matter: On the Discursive Limits of "Sex."* New York: Routledge, 1993.

———. *Gender Trouble: Feminism and the Subversion of Identity*. New York: Routledge, 1989.

Butor, Michel. *Scènes de la vie féminine: improvisations sur Balzac III*. Paris: Éditions de la Différence, 1998.

Campbell, Colin. *The Romantic Ethic and the Spirit of Modern Consumerism.* New York: Basil Blackwell, 1987.

———. "Shopping, Pleasure, and the Sex War." In *The Shopping Experience,* edited by Pasi Falk and Colin Campbell, 166–76. London: Sage Publications, 1997.

Cannon, Aubrey. "The Cultural and Historical Contexts of Fashion." In *Consuming Fashion: Adorning the Transnational Body,* edited by Anne Brydon and Sandra Niessen, 23–38. New York: Berg, 1998.

Castro, Chantal-Sophie. "Le Vêtement dans *Pot-Bouille* et *Au Bonheur des Dames*: De l'art de la seduction à la manipulation." In *L'Écriture du féminin chez Zola et dans la fiction naturaliste/Writing the Feminine in Zola and Naturalist Fiction,* edited by Anna Gural-Migdal, 145–67. Bern, Switzerland: Peter Lang, 2003.

Chapus, Eugène. *Manuel de l'homme et de la femme comme il faut.* New ed. Paris: Bourdilliat et Cie, 1862.

Chateaubriand, François-René de. *Atala,* edited by Pierre Moreau. Paris: Gallimard, 1971.

———. *Atala,* translated by Irving Putter. Berkeley: University of California Press, 1952.

Chaudhuri, Nupur. "Shawls, Jewelry, Curry and Rice in Victorian Britain." In *Western Women and Imperialism: Complicity and Resistance,* edited by Nupur Chaudhury and Margaret Strobel, 231–46. Bloomington: Indiana University Press, 1992.

Chenoune, Farid, ed. *Le Cas du sac: histoires d'une utopie portative.* Paris: Hermès, 2004.

Chollet, Louis. *Monsieur Parapluie et Mademoiselle Ombrelle.* Tours: Maison Mame et Fils, 1912.

Clancy-Smith, Julia. "Woman without her Distaff." In Meriwether and Tucker.

Coffignon, Ali. "Accessoires féminins." In *Paris-vivant: les coulisses de la mode,* 231–38. Paris: Librairie illustrée, 1888.

Coffin, Judith. *The Politics of Women's Work: The Paris Garment Trades, 1750–1915.* Princeton, N.J.: Princeton University Press, 1996.

Cohen, William. *The French Encounter with Africans: White Response to Black, 1530–1880.* Bloomington: Indiana University Press, 1980.

Corbin, Alain. *L'Avènement des loisirs, 1850–1960.* Paris: Aubier, 1995.

———. *Les filles de noces: misère sexuelle et prostitution aux dix-neuvième et vingtième siècles.* Paris: Aubier Montaigne, 1978.

Cosnier, Colette. *Le Silence des filles: de l'aiguille à la plume.* Paris: Fayard, 2001.

Crick, Rosemary Peters. "For the Pleasure of the Ladies: Theft, Gender and

Object Relations in *Au Bonheur des Dames*." In *L'Écriture du féminin chez Zola et dans la fiction naturaliste/Writing the Feminine in Zola and Naturalist Fiction*, edited by Anna Gural-Migdal, 471–87. Bern, Switzerland: Peter Lang, 2003.

Crouzet, Michel. "Passion et politique dans *L'Éducation sentimentale*." In *Flaubert, la femme, la ville*, edited by Marie-Claire Bancquart, introduction by Armand Lanoux, 39–71. Paris: Presses Universitaires de France, 1982.

Curtis, Sarah. "Charitable Ladies: Gender, Class and Religion in Mid Nineteenth-Century Paris." *Past and Present* 177 (2002): 121–56.

Czyba, Lucette. "Paris et la lorette." In *Paris au XIXe siècle: aspects d'un mythe littéraire*, edited by Roger Bellet, 107–22. Lyon: Presses Universitaires de Lyon, 1984.

Dauvergne, Geneviève Lafosse. *Mode et fétichisme*. Paris: Éditions alternatives, 2002.

DeJean, Joan. *The Essence of Style: How the French Invented High Fashion, Fine Food, Chic Cafés, Style, Sophistication, and Glamour*. New York: Free Press, 2005.

Delaney, Susan. "*Atala* in the Arts." In *The Wolf and the Lamb: Popular Culture in France from the Old Regime to the Twentieth Century*, edited by Jacques Beauroy, Marc Bertrand, and Edward T. Gargan, 209–31. Saratoga, Calif.: Anma Libri, 1977.

Delpierre, Madeleine. *L'Éventail, miroir de la Belle Époque: 24 Mai-27 Octobre 1985, Palais Galliéra, Paris*, exhibition catalogue. Paris: Musée de la Mode et du Costume, 1985.

——. *Indispensables accessoires: XVI–XXe siècle*. Exhibition catalogue. Musée de la Mode et du Costume. Paris: Galliéra, 1983–84.

d'Harcourt, Claire. *Les Habits*. Paris: Seuil, 2001.

Dictionnaire de l'Académie française. 6th ed., 1835. ARTFL Project.

Diderot, Denis. *Les Bijoux indiscrets*, edited by Jacques Rustin. Paris: Gallimard, 1981.

Dolan, Therese. "Guise and Dolls: Dis/covering Power, Re/Covering Nana." *Nineteenth-Century French Studies* 26:3–4 (1998): 368–86.

Donaldson-Evans, Mary. "Pricking the Male Ego: Pins and Needles in Flaubert, Maupassant and Zola." *Nineteenth-Century French Studies* 30:3–4 (2002): 254–65.

Dorlin, Elsa. *La Matrice de la race*. Paris: Éditions la Découverte, 2006.

Droz, Gustave. *Entre nous*. Paris: Havard, 1883.

Dubois, J.-B. *Le Cachemire, ou l'étrenne à la mode, comédie anecdotique, en un acte et en prose*. Paris: Barba, 1811.

Dufaux de la Jonchère, Ermance. *Le Savoir-vivre dans la vie ordinaire et dans les cérémonies civiles et religieuses*. 6th ed. Paris: Garnier frères, 1883.

Duguet, Camille. "Du réticule à la trousse." *Fémina* (April 1908): 148–49.

Dumas, Alexandre père. *Filles, lorettes et courtisanes*. Paris: Flammarion, 2000.

Dumas, Alexandre fils. *La Dame aux camélias*. Paris: Pocket, 1994.

———. *Le Demi-Monde, comédie en cinq actes, en prose*. In *Théâtre complet d'Alexandre Dumas*. Vol. 2. Paris: Calmann Lévy, 1896.

———. *Théâtre complet avec préfaces inédites*. Paris: Calmann-Levy, 1900.

Dupin, Henri. *Le Cachemire, comédie en un acte et en prose*. Paris: Masson, 1810.

Dupuis, Danielle. "La Mode feminine dans les romans de mœurs d'Honoré de Balzac." Ph.D. diss. Université de Paris, Sorbonne, 1988.

Duranty, Edmond. *Le Malheur d'Henriette Gérard*, preface by Jean Paulhan. 1860; reprint, Paris: Gallimard, 1981.

Dyer, Richard. *White*. New York: Routledge, 1997.

Elias, Norbert. *The Civilizing Process: Sociogenetic and Psychogenetic Investigations*. Rev. ed., edited by Eric Dunning, Johan Goudsblom, and Stephen Mennell, translated by Edmund Jephcott. Malden, Mass.: Blackwell, 2000.

Elliott, Dorice Williams. *The Angel out of the House: Philanthropy and Gender in Nineteenth-Century England*. Charlottesville: University Press of Virginia, 2002.

Emery, Marie. "Une Corbeille." *Le Journal des demoiselles* 37:3 (1869): 79–85.

Exposition universelle. *Travaux de la commission française sur l'industrie des nations*. 12 vols. Paris: Imprimerie impériale, 1854–67. Vol. 7, *Exposition universelle de 1851*, introduction by M. le baron Charles Dupin.

Fairchilds, Cissie. "Fashion and Freedom in the French Revolution." *Continuity and Change* 15:3 (2000): 419–33.

Fanchon. "Fanfreluches." *Fémina* (February 1901): 15.

Farrell, Jeremy. *Umbrellas and Parasols*. London: Batsford, 1985.

Feldman, Jessica. *Gender on the Divide: The Dandy in Modernist Literature*. Ithaca, N.Y.: Cornell University Press, 1993.

Felski, Rita. *The Gender of Modernity*. Cambridge, Mass.: Harvard University Press, 1995.

Ferguson, Priscilla Parkhurst. *Accounting for Taste: The Triumph of French Cuisine*. Chicago: University of Chicago Press, 2004.

———. "Mobilite et modernité: Le Paris de *la Curée*." *Les Cahiers Naturalistes* 67 (1993): 73–81.

Finn, Michael R. "Proust and Dumas *Fils*: Odette and La Dame aux camélias."

French Review: Journal of the American Association of Teachers of French 47 (February1974): 528–42.

Flaubert, Gustave. *L'Éducation sentimentale*, edited by Pierre-Louis Rey. Paris: Pocket, 1998.

———. *Madame Bovary*, edited by Pierre-Marc de Biasi. Paris: Seuil, l'école des lettres, 1992.

———. *Madame Bovary*, edited and translated by Geoffrey Wall. New York: Penguin, 1992.

———. *Sentimental Education*, edited and translated by Robert Baldick. New York: Penguin Books, 1964.

Foley, Susan. *Women in France Since 1789*. New York: Palgrave MacMillan, 2004.

Fonssagriues, J.-B. *Dictionnaire de la santé ou répertoire d'hygiène pratique à l'usage des familles et des écoles*. Paris: Librairie Charles Delagrave, 1876.

Fortassier, Rose. *Les Écrivains français et la mode*. Paris: Presses Universitaires de France, 1988.

Foucault, Michel. *The History of Sexuality*, translated by Robert Hurley. Vol. 1. New York: Vintage Books, 1980.

Frappier-Mazur, Lucienne. "Lecture d'un texte illisible: *Autre étude de femme* et le modèle de la conversation." *Modern Language Notes* 98:4 (1983): 712–27.

Freedgood, Elaine. *The Ideas in Things: Fugitive Meaning in the Victorian Novel*. Chicago: University of Chicago Press, 2006.

Freud, Sigmund. *Dora: An Analysis of a Case of Hysteria*, edited by Philip Rieff. New York: Touchstone. 1997.

Frølich, Juliette. *Des hommes, des femmes et des choses: langages de l'objet dans le roman de Balzac à Proust*. Vincennes: Presse Universitaires de Vincennes, 1997.

Frost, Linda. "The Circassian Beauty and the Circassian Slave: Gender, Imperialism, and American Popular Entertainment." In *Freakery: Cultural Spectacles of the Extraordinary Body*, edited by Rosemary Garland Thomson, 248–64. New York: New York University Press, 1996.

Furbank, P. N., and A. M. Cain. "*La Dernière Mode* and Its Pre-History." In *Mallarmé on Fashion: A Translation of the Fashion Magazine* La Dernière Mode *with Commentary*, edited and translated by P. N. Furbank and Alex Cain, 3–13. New York: Berg, 2004.

Gabriel and Armand (MM). *La Féerie des arts, ou le sultan de cachemire (folie féerique, vaudeville en un acte)*. Paris: Huet-Masson, 1819.

Gaite, Carmen Martin. *Love Customs of Eighteenth-Century Spain*, translated by Maria G. Tomsich. Berkeley: University of California Press, 1991.

Gardot, Maurice. "Parasol et parapluie." *Journal des demoiselles* 51:12 (1883): 317–320.

Garelick, Rhonda K. *Rising Star: Dandyism, Gender, and Performance in the Fin de Siècle.* Princeton, N.J.: Princeton University Press, 1998.

Gavarni, Paul, et al. *Le Diable à Paris: Paris et les parisiens à la plume et au crayon.* Paris: Hetzel, 1868.

Gelbart, Nina Rattner. *Feminine and Opposition Journalism in Old Regime France.* Berkeley: University of California Press, 1987.

George, Ken. "'Le Monde à demi et le demi-monde': Half-Measures in French." *French Studies Bulletin: A Quarterly Supplement* 61 (1996): 1–3.

George, Lisa Rengo. "Reading the Plautine *Meretrix*." Ph.D. diss., Bryn Mawr College, 1997.

Gilman, Sander. *Difference and Pathology: Stereotypes of Sexuality, Race, and Madness.* Ithaca, N.Y.: Cornell University Press, 1985.

Girardin, Madame de. *Lettres parisiennes du vicomte de Launay.* 2 vols. Le Temps retrouvé series. Paris: Mercure de France, 1986.

Godard, Jean-Luc. *Week-end.* DVD. Directed by Jean-Luc Godard. Paris: Les Films Coperenic, 1967.

Goncourt, Edmond de. *La Fille Élisa.* Paris: Zulma, 2004.

Goncourt, Edmond and Jules de. *La Femme au dix-huitième siècle.* Elibron Classics Series, Adamant Media Corporation, 2006.

———. *La Lorette*, edited by Alain Barbier Sainte Marie. Tusson: Éditions du Lérot, n.d.

Goody, Jack, and S. J. Tambiah. *Bridewealth and Dowry.* Cambridge: Cambridge University Press, 1973.

Gordon, Rae Beth. *Ornament, Fantasy, and Desire in Nineteenth-Century French Literature.* Princeton, N.J.: Princeton University Press, 1992.

Granger, Alice. "Le Contrat de mariage, Honoré de Balzac." http://www.e-literature.net/publier/spip/article.php3?id_article=147.

Grauby, Françoise. "Corps privé et vêtement public: les jeux et les enjeux du costume féminin dans L'Éducation sentimentale de Flaubert." *New Zealand Journal of French Studies* 18:1 (1997): 5–19.

———. "Le Parfum de l'homme en noir: Mallarmé et *La Dernière Mode* (1874)," *Australian Journal of French Studies* 41:1 (2004): 102–20.

Green, Nancy L. "Art and Industry: The Language of Modernization in the Production of Fashion." *French Historical Studies* 18:3 (Spring 1994): 722–48.

Greene, John Patrick. "Balzac's Most Helpless Heroine: The Art Collection in *Le Cousin Pons.*" *French Review: Journal of the American Association of Teachers of French* 69: 1 (October 1995): 13–23.

Greimas, Algirdas Julien. *La Mode en 1830: langage et société, écrits de jeunesse*, edited by Thomas F. Broden and Françoise Ravaux-Kirkpatrick. Paris: Presses Universitaires de France, 2000.

Gronow, Jukka. *The Sociology of Taste*. New York: Routledge, 1997.

Guillemard, Colette. *Les Mots du costume*. Paris: Belin, 1991.

Gyp (pseudonym of Sibylle Aimée Marie Antoinette Gabrielle de Riquetti de Mirabeau, Comtesse de Martel de Janville). *Pauvres petites femmes*. Paris: Calmann Lévy, 1888.

Harrow, Susan. "Exposing the Imperial Cultural Fabric: Critical Description in Zola's *La Curée*." *French Studies* 54: 4 (2000): 439–52.

Hart, Avril, and Emma Taylor. *Fans*. London: V&A Publications, 1998.

Hartzman, Marc. *American Sideshow: An Encyclopedia of History's Most Wondrous and Curiously Strange Performers*. New York: Penguin, 2005.

Harvey, David. *Paris, Capital of Modernity*. New York: Routledge, 2003.

———. *The Urban Experience*. Baltimore: John's Hopkins University Press, 1989.

Hayem, Julien, Licencié ès-lettres, Avocat à la Cour impériale. *M. X*** contre Mlle Z***, Plaidoyer prononcé à la chambre du tribunal civil de la Seine pour un Cachemire des Indes*. Paris: Chaix, 1868.

Heller, Sharon. *Freud A to Z*. Hoboken, N.J.: Wiley, 2005.

Hiner, Susan. "Lust for *Luxe*: Cashmere Fever in Nineteenth-Century France." *Journal of Early Modern Cultural Studies* 5.1 (2005) 76–98.

Houbre, Gabrielle. *La Discipline de l'amour: l'éducation des filles et des garçons à l'âge du romantisme*. Paris: Plon, 1997.

Howells, Bernard. *Baudelaire: Individualism, Dandyism and the Philosophy of History*. Oxford: Legenda, European Humanities Research Centre, 1996.

Hulme, Peter. "Balzac's Parisian Mystery: *La Cousine Bette* and the Writing of Historical Criticism." *Literature and History* 11:1 (Spring 1985): 47–64.

Huyssen, Andreas. *After the Great Divide: Modernism, Mass Culture, Postmodernism*. Bloomington: Indiana University Press, 1986.

Irwin, John. *Shawls: A Study of Indo-European Influences*. London: Her Majesty's Stationery Office, 1955.

Janin, Jules. "L'Éventail." In *Almanach de la littérature, du théâtre, et des beaux-arts* (1853–69), 88–90. Paris: Pagnerre, 1862.

Jones, Jennifer. "Coquettes and Grisettes: Women Buying and Selling in Ancien Régime France." In *The Sex of Things: Gender and Consumption in Historical Perspective*, edited by Victoria de Grazia, 25–53. Berkeley: University of California Press, 1996.

———. *Sexing la mode: Gender, Fashion and Commercial Culture in Old Regime France*. Oxford: Berg, 2004.

Jouy, Étienne de. *L'Hermite de la Chaussée d'Antin ou observations sur les mœurs et les usages parisiens au commencement du XIXe siècle*. 6th ed. 2 vols. Paris: Pillet, 1815.

Jullien, Dominique. "Cendrillon au grand magasin: *Au Bonheur Des Dames* et le rêve." *Les Cahiers naturalistes* 67 (1993): 97–105.

Kahanov, Alfred. "Une Icône dans l'oeuvre de Zola: Le portrait de Mme Hédouin dans *Au Bonheur Des Dames.*" *Les Cahiers naturalistes* 41:69 (1995): 127–38.

Kelly, Dorothy. *Fictional Genders: Role and Representation in Nineteenth-Century French Narrative*. Lincoln: University of Nebraska Press, 1989.

Kessler, Marni Reva. *Sheer Presence: The Veil in Manet's Paris*. Minneapolis: University of Minnesota Press, 2006.

Kingery, W. David. Introduction to *Learning from Things: Method and Theory of Material Culture Study*, edited by W. David Kingery, 1–15. Washington, D.C.: Smithsonian Institution Press, 1996.

Kleinart Annemarie. *Le "Journal des dames et des modes" ou la conquête de l'Europe féminine, 1797–1839*. Stuttgart: Jan Thorbecke Verlag, 2001.

Labiche, Eugène. *Le Cachemire X.B.T.* In *Théâtre complet*, vol. 6, 1–6. Paris: Calmann Lévy, 1885.

Lamartine, Alphonse de. "Le Lac." In *Méditations poétiques*, 1: 157–59. Paris: Hachette, 1915.

Lanskin, Jean Michel. "Cocottes à la ville et colombes aux champs: dichotomie spatiale dans *La Dame aux camélias* et *Nana* ou l'écologie de deux demi-mondaines." *French Literature Series* 22 (1995): 105–18.

Laparra, Camille."L'Aristocratie dans *La Comédie humaine* de Balzac: ses pluralismes." *French Review* 68:4 (March 1995): 602–14.

Laver, James. *Fashion, Art, and Beauty*. New York: Metropolitan Museum of Art, 1967.

Laverrière, Stéphane. "Le Sac à ouvrage, accessoire de la femme vertueuse." In Chenoune, 154–63.

Le Bail, Stéphanie. "*Au Bonheur Des Dames*: le magazine féminin d'un magasin imaginaire." *Les Cahiers naturalistes* 73 (1999): 195–97.

Lecercle, Jean-Pierre. *Mallarmé et la mode*. Paris: Librairie Séguier, 1989.

Lehmann, Ulrich. *Tigersprung: Fashion in Modernity*. Cambridge, Mass.: MIT Press, 2000.

Leslie, Catherine Amoroso. *Needlework Through History: An Encyclopedia*. Westport, Conn.: Greenwood, 2007.

Lester, Katherine, and Bess Viola Oerke. *Accessories of Dress: An Illustrated Encyclopedia*. Mineola, N.Y.: Dover Publications, 2004.

Lévi-Strauss, Monique. *Cachemires parisiens 1810–1880 à l'école de l'Asie*. Paris: Éditions des Musées de la Ville de Paris, 1998.

Lipovetsky, Gilles. *The Empire of Fashion: Dressing Modern Democracy*. Princeton, N.J.: Princeton University Press, 1994.

Lipovetsky, Gilles, and Elyette Roux. *Le Luxe éternal: de l'âge du sacré au temps des marques*. Paris: Gallimard, 2003.

Littré, Émile. *Dictionnaire de la langue française*, 1872–77, ARTFL Project.

Lowe, Lisa. *Critical Terrains: French and British Orientalisms*. Ithaca, N.Y.: Cornell University Press, 1991.

Lucey, Michael. "Balzac's Queer Cousins and Their Friends." In *Novel Gazing: Queer Readings in Fiction*, edited by Eve Kosofsky Sedgwick, 167–98. Durham, N.C.: Duke University Press, 1997.

———. *The Misfit of the Family: Balzac and the Social Forms of Sexuality*. Durham, N.C.: Duke University Press, 2003.

Lyu, Claire. "Stéphane Mallarmé as Miss Satin: The Texture of Fashion and Poetry." *Esprit Créateur* 40:3 (Fall 2000): 61–71.

Magubane, Zine. "Which Bodies Matter? Feminism, Poststructuralism, Race, and the Curious Theoretical Odyssey of the 'Hottentot Venus.'" *Gender and Society* 15:6 (2001): 816–34.

Maignan, Michel. *L'Éventail à tous vents: du XVI au XXe siècle*. Paris: Le Louvre des Antiquaires, 1989.

Mainardi, Patricia. *Husbands, Wives, and Lovers: Marriage and Its Discontents in Nineteenth-Century France*. New Haven, Conn.: Yale University Press, 2003.

Majewski, Henry. *Transposing Art into Texts in French Romantic Literature*. Chapel Hill: University of North Carolina Press, 2002.

Marc, Gabriel. "L'Éventail." In *Sonnets parisiens*, 83–84. Paris: Lemerre, 1875.

Marcadé, V. *Explication théorique et pratique du Code Napoléon*. 6th ed. Paris: Garnier, 1869.

Marcus, Sharon. *Apartment Stories: City and Home in Nineteenth-Century Paris and London*. Berkeley: University of California Press, 1999.

———. "Reflections on Victorian Fashion Plates." *differences: A Journal of Feminist Cultural Studies* 14:3 (Fall 2003): 4–33.

Margadant, Jo Burr, ed. *The New Biography: Performing Femininity in Nineteenth-Century France*. Berkeley: University of California Press, 2000.

Martin-Fugier, Anne. *La Bourgeoise: Femme au temps de Paul Bourget*. Paris: Grasset, 1983.

———. *La Vie élégante, ou, la formation du Tout-Paris, 1815–1848*. Paris: Fayard, 1990.

Maskiell, Michelle. "Consuming Kashmir: Shawls and Empires, 1500–2000." *Journal of World History* 13:1 (2002): 27–65.

Matlock, Jann. *Scenes of Seduction: Prostitution, Hysteria, and Reading Differ-*

ence in Nineteenth-Century France. New York: Columbia University Press, 1994.

Mauss, Marcel. *The Gift: Forms and Functions of Exchange in Archaic Societies,* translated by Ian Cunnison, introduction by E. E. Evans Pritchard. New York: Norton, 1967.

Maza, Sarah. "Uniforms: The Social Imaginary in Balzac's *La Cousine Bette.*" *French Politics, Culture and Society* 19 (Summer 2001): 21–42.

McCallum, E. L. *Object Lessons: How to Do Things with Fetishism.* Albany: State University of New York Press, 1999.

McMillan, James F. *France and Women, 1789–1914: Gender, Society and Politics.* New York: Routledge, 2000.

Meriwether, Margaret Lee, and Judith E. Tucker. *Social History of Women and Gender in the Modern Middle East.* Boulder, Colo.: Westview, 1999.

Michel, Arlette. *Le Mariage chez Balzac: amour et féminisme.* Paris: Société des Éditions "Les Belles Lettres,"1978.

Moers, Ellen. *The Dandy: Brummell to Beerbohm.* New York: Viking, 1960.

"Monologue du Cachemire." *La Silhouette: journal des caricatures* 3, 1830.

Morgan, Lady. *Le Livre du boudoir.* Vol. 2, translated by A.-J.-B. Defauconpret. Paris: Gosselin, 1829.

Moses, Claire Goldberg. *French Feminism in the Nineteenth Century.* Albany: State University of New York Press, 1984.

Munich, Adrienne. "Jews and Jewels on the South African Diamond Fields." In *The Jew in Late-Victorian and Edwardian Culture: Between the East End and East Africa,* edited by Eitan Bar-Yosef and Nadia Valman, 28–44. New York: Palgrave-MacMillan, 2009.

Murger, Henry. *Scènes de la vie de bohème,* edited by Loïc Chotard. Paris: Gallimard, 1988.

Musée de la Mode et du Costume. *Indispensables accessoires: XVI–XXe siècle.* Exhibition catalogue. Paris: Galliera, 1983–84.

Nava, Mica. "Modernity's Disavowal: Women, the City, and the Department Store." In *The Shopping Experience,* edited by Pasi Falk and Colin Campbell, 56–87. London: Sage, 1997.

Nelson, Brian. "Désir et consommation dans *Au Bonheur Des Dames.*" *Les Cahiers naturalistes* 42:70 (1996): 19–34.

———. "Zola and the Counter Revolution: Au Bonheur Des Dames." *Australian Journal of French Studies* 30:2 (1993): 233–40.

Nesci, Catherine. *La Femme mode d'emploi: Balzac de "La Physiologie du marriage" à "La comédie humaine."* French Forum Monographs. Lexington, Ky.: French Forum, 1992.

———. *Le Flâneur et les flâneuses: les femmes et la ville à l'époque romantique*. Bibliothèque stendhalienne et romantique. Grenoble: ELLUG, Université Stendhal, 2007.

Nevinson, J. L. *Origin and Early History of the Fashion Plate*. Washington, D.C: Smithsonian Press, 1967.

Offen, Karen. *European Feminisms, 1700–1950: A Political History*. Palo Alto, Calif.: Stanford University Press, 2000.

Olds, Marshall C. "Value and Social Mobility in Flaubert." In *Moving Forward, Holding Fast: The Dynamics of Nineteenth-Century French Culture*, edited by Barbara T. Cooper and Mary Donaldson-Evans, 81–90. Amsterdam, Netherlands: Rodopi, 1997.

O'Neill, John. "Psychoanalytic Jewels: The Domestic Drama of Dora and Freud." In *The Socialness of Things: Essays on the Socio-Semiotics of Objects*, edited by Stephen Harold Riggins, 451–69. New York: Mouton de Gruyter, 1994.

Orr, Mary. "Reflections on 'Bovarysme': The Bovarys at Vaubyessard." *French Studies Bulletin: A Quarterly Supplement* 61 (Winter 1996): 6–8.

Outka, Elizabeth. *Consuming Traditions: Modernity, Modernism, and the Commodified Authentic*. New York: Oxford University Press, 2009.

Owen-Hughes, Diane. "From Brideprice to Dowry in Mediterranean Europe." In *The Marriage Bargain: Women and Dowries in European History*, edited by Marion Kaplan, 13–58. New York: Harrington Park, 1985.

Parent-Duchâtelet, Alexandre. *La Prostitution à Paris au XIXe siècle*, edited by Alain Corbin. Paris: Seuil, 1981.

Parkins, Wendy. *Fashioning the Body Politic: Dress, Gender, Citizenship*. Oxford; New York: Berg, 2002.

Pedraza, Jorge. "Le Shopping d'Emma." In *Emma Bovary*, edited by Alain Buisine, 100–121. Paris: Éditions Autrement, 1997.

Peiss, Kathy. "Masks and Faces." In *Hope in a Jar: The Making of America's Beauty Culture*. New York: Holt, 1998.

Perrot, Michelle, and Alain Paire. *Writing Women's History*. Oxford: Blackwell, 1992.

Perrot, Philippe. *Fashioning the Bourgeoisie: A History of Clothing in the Nineteenth Century*, translated by Richard Bienvenu. Princeton, N.J.: Princeton University Press, 1994.

———. *Le Travail des apparences, ou, les transformations du corps féminin, VIII–XIXe siècle*. Paris: Éditions du Seuil, 1984.

Perthuis, Françoise de, and Vincent Meylan, *Éventails*. Paris: Éditions Hermé, 1989.

Pollack, Griselda. *Vision and Difference: Femininity, Feminism and the Histories of Art*. New York: Routledge, 1988.

Pratt, Mary Louise. *Imperial Eyes*. New York: Routledge, 1992.

Proust, Marcel. *À la recherche du temps perdu*. Paris: Gallimard-Pléiade, 1954.

———. *La Prisonnière*, ed. Pierre-Edmond Robert. Paris: Gallimard, 1989.

———. *Remembrance of Things Past*. Vol. 3, translated by C. K. Scott Moncrieff and Terence Kilmartin. New York: Vintage Books, 1982.

———. *Swann's Way*, translated by C. K. Scott Moncrieff and Terence Kilmartin. New York: Vintage, 1989.

———. *Time Regained*, translated by Andreas Mayor and Terence Kilmartin. New York: Random House, 1993.

Purdy, Daniel L., ed. *The Rise of Fashion: A Reader*. Minneapolis: University of Minnesota Press, 2004.

Raisson, Horace. *Le Code de la toilette: manuel complet d'élégance et d'hygiène, contenant les lois, règles, applications et exemples de l'art de soigner sa personne et de s'habiller avec goût et méthode*. Paris: Roret, 1829.

Reed, Arden. *Manet, Flaubert, and the Emergence of Modernism: Blurring Genre Boundaries*. Cambridge: Cambridge University Press, 2003.

Restif de la Bretonne. *Le Palais-Royal*. Paris: Louis-Michaud, 1908.

Ribeiro, Aileen. *The Art of Dress: Fashion in England and France 1750–1820*. New Haven, Conn.: Yale University Press, 1995.

———. *Ingres in Fashion: Representations of Dress and Appearance in Ingres's Images of Women*. New Haven, Conn.: Yale University Press, 1999.

Richardson, Joanna. *The Courtesans; the Demi-Monde in Nineteenth-Century France*. London: Weidenfeld and Nicolson, 1967.

"Le ridicule." *Almanach des ridicules, pour l'année 1801*. Paris: Imprimerie des Sourds-Muets, 1801), 108.

Rifelj, Carol. "'Ces Tableaux Du Monde': Keepsakes in Madame Bovary." *Nineteenth-Century French Studies* 25:3–4 (1997): 360–85.

———. "The Language of Hair in the Nineteenth-Century Novel." *Nineteenth-Century French Studies* 32:1–2 (2003): 83–96.

Rifkin, Adrian. "Total Ellipsis: Zola, Benjamin and the Dialectics of Kitsch." *Parallax: A Journal of Metadiscursive Theory and Cultural Practices* 2 (1996): 101–13.

Riggs, Larry. "Semiotics, Simulacra and Consumerist Rhetoric of Status in Molière's Cérémonie Turque and Flaubert's Château de la Vaubyessard." *Cincinnati Romance Review* 14 (1995): 44–50.

Robb, Graham. *Balzac: A Biography*. New York: Norton, 1996.

Roberts, Mary Louise. "Acting Up: The Feminist Theatrics of Marguerite Durand." In Margadant, 171–217.

———. *Disruptive Acts: The New Woman in Fin-de-Siècle France*. Chicago: University of Chicago Press, 2002.

Roche, Daniel. *La Culture des apparences: une histoire du vêtement (XVIIe–XVIIIe siècle)*. Paris: Fayard, 1991.

Rossum-Guyon, Françoise van, and Michiel van Brederode. *Balzac et les parents pauvres: Le Cousin Pons, La Cousine Bette*. Paris: SEDES, 1981.

Sagalow, Annie. "L'Ombrelle." In *Les Accessoires du temps: ombrelles et parapluies*. Exhibition catalogue, edited by Catherine Join-Diérterle, 16–45. Paris: Paris Galliera, 1989–90.

Said, Edward. *Culture and Imperialism*. New York: Knopf, 1993.

Saillard, Olivier. "À bout portant: modernités du sac." In Chenoune, 32–49.

Saverny, Marie de. *La Femme chez elle et dans le monde*. Paris: Au Bureau du journal *La Revue de la mode*, 1876.

Schloesser, Pauline. *The Fair Sex: White Women and Racial Patriarchy in the Early American Republic*. New York: New York University Press, 2002.

Schneider, Jane. "Trousseau as Treasure: Some Contradictions of Late Nineteenth-Century Change in Sicily." In *The Marriage Bargain: Women and Dowries in European History*, edited by Marion Kaplan, 81–119. New York: Harrington Park, 1985.

Schor, Naomi. "Devant le château: femmes, marchandises et modernité dans *Au Bonheur des Dames*." In *Mimesis et semiosis: littérature et représentation, miscellanées offertes à Henri Mitterand*, edited by Philippe Hamon and Jean-Pierre Leduc-Adine, 179–86. Paris: Nathan, 1992.

———. *Reading in Detail: Aesthetics and the Feminine*. New York: Routledge, 1987.

———. "*Triste Amérique: Atala* and the Construction of Post-Revolutionary Femininity." In *Bad Objects: Essays Popular and Unpopular*, 132–48. Durham, N.C.: Duke University Press, 1995.

Schuerewegen, Franc. "Muséum ou croutéum? Pons, Bouvard, Pécuchet et la collection." *Romantisme: revue du dix-neuvieme siècle* 17:55 (1987): 41–54.

Sieburth, Richard. "Une Idéologie du lisible: le phenomène des 'physiologies.'" *Romantisme* 47 (1985): 39–60.

Silverman, Debora L. *Art Nouveau in Fin-de-Siècle France: Politics, Psychology, and Style*. Berkeley: University of California Press, 1989.

Silverman, Kaja, and Harun Farocki. *Speaking About Godard*. New York: New York University Press, 1998.

Silverman, Willa Z. *The New Bibliopolis: French Book Collectors and the Culture of Print, 1880–1914*. Toronto: University of Toronto Press, 2008.

Simmel, Georg. "Fashion." In Purdy, 289–309.

———. "On Fashion." In *On Individuality and Social Forms*, edited by Donald Levine, 294–323. 1904; reprint, Chicago: University of Chicago Press, 1971.

Smith, Bonnie. *Ladies of the Leisure Class: The Bourgeoises of Northern France in the Nineteenth Century.* Princeton, N.J.: Princeton University Press, 1981.

Smith, Woodruff D. *Consumption and the Making of Respectability 1600–1800.* New York: Routledge, 2002.

Soulier, Vincent. *Presse féminine: la puissance frivole.* Paris: L'Archipel, 2008.

Staffe, La Baronne. *Les Hochets féminins: les pierres précieuses, les bijoux, la dentelle, la broderie, l'éventail, quelques autres superfluités.* Paris: Flammarion, 1902.

——. *Mes secrets pour plaire et pour être aimée.* Paris: Les Éditions 1900, 1990.

——. *Usages du monde: Règles du savoir-vivre dans la société moderne.* Paris: Havard, 1891.

Steele, Valerie. *The Corset: A Cultural History.* New Haven, Conn.: Yale University Press, 2001.

——. *The Fan: Fashion and Femininity Unfolded.* New York: Rizzoli International Publications, 2002.

——. *Fashion and Eroticism: Ideals of Feminine Beauty from the Victorian Era to the Jazz Age.* New York: Oxford University Press, 1985.

——. "Fashion, Fetish, Fantasy." In *Masquerade and Identities: Essays on Gender, Sexuality and Marginality*, edited by Tseelon Efrat, 73–82. London: Routledge, 2001.

——. *Fetish: Fashion, Sex and Power.* New York: Oxford University Press, 1996.

——. *Paris Fashion: A Cultural History.* New York: Berg, 1999.

Sue, Eugène. *Les Mystères de Paris.* Paris: Éditions Robert Laffont, 1989.

Sullivan, Courtney, A. "'Cautériser la plaie': The *Lorette* as Social Ill in the Goncourts and Eugène Sue." *Nineteenth-Century French Studies* 37:3–4 (2009): 247–61.

Summers, Leigh. *Bound to Please: A History of the Victorian Corset.* New York: Berg, 2001.

Tadié, Jean-Yves. *Marcel Proust*, translated by Euan Cameron. New York: Viking Penguin, 2000.

Tanner, Tony. *Adultery and the Novel: Contract and Transgression.* Baltimore: Johns Hopkins University Press, 1981.

Tata, Michael Angelo. "Post-Proustian Glamour." *Rhizomes: Cultural Studies in Emerging Knowledge* 5 (2002), http://www.rhizomes.net/issue5/tata.html#1.

Taylor, Lou. *Establishing Dress History.* New York: Palgrave, 2004.

Thesen, Doreen. *The Function of Gift Exchange in Stendhal and Balzac.* New York: Peter Lang, 2000.

Thomas, Chantal. *La Reine scélérate: Marie-Antoinette dans les pamphlets.* Paris: Seuil, 1989.

Thomas, Dana. *Deluxe: How Luxury Lost Its Luster.* New York: Penguin, 2007.

Thompson, Hannah. *Naturalism Undressed: Identity and Clothing in the Novels of Émile Zola.* Oxford: Legenda, 2004.

Thompson, Victoria. *The Virtuous Marketplace: Women and Men, Money and Politics 1830–1870.* Baltimore: Johns Hopkins University Press, 2000.

Trouvé, MM Arsène and Eugène. *Une Ombrelle compromise par un parapluie: vaudeville en un acte.* In *Théâtre contemporain illustré*, vol. 5, no. 41. Paris: Michel Lévy frères, 1861.

Uzanne, Octave. *La Femme et la mode: métamorphoses de la Parisienne de 1792 à 1892.* Paris: May, 1892.

Uzanne, Octave, and Paul Avril, illus. *L'Éventail.* Paris: Quantin, 1882.

———. *L'Ombrelle, le gant, le manchon.* Paris: A. Quantin, 1883.

Valis, Noël. *The Culture of Cursilería: Bad Taste, Kitsch, and Class in Modern Spain.* Durham, N.C.: Duke University Press, 2002.

Vannier, Henriette. "La Mode sous le consulat et l'empire." *Miroir de l'histoire* 98 (1958): 204–9.

Veblen, Thorstein. *Conspicuous Consumption.* New York: Penguin, 2006.

———. *The Theory of the Leisure Class*, edited by Robert Lekachman. New York: Penguin Classics, 1994.

Verardi, Louis M. *Manuel du bon ton et de la politesse française: nouveau guide pour se conduire dans le monde.* Paris: Passard, 1850–59.

Vesseron, Henry. *Études et souvenirs.* Sedan: Tellier, 1870.

Vinken, Barbara. *Fashion Zeitgeist,* translated by Mark Hewson. New York: Berg, 2005.

Waller, Margaret. "Disembodiment as a Masquerade: Fashion Journalists and Other 'Realist' Observers in Directory Paris." *Esprit Créateur* 37:1 (1997): 44–54.

Watson, Janelle. *Literature and Material Culture from Balzac to Proust.* New York: Cambridge University Press, 1999.

Weber, Caroline. *Queen of Fashion: What Marie Antoinette Wore to the Revolution.* New York: Holt, 2006.

Werther, Betty. "Paisley in Perspective: The Cashmere Shawl in France," *American Craft* 58 (February–March 1983): 6–8, 88.

Westbrook, John. "Digesting Godard Filming Bataille: Expenditure in 'Weekend.'" *Contemporary French and Francophone Studies* 9:4 (December 2006): 345–52.

Wilkinson, Lynn R. "Le Cousin Pons and the Invention of Ideology." *PMLA:*

Publications of the Modern Language Association of America 107:2 (1992): 274–89.

Williams, Rosalind. *Dream Worlds: Mass Consumption in Late Nineteenth-Century France.* Berkeley: University of California Press, 1982.

Wilson, Elizabeth. *Adorned in Dreams: Fashion and Modernity.* 1985; reprint, New Brunswick, N.J.: Rutgers University Press, 2003.

Wilson, Elizabeth, and Lou Taylor. *Through the Looking Glass: A History of Dress from 1860 to the Present Day.* London: BBC Books, 1989.

Woestelandt, Evelyne. "Le Corps vénal: Rosanette dans *L'Éducation sentimentale.*" *Nineteenth Century French Studies* 16:1–2 (1987): 120–31. ———. "Système de la mode dans *L'Éducation sentimentale.*" *French Review* 58: 2 (December 1984): 244–54.

———. "Un Corps parlant: Madame Arnoux dans *L'Éducation sentimentale.*" *Modern Language Studies* 19:4 (1989): 66–74.

Wollen, Peter. "The Concept of Fashion in *The Arcades Project.*" *boundary 2* 30:1 (2003): 131–42.

Wrigley, Richard. *The Politics of Appearances: Representations of Dress in Revolutionary France.* Oxford: Berg, 2002.

Yates, Susan. "Women in the Discourse of Balzac's Horace Bianchon." *Australian Journal of French Studies* 36:2 (1999): 173–87.

Yeatman, Rannveig. "Le Château de la Vaubyessard: L'enchantement d'Emma Bovary." *Dalhousie French Studies* 29 (1994): 169–80.

Yeazell, Ruth. *Harems of the Mind: Passages of Western Art and Literature.* New Haven, Conn.: Yale University Press, 2000.

Zaragoza, Georges. "Le Coffret de Madame Arnoux ou l'achèvement d'une éducation." *Revue d'histoire littéraire de la France* 89:4 (July–August 1989): 674–88.

Zdatny, Steven. "Fashion and Class Struggle: The Case of Coiffure." *Social History* 18:1 (1993): 53–72.

Zizek, Slavlov. *The Plague of Fantasies.* New York: Verso, 1997.

Zola, Émile. *Au Bonheur des Dames,* edited by Robert Sctrick and Claude Aziza. Paris: Pocket, 1990.

———. *The Ladies' Paradise,* edited and translated by Brian Nelson. New York: Oxford University Press, 2008.

———. *Nana,* edited by Marie-Ange Voisin-Fougère. Paris: Flammarion, 2000.

———. *Nana,* translated by Burton Rascoe, edited by Luc Sante. New York: Barnes and Noble Classics, 2006.

———. *Pot-Bouille,* edited by Marie-Ange Voisin-Fougère. Paris: Librairie Générale Française, 1998.

———. *Pot-Bouille*, translated by Percy Pinkerton, edited by Robert Leth-bridge. London: Dent, 2000.

Zutshi, Chitralekha. "'Designed for Eternity': Kashmiri Shawls, Empire, and Cultures of Production and Consumption in Mid-Victorian Britain." *Journal of British Studies* 48 (April 2009): 420–40.

PERIODICALS

L'Almanach des modes
Le Bon Ton
Le Cabinet des modes
La Corbeille
Fémina
Le Follet
La Fronde
La Gazette rose
Le Journal des dames et des demoiselles
Le Journal des dames et des modes
Le Journal des demoiselles
Le Journal des femmes
L'Illustration
Le Magasin pittoresque
Le Miroir de la mode
La Mode
La Mode illustrée
Le Moniteur de la mode
Le Petit courrier des dames
Le Petit écho de la mode
Psyché
La Silhouette: journal des caricatures
La Vie parisienne

INDEX

accessory, as term, 2–3
adultery, 127, 147
aesthetics
    and commodification, 161, 163–66, 171, 176
    feminist, 212–13
    Western, 110–11, 131, 143
Algeria, 79, 94, 197–98
Alhoy, Maurice, *Physiologie de la lorette*, 38–40
Ancien Régime. See Old Regime
aristocracy, 24, 26, 147, 149–50, 159–60, 175
    See also identity, essential; Old Regime
Atala (Chateaubriand), 133–34, 235nn34–35
aumônière, 61, 179, 187–90, 191, 195
    See also bourse de la mariée; sac à main
authenticity, 29–30, 82, 91, 103, 161–71, 219n29
    See also social mobility
Autre étude de femme (Balzac), 9, 21–26, 29, 43, 104
Avant-Propos (Dumas *fils*), 12–13
Avril, Paul, 112–13

ballantine, 200
balls. *See éventail*, and balls
Balzac, 9–10, 12–13, 217n10, 219n26, 225nn20–21, 229n14, 242n37, 243n54
    Autre étude de femme, 20–22, 23, 29, 43, 104
    La Bourse, 199–200
    Le Contrat de mariage, 61–70, 73
    Le Cousin Pons, 162–71, 243n53, 244n55
    La Cousine Bette, 94–98, 197–98, 229n19
    Ferragus, 27–29

Le Lys dans la vallée, 135–38, 236n39
Baronne Staffe, 57, 60, 65, 115, 159, 211–13, 239n13, 252n3
    Les Hochets féminins, 211–12
    Secrets pour plaire et pour être aimée, 195
Barthes, Roland, 15, 19, 222
Baudelaire, Charles, 15–16, 139, 220n36
beauty. *See* aesthetics
Benjamin, Walter, 15–16, 30, 81
Au Bonheur des Dames (Zola), 119–120, 171–73, 176, 181, 191, 194, 202–6, 251n45
Bourdieu, 15, 18, 97
bourgeois *visage*, 133, 139
    See also whiteness
bourgeoise, 25, 104, 131, 189
La Bourse (Balzac), 199–200
bourse de la mariée, 179, 184–87, 197, 202.
    See also aumônière; sac à main
brideprice, 60-61, 187, 224n18

cachemire
    and colonialism, 5–6, 79–83, 96, 105–6, 228nn9, 11
    and *corbeille de mariage*, 75, 84, 88
    and distinction. *See* distinction, and *cachemire*
    and the domestic, 80, 83–84, 86, 228n11
    and economic associations, 79, 86, 90
    and eroticism, 80–84, 86, 99, 103
    and the exotic, 79–81, 83–84, 95
    history of, 83–91
    and male power, 80, 81–82, 86
    and marriage, 88–89, 102
    and moral associations, 79, 84, 88
    office of verification of, 91

ACKNOWLEDGMENTS

Several years back while sitting in a hair salon preparing Balzac's *La Cousine Bette*, which I was teaching, I found myself sneaking glimpses at the fashion magazines instead. Finally, I picked one up and became engrossed in an article about wealthy women fined for importing the status symbol of the day—exquisite, but illegal, scarves made from the belly hairs of an endangered species of a rare Kashmiri goat. Because my husband had just given me a soft green pashmina, I was queasy for a split second as I wondered if I was implicated. But I remembered Bette's shawl and turned my mind back to the book, speculating what cashmere might mean there. This happy coincidence of the intellectual, the personal, and the everyday opened the door to this book.

That "happy coincidence" though was the result of fundamental influences that continue to shape my thinking. I thank first my parents, Lucian and Mary Elizabeth Hiner, without whose steadfast encouragement and curiosity about my work from earliest days I would not have dreamed it possible to write a book. My mother instilled in me a passion for the untold histories of familiar stories as well as a reverence for the power of objects to reveal those histories. My father did not live to see the publication of this book, but his pride and interest in the project remain with me now.

I am grateful to my home institution, Vassar College, and to the many fine people there who have contributed to this project: my students, both in French and in Women's Studies, who have shared in the evolution of the book; my colleagues in the Department of French and Francophone Studies, in particular, Thomas Parker, who organized a departmental Salon surrounding an early chapter draft and generously listened over the years as I worked through my ideas, and Kathleen Hart for her meticulous comments on earlier drafts of some chapters;

the staff at the Library, in particular, Martha Connors and the Interlibrary Loan Office; Vassar's technology staff, Baynard Bailey, John McCartin, Cristian Opazo, and Steve Taylor; Raluca Besliú and Lindsay Cook, my dependable research assistants; the Grants Office, for its help processing research grants, and the funding institutions that provided them-the Mellon Foundation, for a Mellon Faculty New Directions Grant through Vassar, the Gabrielle Snyder Beck Fund and the Florence Donaldson White Fund; the Dean of the Faculty, Jon Chenette, for generously funding portions of the book's production; my colleagues in other departments, Holly Hummel, Arden Kirkland, and Mita Choudhury; my colleagues in the Women's Studies Program, in particular, Kristin Sánchez Carter, Diane Harriford, Lydia Murdoch, and Susan Zlotnick. I also express my gratitude to my writing group for pushing me, critiquing me, and rereading the manuscript many times over. Their exemplary standards, generosity and intelligence made for intellectual comradeship of the highest caliber: Eva Woods Peiró, Jeffrey Schneider, Elliot Schreiber, and Joshua Schreier.

I also owe a debt of gratitude to many people beyond Vassar College: Milton and Vias Fellas, Lisa Rengo George, Pauline LeVen, Martha Matthews, Suzanne Nagy-Kirchhofer, Monique Nathan, and Karen Sawdey; the staffs of several libraries, museums, and presses both in Paris and in the United States where the research for this book was conducted: the Bibliothèque nationale de France, the Bibliothèque des arts décoratifs, and the Bibliothèque historique de la ville de Paris; the Pierpont Morgan Library in New York City, the University of Florida George A. Smathers Libraries, the Washington University Libraries, the University of Washington Libraries, the Museum of Fine Arts, Boston, Dover Publications, the Baschet family, Karen Cannell of the Gladys Marcus Library at the Fashion Institute of Technology, the Bard Graduate Center, and the Cora Ginsberg Gallery in New York City.

Earlier portions of some chapters appeared in journal articles: portions of Chapter 2 in *Dix-Neuf: Journal of the Society of Dix-Neuviémistes* (2008); portions of Chapter 5 in *Romance Studies* (2007); and portions of Chapter 3 in *The Journal of Early Modern Cultural Studies* (2005). I thank the editors of these journals for permission to reprint them. I wish also to thank the anonymous readers of the manuscript and the staff at the University of Pennsylvania Press, especially Jerry Singerman, whose early enthusiasm for my project, humor, and professionalism made him the ideal editor. I wish also to thank Andrea Goulet for her precise and thoughtful reading of the manuscript. I thank

Tim Roberts, managing editor of the Modern Language Initiative, and Robert Milks, who copyedited the final manuscript. I also thank Michèle Majer of the Bard Graduate Center, who graciously allowed me to sit in on her costume history class when I was in the early stages of this project and who has since helped me immeasurably with leads on texts and images, and Marina van Zuylen for her brilliant suggestions in the book's later stages..

I owe my deepest debt to those who have left their mark in incalculable ways: my friend and editor, Kalbryn A. McLean, with whom I was felicitously reunited over the course of writing this book—our shared *apprentissage* under the magnificent Millicent K. Ruddy made her my perfect reader, and without her keen skill and thorough understanding, the book would be much the poorer; Michael Riffaterre, whose virtuoso performances made textual analysis integral to my work; John Anzalone, for the mentorship he has offered me these many years; Masha Belenky, whose advice and perceptive readings were always invaluable; Marni Kessler, whose first book was an inspiration, and whose insights and expertise made my work infinitely better; Carolyn Betensky, whose honest and brilliant observations helped me see the forest through the trees many times over; Priscilla Ferguson, most generous friend and counselor and an infinite resource for all things nineteenth-century; and Lise Schreier, who perfected my translations, read and reread the manuscript in its many forms, navigated the archives of Paris with me, and enriched the book in ways I cannot quantify.

I want to thank my friends and family, in particular, my niece, Virginia Douglas Hiner, for accompanying me to Paris several times to care for my then-young daughter so I could conduct research. I offer my deepest thanks and love to my husband, John Fellas, whose gift initiated this book, and whose steady strength, intelligence, and engagement sustained me throughout this project and so much more, and to my beloved daughter Nora, always elegant and rarely proper.

I dedicate this book to the memory of my dear friend Rose Shapiro.

DATE DUE
